A *Jerry Baker* Good Health Book

Cut Your
HEALTH
CARE
BILLS
in Half!

www.jerrybaker.com

Other Jerry Baker Books:

A *Jerry Baker* Good Health Book

Cut Your
HEALTH
CARE
BILLS
in Half!

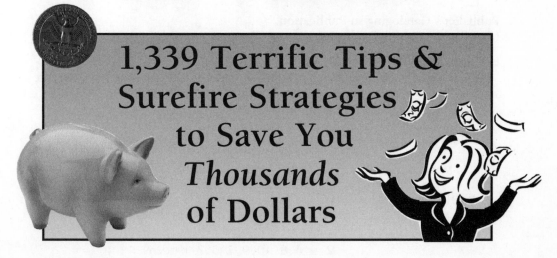

1,339 Terrific Tips &
Surefire Strategies
to Save You
Thousands
of Dollars

Copyright © 2005 by Jerry Baker

NOTICE

Published by American Master Products, Inc./Jerry Baker

Kim Adam Gasior, Publisher

A Jerry Baker Good Health Book and a Blackberry Cottage Production
Editorial: Ellen Michaud, Blackberry Cottage Productions, Ltd.
Design: Nest Publishing Resources

Editor: Mathew Hoffman
Book Composition: Wayne F. Michaud
Copy Editor: Jane Sherman

Printed in the United States of America

Publisher's Cataloging-in-Publication
(*Provided by Quality Books, Inc.*)

Hoffman, Matthew, 1959-
    Jerry Baker's cut your health care bills in half : 1,339 terrific tips and surefire strategies to save you thousands of dollars. / Matthew Hoffman.
    p. cm. — (Jerry Baker's good health series)
    Includes index.
    ISBN 0–922433–58–5

    1. Medicine, Popular.   I. Baker, Jerry.   II. Title

RC81.H686 2004   616.02'4
                         QB104-200188

2 4 6 8 10 9 7 5 3 hardcover

Contents

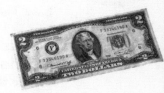

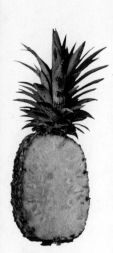

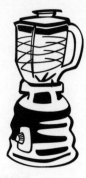

Contents

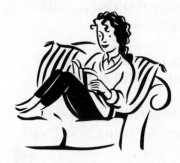
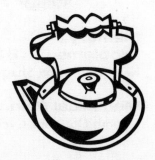

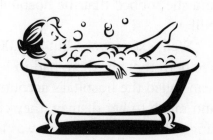

Foreword

Every summer, I invite the whole neighborhood over for my annual Baker Barbecue and stuff every last one of my neighbors with barbecued short ribs, potato salad, baked beans, coleslaw, watermelon, ice cream, and Grandma Putt's amazing lemon pound cake. But no sooner had the feeding frenzy died down this year than I noticed my neighbor Jean hunched over with a pained look on her face. I went over to see what was wrong and discovered that she was having terrible pain in her right side. I ran and called 911, and several minutes later, Jean was whisked away in an ambulance.

It turned out that Jean's pain was nothing more than a little indigestion—thanks to her recent overindulgence in my spicy ribs. She was in the hospital for a few days while the doctors checked her out, but they released her with a prescription for a tummy soother and an admonition not to eat so many ribs at next year's barbecue.

A few weeks later, when I was out for a walk, I noticed Jean on her front porch—practically in tears. I asked her what was wrong, and she sobbed that the hospital had slapped her with a $13,000 bill!

Well, excuse me...but $13,000 for indigestion!? We both thought there had to be some mistake. Jean called the hospital's accounting department, and much to her dismay, they claimed that every single dime on the invoice was legit. Apparently, she said, that ambulance had just stopped by the hospital on a one-way trip to the poorhouse!

What was poor Jean to do? I decided to head over to my friend George's place to ask his advice. Instead of offering any reassurance, though, George just shuffled off to his office and emerged carrying a fistful of papers. It was a bunch of bills—$129 for his arthritis medicine, $93.87 for his cholesterol-lowering medicine, $90 for his diabetes medicine, $53 for his stomach-soothing medicine, and $70.59 for four tiny pills that prevent the bone loss of osteoporosis. I added it up and realized that he was paying $436.46 for a single month's worth of medicine!

I couldn't believe it.

That's when I decided to call a friend of mine, Matthew Hoffman. Matt has published lots of health books over the years, and I figured if anyone could find ways to save folks from politicians, government bureaucracies, hospital moneymen, and big insurance companies, he could. Matthew was more than happy to look into the problem to see what he could find. He spent months tearing into each and every resource he could dig up, and he uncovered a boatload of cost-cutting, health-improving secrets—remedies that can ease hundreds of different ailments while chopping those whopping health care bills down to size.

So we took Matt's research, added some old-fashioned, tried-and-true home remedies from the best of our health books—blockbusters like *Jerry Baker's Amazing Antidotes* and *Jerry Baker's Anti-Pain Plan*—and packed 1,339 cures for more than 105 common ailments and health problems into this book. No matter whether you're aching with arthritis or fighting the flu, have a nagging case of heartburn, or are coping with another common complaint, you'll find fast, fun, easy, and (best of all) cheap ways to ease your discomfort—all at your fingertips! Whether your concern is major health problems like high blood pressure and osteoporosis or more minor complaints like dandruff and nausea, we've got it covered.

Looking for some cut-rate relief? Our "25¢ Specials" and

"$2 Deals" offer quick-'n-easy treatments that are available for pocket change. Need speed? Our "Fast Fixes" show you the secrets of on-the-spot relief. How about meals that heal? Our "Food Pharmacy" features reveal the healing power of Mother Nature's finest. And, if you really need serious medical attention, have no fear—"Holler for Help" will point you in the right direction.

Thanks to the amazing advice in this book, George, Jean, and I have been able to cut our crazy medical bills in half. Instead of struggling to keep drug company CEO's on their sailboats, we're saving money, feeling healthier, and living the good life again.

So check out the quick, simple, and effective solutions inside, then talk to your doctor about them. If you're feeling as if you have to choose between taking up residence in the poorhouse and suffering from debilitating aches and pains or the effects of conditions like high cholesterol, arthritis, and diabetes, the hundreds of feel-good secrets in this book can change your life—just like they did for George, Jean, and me!

Jerry Baker

P.S. Worry about health care costs can kill. As this book goes to press, the American Heart Association has just released a study of more than 2,000 people that revealed that those who undergo heart bypass surgery and have to worry about paying their medical bills are twice as likely to die within the next year as people who don't have that problem. So make sure you're not one of the ones who need to worry. Talk to your doctor about all the money-saving strategies in this book—and pay close attention to the tips in our chapters on angina, high cholesterol, and high blood pressure. We want to see you in the garden next spring!

Acne

Best Bets to Banish Blemishes

No matter how much you hate pimples, you have to give them credit for timing. You may go months or years without an outbreak, but as soon as you want to look your best—for your 15-year high school reunion or a meeting with the company hotshots, for example—they make a sudden appearance.

Here's where the problem begins. Periodically, the sebaceous glands under your skin work overtime and produce more oil than your skin needs or your oil ducts can handle. The excess collects under the skin's surface. Add some dead skin cells to the mix, and a hard plug forms. If it stays under the skin, it's a whitehead. If it enlarges and pushes out to the surface, it's a blackhead. If it ruptures the wall of a pore, invading

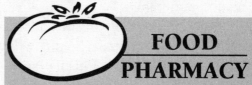

FOOD PHARMACY

Soothing Spuds

White potatoes contain natural chemicals that seem to help pimples and boils drain. Grate a potato and apply it directly to the area. Leave it on for 10 to 20 minutes, then wash the area well. You can repeat the treatment once or twice a day.

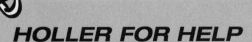

HOLLER FOR HELP

Beware of Boils

Boils are similar to pimples in some ways. They appear as red or pinkish, pus-filled bumps on the skin, sometimes with a white or yellow spot in the center. They're unsightly, but that's not why they're worrisome. When bacteria colonize a hair follicle (a tiny chamber from which a single hair grows), they have the potential to multiply to harmful levels. The immune system tries to keep them in check, but if it fails, the organisms can trigger a potentially serious infection. At the very least, they can cause boils, along with a lot of inflammation and pain.

If you're generally healthy, a boil is unlikely to be serious. The pus will usually drain on its own, and the boil should disappear within one to two weeks, says Lisa Arnold, N.D. Large or painful boils should always be treated by a doctor, especially if you have other signs of infection, such as a fever, chills, or fatigue. Minor boils are relatively easy to treat at home—by keeping the area clean and helping them drain in the same way you take care of bad pimples, says Dr. Arnold.

bacteria jump in, and there's your zit. If more than one zit erupts—and let's face it, zits travel in groups—there's an acne breakout.

BLAME INTERNAL CHEMISTRY

Acne usually results from the increased hormonal activity of adolescence—specifically, the surge of androgens that stimulate the growth of body hair. Unfortunately, this process sometimes ends up clogging pores and blocking the flow of sebum. In grownups, the sudden appearance of acne is often a sign of a hormone imbalance or a side effect of certain drugs, such as steroids, lithium, anticonvulsants, and medications with iodine. If you take any of these medications, ask your doctor if you can change prescriptions.

Thankfully, most acne is more of an embarrassment than a serious medical problem. If it persists past adolescence or is particularly severe, however, you may need medical treatment to prevent scarring. The most effective medications—for both topical and oral use—are derivatives of vitamin A. These drugs are safe when used under the supervision of a dermatologist, but they shouldn't be taken casually, because they can be irritating and toxic. Likewise, since infection isn't the primary cause of acne, long-term treatment with tetracycline and other antibiotics should be avoided.

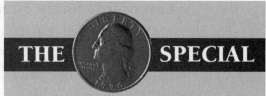

THE ☐ SPECIAL

Nature's Bacteria Killer

Tea tree oil, available at health food stores, is one of the most powerful herbal oils for killing the bacteria that make pimples painful. Add a few drops of oil to a cup of warm water. Moisten a washcloth with the water and hold it on the pimple for about 10 minutes several times a day.

KEEP YOUR SKIN CRYSTAL CLEAR

You can't prevent acne entirely, but there are a number of very effective strategies for keeping outbreaks under control and preventing them from coming back. So before you hand over your bank account to a dermatologist, here are a few things to try.

Baby your skin. All the scrubbing in the world won't make those zits disappear—in fact, it may just cause them to spread. Wash your skin gently.

Be a clean machine. Pimples can literally overflow with bacteria, and the last thing you need is for stray germs to cause an infection elsewhere. The most important home treatment is to keep pimples and the surrounding skin clean and dry. Wash the area with soap and water a few times a day. If you touch a pimple, wash your hands immediately afterward.

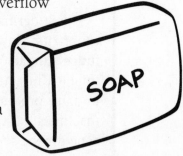

Lavender is lovely. Steam your pores open and prevent acne with an herbal antiseptic. Just place 1 tablespoon of lavender flowers in a pot of hot, steaming water. Place a towel over your head to trap the steam, then bend over the pot (but not so close that you burn your face). Let the lavender vapors steam your face for 15 minutes, then rinse with cool water and pat dry.

Stay cool and calm. Try to arrange your life so you're under as little stress as possible (easier said than done, we know!). Stress alters hormone levels, which can trigger zit outbreaks.

Erase 'em with eggs. Egg white draws out the oils from your skin, so when a nasty pimple appears, use a cotton swab to apply a little to the area. Egg whites are mild astringents and may contain some anti-inflammatory proteins as well.

Refresh with an herbal rinse. Calendula's bright orange flowers can be made into a refreshing facial wash. Just steep 1 teaspoon of flowers in 1 cup of hot water for 10 minutes, then strain and let cool. After cleansing your face as usual, rinse with the calendula solution.

Wash with the witch. Witch hazel, an excellent oil remover, has long been a popular item in medicine cabinets.

Say Goodbye to Iodine

Most dermatologists insist that chocolate and pizza don't cause zits. However, doctors do warn that the iodine in a hot fudge sundae or a slice of anchovy and extra-cheese pizza just might. Known to trigger angry red pimples, iodine is abundant in dairy products because iodine cleansers are used on milking machines. Fast food, salty foods, and shellfish can aggravate acne for the same reason.

Use a clean cotton ball to dab some on your skin to help keep it oil-free.

Tame them with tea. One of the most effective remedies for a painful pimple is to cover it with a tea bag. Black tea contains tannins, chemical compounds that help pimples drain. Soak a tea bag in hot water just long enough to soften it. Let it cool slightly, then hold it on the pimple for 10 minutes or so, says Lisa Arnold, N.D., a naturopathic physician in Orleans, Massachusetts.

Apply a sweet soother. Add 1 teaspoon of onion juice to 2 tablespoons of honey. Mix well, apply it to your face, and leave it on for 10 to 15 minutes. Rinse with warm water followed by cool water. This combination has a soothing effect on irritated skin.

Drain away infection. Buy some dried yarrow, an astringent herb, from a local herbalist or health food store. Crumble the leaves, add a little water to make a paste, and apply it to the pimple. Leave it on for about 20 minutes, then wash the area well, says Dr. Arnold.

Get over-the-counter help. Over-the-counter acne creams contain ingredients, such as benzoyl peroxide and salicylic acid, that can be helpful in reducing acne flare-ups in some people. Use a cream at night and, after a week or so, add a morning application. You should notice an improvement in about three weeks.

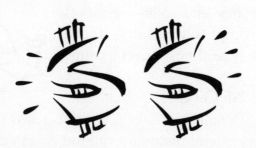

Age Spots

Watch Them Fade

You already know that unrestrained sunbathing can trigger the development of premature wrinkles. What you may not know is that the sun's strong rays can also produce a bunch of flat, freckle-like age spots that make you look like a freckled frog. Technically, they're called lentigines, although folks sometimes call them (wrongly) liver spots.

While lentigines usually debut—often on the hands, face, or shoulders—around age 40, they're a long time in the making. If you spend years enjoying the sun's golden rays, your body tries to protect your skin from solar damage by producing an excess of protective melanin. Over time, however, the melanin turns to cellular debris that bunches up in irregular patches, and voilà—age spots! While they're completely harmless, much like freckles, they're almost never as cute.

NO MORE SPOTS

If you want to fade your spots, your doctor is likely to suggest that you try one of the many vitamin A skin creams, called retinoids, that peel off the top layer of skin and possibly those vexing spots.

If over-the-counter retinol products don't do the job, you may need to up the ante and use a prescription-strength retinoid such as tretinoin (Retin-A). These drugs slough off old age spots and stop new ones from forming. Their only drawback is that they can be quite harsh, especially if you have very fair skin. In fact, if you use a prescription-strength retinoid, you may trade your age spots for a nasty sunburn with the slightest exposure to the sun, warns Jeanette Jacknin, M.D., a dermatologist in Scottsdale, Arizona. And wasn't it too much sun that sent you scurrying for the stuff in the first place?

If, despite your best efforts, you find yourself applying your foundation with a putty knife, you may want to consider pulling out all the stops with one or more skin-stripping medical procedures. Your doctor may suggest removing your spots with a chemical peel, which uses strong acids to dissolve the skin surface; a liquid nitrogen peel, which "freezes" spots for easier removal; or a laser peel, in which your doctor actually lifts off age spots using a high-intensity light. All of these methods can erase age spots as completely as paint stripper peels off unwanted varnish— but they're expensive, and the recovery can be painful.

In truth, you probably don't

Tea Time

Fade Spots from the Inside Out

Traditional herbal blood purifiers are said to clear the skin of blemishes and spots. To try one, mix equal parts of the dried root of burdock, yellow dock, and dandelion. Bring 1 cup of water to a boil and steep 1 tablespoon of the mixture for 20 minutes, then strain and drink. You can add honey and lemon to taste. Caution: Dandelion greens should not be used if you're taking diuretics or potassium supplements. Consult your doctor if you have any concerns.

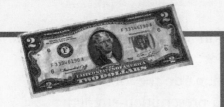

The $2 Deal

Save Your Skin with C

Topical vitamin C penetrates the outer layers of the skin, and encourages shedding of old skin cells, including those that contain melanin. Plus, it reduces what's called free radical damage—one of the consequences of too much sun exposure, says Jeannette Jacknin, M.D.

Why not just drink a glass of OJ? Because you can find creams and lotions that provide a whopping 30 times more C than oral forms, explains Dr. Jacknin. Start by applying topical C to spots every other day, but never use it more than twice a day. The higher the concentration of vitamin C, the better the lightening power.

have to spend a lot of money to get rid of age spots. Sometimes the very best remedies are the most basic. Here are some low-tech but highly effective ways to coax those pesky spots into the background.

Do the fade. There is a variety of acid-based remedies that act as exfoliants. That is, they slough off the top layer of your skin, along with the lentigines. The spots will seem lighter on the underneath layers, and eventually, as skin layers are replaced, the lentigines will no longer be there.

Most dermatologists recommend alpha hydroxy acids, commonly known as AHAs. These 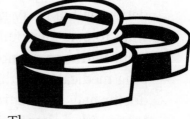 natural acids come from milk (lactic acid), sugarcane (glycolic acid), and fruit (citric acid). The glycolic acid in sugarcane is the most common AHA. It loosens those dead cells and motivates new cells from lower layers of the epidermis to get busy and grow some new skin. In other words, they exfoliate—or remove—superficial pigmentation.

Cream 'em with kinerase. This plant growth hormone stops leaves from turning brown—and it may help diminish brown spots on your skin with little or no irritation, notes Phillip Shenefelt, M.D., associate professor of dermatology at the

University of South Florida in Tampa. Look for it in over-the-counter lotions, then use it twice a day.

Wash your face with flowers. Elderflowers, known for keeping the complexion clear and free of blemishes, have their origins in folk medicine and are still used today in many commercial skin creams. Make your own elderflower water by steeping 1 ounce of fresh flowers in 1 pint of distilled water overnight. Strain, then use as a rinse after your daily cleansing regimen. Refrigerated, the solution will keep for four or five days.

Erase them with aloe. Best known for its ability to heal burns, aloe gel may help fade skin spots by boosting cell turnover so the pigmented cells eventually slough off. Apply the gel directly to the spots twice a day for a month or two. The smell's a bit pungent, but the results are well worth it.

Make room for mushrooms. Their juice contains kojic acid, a lightening agent that has been found to block the overproduction of melanin. It's just as effective as over-the-counter creams for fading age spots without overlightening or irritating skin, according to Dr. Jacknin.

Mind you, juice from your portobello burger probably won't do the trick, but any over-the-counter skin lotion that contains kojic acid will. Simply apply it twice daily, and your age spots

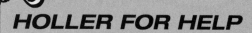

HOLLER FOR HELP

Spots to Watch

While age spots are harmless, precancerous lesions may not be. Consult a dermatologist immediately if one of your age spots suddenly darkens to a deep brown or black, changes shape, becomes raised, or bleeds.

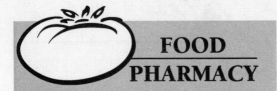

FOOD PHARMACY

Bet On Buttermilk

The next time you grocery shop, grab a quart of buttermilk. For ages, women have enjoyed lolling in milk baths and, more specifically, in buttermilk baths because of buttermilk's high lactic acid content. A tubful would probably mean you'd need your own cow, but many women simply bathe their faces or hands in buttermilk once or twice a day.

may fade significantly in less than two months.

Mix up some 'radish. The enzyme activity of horseradish and yogurt may help decrease age spots. Mix 1 tablespoon of grated horseradish in 1/4 cup plain yogurt, then refrigerate. Dab on the mixture daily until you see your spots fade. Follow each application with a smear of vitamin E oil or wheat-germ oil.

Get some lemon aid. Lemon is a mild bleaching aid that works as well on age spots as it does on stains in fabrics. Mix equal parts lemon juice and water and apply to each spot. Leave it on for 5 minutes before rinsing. Repeat three times a week, and the brown spots may fade to taupe, says Dr. Jacknin. Add more lemon juice and less water as your skin gets used to the preparation. Your goal is to be able to apply the juice "straight up."

Save your skin with sunscreen. By far, the best way to prevent age spots is to apply sunscreen every time you go outside. Be sure to slather it on all exposed skin—not only your face but also your legs, arms, and hands. If you have a fetching short haircut, don't forget your ears! And reapplying sunscreen every time you wash your hands really makes a difference, so always carry a small bottle with you.

Avoid the danger times. The sun is most damaging at its highest peak. The force of ultraviolet (UV) rays is 10 times stronger at noon than it is 3 hours earlier or later.

Even if you spend all day out in the sun, you'll get the biggest dose of UV radiation from 11:00 A.M. to 1:00 P.M.—when the sun is directly overhead.

Cover your head. Here's your chance to bat your eyelashes under a beautiful brim. A wide-brimmed hat or visor can actually block half the sunlight that would otherwise reach parts of your face. So slap on a chapeau—you'll be stylish and skin savvy, too!

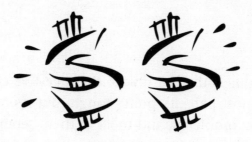

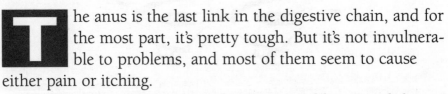

Anal Pain

Banish the Bottom Blues

The anus is the last link in the digestive chain, and for the most part, it's pretty tough. But it's not invulnerable to problems, and most of them seem to cause either pain or itching.

Pain in your nether regions can be caused by several things. Anal fissures, which are small tears in the tissue, are rarely serious, but they can be excruciating for the one to two weeks it takes them to heal. An anal abscess, an infection of a gland inside the anus, can make the area sore and tender. Then there are hemorrhoids, those pesky protuberances that can make sitting an agonizing experience.

It's not a pleasant prospect, but anal pain generally requires a trip to the doctor. Without professional attention, there's really no way to tell what's causing the problem.

Consider anal abscesses. Sometimes, they go away on their own, but other times, the infection gets worse, and the abscess has to be surgically drained. An untreated abscess can also progress to a dangerous, tunnel-like growth called a fistula, which also requires surgery. Even anal fissures, which almost always heal on their own, can cause so much pain that they require a doctor's care.

SOOTHING SOLUTIONS

Here's the bottom line: Call your doctor if you have anal pain accompanied by fever, chills, sweating, or other signs of infection, or if it hurts so much that you can't have a bowel movement. In the meantime, here are some easy remedies that will make your life a lot more comfortable. And you don't have to bust the bank to try 'em.

Soak that bottom. No matter what's making your bottom hurt, soaking in a warm bath for 10 to 20 minutes will almost certainly make you feel better. "It helps soothe the area and relaxes tight muscles," says Michael P. Spencer, M.D., a colon and rectal surgeon and assistant professor of surgery at the University of Minnesota, Twin Cities.

Get over-the-counter help. Don't ignore the benefits of common pain relievers, such as aspirin and ibuprofen. They block chemicals in the body that cause pain, and they help control inflammation.

Drink and keep drinking. No kidding: By the time you're feeling thirsty, your body is already running low on water, which

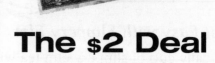

The $2 Deal

Helpful Supplements

If you can't seem to get adequate fiber from foods, take advantage of the fiber supplements that are available at drugstores and health food stores. Just follow the directions on the label. Products that contain psyllium, for example, are loaded with fiber. They make stools soft and slippery and less likely to cause anal pain.

Just be sure not to confuse fiber supplements with stimulant laxatives. They do different jobs, and powerful laxatives should be used only under the supervision of a doctor.

means that you're more likely to have hard stools or other causes of anal pain.

Most people need about 6 glasses of water daily, says Dr. Spencer. If you're active or live in a warm climate, drink 8 to 10 glasses, and don't wait until you're parched. Keep water nearby and sip it throughout the day.

Some like it hot. A little gentle heat makes everything feel better, and your rear end is no exception. Cover a heating pad with a towel, set the heat on low, and sit and relax for as long as it feels comfortable.

Inspect the medicine chest. Some prescription drugs increase the risk of constipation, which can cause or aggravate anal pain. Among the likely suspects are prescription analgesics, antidepressants, tranquilizers, blood pressure drugs, iron and calcium supplements, and antacids. If you've noticed any change in your usual bowel habits, or you're constipated more than occasionally, ask your doctor or pharmacist if any of your medications could be to blame.

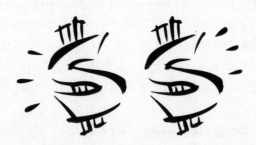

Anemia

Iron Out Fatigue

You may have heard the old joke—told, predictably enough, by old doctors—that the hardest job in medicine is finding a pale patient against a white sheet. Okay, it's not exactly a knee-slapper, but it does make an important point about iron-deficiency anemia. This common condition can drain your color just about as fast as it drains your energy.

You need iron to make hemoglobin, which transports oxygen from your lungs to all the tissues of your body. This is what brings the color to your cheeks. Without iron, hemoglobin production halts, and the body gets too little oxygen. With a drop in hemoglobin, you may be easily fatigued and feel sleepy or even occasionally dizzy. Your brain won't func-

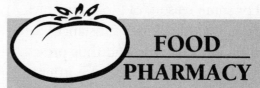

FOOD PHARMACY

A New Wrinkle

All fruits belong in a healthful diet, but if you're fighting anemia, focus on those with lots of wrinkles, such as figs, dates, prunes, raisins, and especially dried peaches and apricots. They're among the best sources of iron.

tion too well, either, so it can be a struggle to concentrate.

This doesn't mean that every mature person who occasionally feels low on energy is low on iron. Sometimes, we all feel as though our get-up-and-go has got-up-and-gone! But iron-deficiency anemia is incredibly common, and it's one of the first things your doctor will look for.

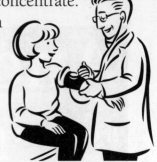

WHERE THE IRON GOES

Iron-deficiency anemia is almost always the result of blood loss from causes such as excessive menstrual flow or intestinal ulcers. It can also be a result of nothing more than not getting enough iron in your diet.

Women are six times more vulnerable than men, at least until the age of 65, when the gender gap narrows to about two to one. Why do men luck out? They have more blood volume than women to begin with, and they're spared the joys of menstruation (blast 'em!).

In the United States, 20 percent of all women of childbearing age have iron-deficiency anemia, compared with 2 percent of adult men. The cause is primarily blood loss during menstruation. When women don't replace the lost iron by eating iron-rich foods, the problem gets worse. If your menstrual periods are particularly heavy or irregular or last seven

---

Tea Time

Bitter Is Better

For some reason, old folk remedies often included bitter substances to stimulate digestion and thus promote better absorption of nutrients. Gentian is a bitter herb that's popular in Europe to treat a number of ailments, including iron-deficiency anemia. *Gentiana lutea* is the botanical name of this herb, which you can find at health food stores. Follow the package directions to brew a tea, then drink it before meals to aid digestion.

Acidic foods such as tomato-based sauces leach iron out of cast-iron pots, and every little bit counts when you tally your iron gains for the day. So whether you're making spaghetti, bowties, rotini, or shells, cook the sauce in an iron pot.

days or more, you have a greater risk of iron-deficiency anemia.

Once they begin menstruating in their teens, some girls fail to understand that they need to make up for the iron they lose in the process. Along with menstrual blood loss, a steady diet of junk food, irregular hours, and the emotional chaos of adolescence mean that teenage girls often neglect their iron needs. This is also the time many girls decide to go vegetarian or embark on total fasts to lose a pound and a half to fit into their skinny jeans. The trouble is, they do this without giving much thought to their health.

Because anemia can lead to serious illness and can have several causes, don't treat it by yourself until you see your doctor for a blood test. A complete blood count (CBC) will determine if the number of red blood cells and amount of hemoglobin in your blood are abnormally low. If they are, further diagnostic tests can pin down the cause so you can get treatment.

HOLLER FOR HELP

Beware of Blood Loss

Iron-deficiency anemia is usually easy to reverse with home care—but not always. You could be losing blood internally—from an ulcer, a kidney or ovarian tumor, or even colon cancer. Call your doctor immediately if you notice blood in your urine or stools, or if your energy has taken a sudden nosedive for no good reason.

MAXIMIZE THE MINERAL

Once you know you have iron-deficiency anemia, it's very easy to reverse. You don't need expensive supplements. In fact, most doctors today don't want you to take iron supplements, since they can be life-threatening. High levels of iron in the blood may increase your risk of heart attack as well as cause seizures, jaundice, or gastrointestinal problems.

All you have to do is eat more iron-rich foods or increase your iron absorption. Here's how.

Have more cow chow. Most research shows that meat sources of iron are easier to absorb than vegetable sources. Meat also boosts the absorption of iron from other foods. Lean red meat and beef liver are good iron sources. Organ meats such as brains and kidneys are especially rich in the mineral, and poultry, fish, and oysters are next in line.

Because meat and fish are such major sources of iron in most people's diets, vegetarians need to be especially careful to eat fruits, vegetables, and grains that offer high amounts, such as green leafy vegetables, dried fruit, legumes, and whole grain breads.

Dandelions are dandy. Lawn lovers may despise pesky dandelions, but they're super sources of iron and are gentle to the liver, points out Ryan Drum, Ph.D., a medical herbalist in Washington State. Plus, they taste great—a little like arugula, a nutty, spiky-leaved salad green. It's the leaves at the crown of the dandelion plant that you want. Just be sure to pick them from an area that you're sure is free of pesticides and other chemicals, then rinse them thoroughly and toss into salads. Also, don't eat a lot of dandelion if you're taking diuretics or potassium supplements.

Pump up with sushi. Forget the avocado and other enticing ingredients inside that little roll. Nori, the black, paper-thin seaweed that holds the roll together, contains more iron than any land plant, says Dr. Drum. If sushi isn't your style, simply pick up some dried nori at a health food store and crumble it into your favorite salad.

Lift iron with lemon. Ever wonder about the Southern habit of spicing up greens with vinegar? Sprinkled on greens, acidic condiments such as vinegar and lemon juice help liberate minerals, making iron more easily absorbed by your body.

Add green to your plate. As many as one-fifth of all vegetarian women are anemic. If you don't eat meat, try your best not to be one of them by loading up on salads made with iron-rich kale, beet greens, collard greens, chard, and parsley.

Beat it with blackstrap. The syrupy substance that remains after sugarcane is processed—blackstrap molasses—is a great source of iron. In the old days, folks often slathered it on whole grain bread for breakfast. If you enjoy the taste, you can simply swallow 2 tablespoons of molasses. This amount contains about 10 milligrams of iron—nearly 40 percent of the daily requirement—and just 85 calories.

Boost iron with C. Foods high in vitamin C, such as citrus fruits, strawberries, and tomatoes, help your body absorb iron from other foods. Basically, the vitamin moves the iron through the gastrointestinal system and into your bloodstream, so it's not eliminated.

Go the raw route. Heat destroys the protein atom around ferritin, or iron, points out Dr. Drum. Eat produce in its natural, fresh state whenever you can.

Imbibe less. If you're drinking too much wine at dinner or beer at the ballgame, consider what it may be doing to your iron supply. Too much alcohol can affect iron status in several ways. It interferes with your body's ability to absorb folate, a B vitamin that you need for red blood cells. And if the problem is chronic, it usually results in poor nutrition overall.

Lick it with lactic acid. Yogurt and sauerkraut both contain this important substance, which promotes iron absorption. Fermented soy foods such as miso can help, too.

Say hello to yellow. The herb yellow dock, available as capsules or tincture at health food stores, helps your body absorb iron from your diet and is especially recommended for moms-to-be, says Dr. Drum. If you're pregnant, be sure to check with your obstetrician before taking it.

Limit iron robbers. Tannins in black tea inhibit iron absorption. Other thieves include antacids, the food additive EDTA (look for it on food labels), and phosphates in soft drinks and ice cream.

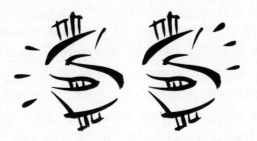

Angina

Help for a Hurting Heart

Your heart is one powerful muscle, but it needs the right fuel to keep on pumping—not just blood, but good old oxygen as well. When the heart doesn't get enough oxygen, it screams "Enough!" the only way it knows how: with sharp chest pains that can make you feel as though someone's sticking daggers into the middle of your chest.

Angina is a lot less serious than a heart attack, but it's nothing to ignore, either. When you first notice symptoms—pain usually comes on during exertion, such as when you're shoveling your car out from under a night's worth of snow or quarreling with your spouse about whose turn it is to do the dishes—call your doctor or 911 immediately. The pain will go away on its own in most cases, but the underlying causes will still be there—and they'll only get worse if you don't take action.

SHORT ON O$_2$

Sudden, heavy chest pressure is a hallmark of angina, and the lack of oxygen that causes it occurs when the arteries that deliver blood to your heart have narrowed. The narrowing is

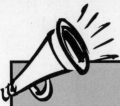

generally a result of either accumulated fatty deposits on the insides of the artery walls (coronary artery disease) or, much more rarely, spasms in the arteries. But angina takes many forms. Sometimes, it's a shooting pain up your arm and other times, it's a sharp, squeezing sensation near your shoulders. In women especially, it can even be super-subtle—say, a tiny twinge that radiates toward your neck—and therefore super-scary.

"Angina is the heart's distress call, but it's not an early warning system," says Peter Brunschwig, M.D., director of Helios Integrated Medicine in Boulder, Colorado. "By the time a person gets angina, his arteries have probably already become narrow and weak from a slow buildup of cholesterol-laden plaque." Anyone with angina, no matter how infrequent or fleeting, should consult a doctor immediately to rule out serious heart disease and an impending heart attack.

OPEN THE GATES

If you've been diagnosed with angina due to coronary artery disease, odds are that your doctor has prescribed nitroglycerin, the drug equivalent of an American Express card—you simply don't leave home without it. Taking nitroglycerin during an angina attack quickly relaxes the arteries, opening them so oxygen-rich blood can flow easily to your heart. Beta-blockers and calcium channel blockers do essentially the same thing.

If your angina persists, and your physician finds that the arteries to your heart are very nearly closed due to a pileup of plaque there, you may need angioplasty—a surgical procedure that involves inflating a balloon to force open blocked vessels—or bypass surgery to shunt blood flow around the narrowed arteries.

These treatments work in the sense that they ease blood flow to the heart, possibly preventing a heart attack. And while that's hugely significant, it's not a cure. "The very best way to control your angina," explains Dr. Brunschwig, "is to adopt a comprehensive program aimed at lowering plaque."

There's no substitute for high-tech medicine if you have angina, but many of the best treatments for the heart are also the easiest and least expensive ways to help prevent angina attacks. Here's what you need to do.

Pace yourself. Exercise is a double-edged sword for people with angina. Because it increases your heart's demand for oxygen, it can bring on an attack. Over time, however, regular exercise improves blood flow and strengthens your heart. Nearly everyone with angina should be on some kind of exercise plan.

Definitely talk to your doctor to find out how much exercise

Save the Skin

Adam and Eve were probably short on knives and peelers, so they undoubtedly ate their apples with the skin on—and that's good. The skins of organic varieties of apples are brimming with quercetin, a much-studied plant chemical that fights heart disease by preventing cholesterol from transforming itself into the muck that plasters itself to your artery walls, narrowing them and setting you up for a heart attack.

you can safely do. Even if your angina is somewhat severe, your doctor will probably advise a daily program of mild activity, such as walking or bicycling. You don't want to rush into anything. Like the fairytale tortoise who raced the hare, you're more likely to be a winner when you make slow and steady progress, says Andrew Parkinson, N.D., a naturopathic physician and faculty member at the Bastyr Center for Natural Health near Seattle.

Take five. Along with taking the medicine your doctor prescribes, the quickest way to halt an angina attack is to stop what you're doing. The pain generally occurs during exertion, when your heart isn't getting enough blood and oxygen. As soon as you relax, your heart slows down and consumes less oxygen, and the pain will almost always subside within a few minutes.

Eat smart. Angina may have put your heart in a half-nelson, but the match isn't over yet. You can avoid getting pinned to the mat by switching to a heart-healthy diet, says Dr. Parkinson. "You want to avoid fried foods and animal fats and replace them with fruits and vegetables," he advises. This and other simple changes, such as getting more fiber in your diet and watching your weight, will lower cholesterol levels in your blood. That way, your arteries won't become more clogged than they already are.

Here's another reason to eat a

Does your breath smell garlicky? It should if you have angina, because garlic has been shown to lower cholesterol. The more raw or cooked garlic you eat, the lower it will go.

healthful diet: Fruits, vegetables, legumes, and other plant foods are rich in antioxidants, chemical compounds that help prevent cholesterol from sticking to artery walls.

Feast on fish. The natural oils in seafood have been shown to help elevate levels of high-density lipoprotein (HDL), the "good" cholesterol. This is important because HDL helps remove artery-clogging low-density lipoprotein (LDL), the "bad" cholesterol, from the blood.

The natural oils, called omega-3 fatty acids, also suppress the inflammation that contributes to the artery-clogging process. For optimal heart protection, eat fish three or four times a week or, as long as you're not taking aspirin or prescription blood thinners, take a teaspoon of fish oil daily.

Make the most of magnesium. This important mineral has a variety of critical functions, among them keeping the heart healthy and strong, says Dr. Parkinson. When you have angina, make an extra effort to get plenty of magnesium. He advises taking supplements; the recommended amount is 500 to 1,000 milligrams a day, divided into two or three doses. But check with your doctor first; this amount of magnesium may cause diarrhea or other, more serious side effects in some people.

The $2 Deal

Stock Up on Sprouts

Laboratory studies suggest that alfalfa sprouts may help dissolve the artery-blocking deposits that cause angina. Research hasn't been done with people, so it's not certain that alfalfa helps, but the evidence is compelling enough that you may want to give it a try. Two caveats: Since it's known that sprouts are frequently contaminated with bacteria, buy from a local grower who's careful to keep his sprouts bacteria-free, and always wash them thoroughly.

Get the mighty duo. Vitamins C and E are powerful antioxidants that help keep harmful oxygen molecules, called free radicals, from damaging artery walls. They also help prevent chemical changes in cholesterol that make it more likely to stick to artery walls. Unless your doctor tells you otherwise, plan on taking at least 500 milligrams of vitamin C daily, preferably divided into two doses to prevent diarrhea or an upset stomach. For vitamin E, the recommended amount is 400 to 800 IU daily. Because angina is such a serious problem, be sure to let your doctor know that you're taking the supplements, since they could interact with other drugs you may be taking.

Cook and cry. Onions may have an eye-watering punch, but they also have a mild blood-thinning effect that can prevent blood clots—a serious risk for people with angina or other heart problems. Add 'em to everything you can.

Sprinkle on plenty of seasonings. If you have angina, keep some pungent ginger in the first row of your spice cabinet. It contains chemical compounds that lower cholesterol and inhibit the formation of blood clots. Along with other spices, such as turmeric and red pepper, ginger inhibits arterial inflammation that may lead to or worsen angina.

Grab some grapes. We can't be certain, but it seems likely that the ancient Romans didn't get

---

Tea Time

Hawthorn for a Healthy Heart

Long before doctors developed nitroglycerin and other drugs for angina, herbalists were treating people with hawthorn. "I've had good results using it to prevent angina pain in my patients," says Andrew Parkinson, N.D. To make hawthorn tea, steep a tablespoon of the dried herb in a cup of boiling water for about 10 minutes, then strain before drinking. If you're taking any other drugs, check with your doctor before using hawthorn.

angina very often. The credit may go to all those grapes they ate while lounging around the Forum. Grapes are loaded with pectin, a type of fiber that removes cholesterol from the blood. They're also rich in bioflavonoids, natural chemicals that have heart-protective effects. So take a tip from the Romans, and eat a bunch!

Get an oil change. "Flaxseed, borage, and walnut oils all contain an omega-3 that is converted to essential fatty acids in the body," says Robert Bonakdar, M.D., director of pain management and heart health at the Scripps Center for Integrative Medicine in La Jolla, California. "They're the next best thing to fish oil." Pour any of the oils over some magnesium-packed leafy greens. Just be sure to use a liberal amount; you need 1 tablespoon a day to get any benefit. If you take aspirin or blood thinners, though, don't use flaxseed oil.

Get plenty of aminos. The mighty amino acid arginine, much like nitroglycerin, helps relax artery walls and keep the vessels open. In fact, supplemental arginine has been shown to prolong the time people can exercise before chest pain kicks in,

Miracle Margarines

Some margarine-like spreads, such as Benecol, contain plant stanols that block the absorption of cholesterol in the intestines, forcing your liver to snatch it from your bloodstream—and keep it away from your heart. In fact, studies show that people who add plant stanols to a low-fat diet can reduce plaque-building cholesterol by 10 to 24 percent. To get the benefits, you'll need three servings a day of 2 tablespoons each. Spread it on toast at breakfast, crackers at lunch, and a dinner roll at supper. But don't go overboard—these spreads still contain fat.

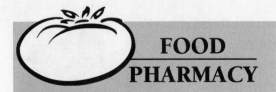

FOOD PHARMACY

Get Nutty

Soy nuts and peanuts—as well as fish, spinach, and organ meats—are packed with a little miracle elixir called coenzyme Q_{10} (CoQ_{10}). "This antioxidant appears to bring oxygen to the heart and may even help curb the damage caused by the lack of oxygen," says Peter Brunschwig, M.D. He recommends taking 100 milligrams a day. You can find CoQ_{10} supplements at health food stores and drugstores.

which is significant because exercise reduces cholesterol, blood pressure, stress, and weight—all risk factors for heart disease.

Arginine's cousin, carnitine, is an amino acid abundant in red meat that may help strengthen the heart muscle. Dr. Bonakdar recommends that people with angina take 500 milligrams of carnitine a day, but since there's no exact dose for arginine, he suggests asking a doctor about a combination formula specifically tailored to their condition.

Tame your temper. Anger releases adrenaline, the "fight or flight" hormone that signals a bump up in blood pressure, heart rate, and blood flow away from the heart and to the muscles (so we can fight or flee). All of these physiologic responses can precipitate angina. To help you manage your anger and sidestep angina, you might seek the help of a support group. To locate one in your area, contact the cardiac rehabilitation unit at your local hospital.

Say sayonara to stress. "The behavior that seems to make the most difference in reducing heart disease is managing stress," notes Dr. Bonakdar. "The outside pressure to, say, head another church committee is absolutely matched by the pressure inside your arteries." The best way to minimize that internal pressure? "Say no to mounting demands," he says. As a bonus, once you're not quite so overcommitted, you'll have time for yoga, deep breathing, or other calming techniques proven to help keep a lid on angina.

Work on your relationship. If you're a husband who feels your wife doesn't show her love, studies show you're twice as likely as husbands with more demonstrative wives to have angina. Likewise, if you're the withholding wife, anger, depression, or even garden-variety stress may have left you feeling stingy with your emotions—and predisposed to your own chest pain. Let a counselor help you sort out the affairs of the heart, and you may ease pain in your life in more ways than one.

Eat beets. Betacyanin, the compound that gives beets their rich color, may help cells take in more oxygen, so eating fresh beets or freshly grated beetroot in salads could give your heart a breath of fresh air.

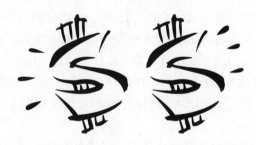

Anxiety

Quick Ways to De-Stress

Anxiety gets a bad rap. The only reason we're even alive today is that our great-great ancestors didn't spend their days all blissed-out with dreamy smiles on their faces. When they saw 400 pounds of fur and claws making a beeline for the cave door, they naturally got distressed. Anxiety signaled their brains to direct their adrenal glands to release a flood of "fight or flight" hormones that primed their muscles for action.

Of course, there's a big difference between sensible worry and chronic, never-ending anxiety. If you never chill out, your muscles and mind remain on high alert and ready to fight or flee, even when you're safe and sound. Your level of "feel good" hormones remains low, which makes you feel jittery, achy, and constantly vigilant. Your immune system becomes depleted, and you're more likely to get sick.

TAKE THE EDGE OFF

Whether you're nagged by niggling worries or chased by heart-pounding panic, you've got plenty of company. "Anxiety is a soaring trend," notes Paul Foxman, Ph.D., director of the Center for Anxiety Disorders in Burlington, Vermont. "And given our jam-packed lifestyles, uncertain economy, and shaky world politics, some worrying is understandable and quite healthy. But when your anxiety is unexplained or overwhelming, you can literally become worried sick."

No one should put up with chronic worry. If anxiety is turning your life upside down, you'll probably want to see a therapist. In addition, there are plenty of cost-free strategies that can make a real difference. Here's a sample.

Get calm with chamomile. Studies show that this herb blocks anxiety-promoting brain chemicals triggered by worry. Simply buy some dried chamomile flowers at a health food store (avoid the weak, prepackaged kind in tea bags) and measure 1 teaspoon into a cup. Fill the cup with freshly boiled water, cover, and steep for 15 minutes. (While you wait, close your eyes and count all the wonderful things you're grateful for.) Sip the strained and cooled tea and feel your worries slip away. One caveat: If you're allergic to ragweed and

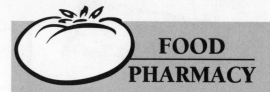

FOOD PHARMACY

Catch Some Serenity

Salmon, tuna, and sardines are filled to the gills with omega-3 essential fatty acids (EFAs), which can powerfully improve your mood, says Hyla Cass, M.D. For the EFAs to have any effect, however, you'll need to eat fish three times a week. If this exceeds your taste for tuna, you can take 1 gram (1,000 milligrams) of fish oil in capsule form a day. Or you can get your EFAs from flaxseed. Take one capsule a day, or check your health food store for flaxseed oil to use in place of salad dressing, for instance. If you take aspirin, other nonsteroidal anti-inflammatory drugs, or prescription blood thinners, avoid fish oil and flaxseed oil until you check with your doctor, since both can thin your blood.

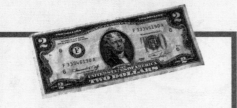

The $2 Deal

De-Stress with Valerian

"Valerian root is a great wind-down herb that relieves tension without dulling the mind," says Heidi Weinhold, N.D. "If you aren't already taking anti-anxiety medication or prescription sleeping pills (if you are, you shouldn't take anything else), I suggest taking two 200- to 300-milligram tablets before bedtime."

other members of the daisy family, don't use chamomile.

Ditch the "what ifs." Are you one of those of those people who always imagine the worst? Do you find yourself saying things like, "What if the bus crashes?" To nip your anxiety in the bud, simply counteract your concern with hard facts. Ask yourself, "What's the probability of being in a bus crash?" Then answer, "Unless I'm an extra in the next *Speed* sequel, it has to be pretty low." In other words, talk yourself free of your spiraling emotions. "Talking back to negative chatter is just as effective as taking anti-anxiety drugs," says Dr. Foxman.

Hit the brakes. When you feel the "what ifs" overwhelming you, try to imagine a stop sign. Say the word "Stop!" out loud to stop the "what ifs" in their tracks. Tell yourself that right now, you are okay.

Turn on your natural drugstore. Exercise will work off anxiety, and many studies have shown how being active changes your body chemistry. When you exercise, your brain releases endorphins, hormones that have a calming effect. Go for a walk, a run, or a bike ride. Go dancing. Anything that gets your body moving will help. Also, getting your heart rate up as a result of exercise rather than because of anxiety makes you feel more in control, says Linda Welsh, Ed.D., director of the Anxiety Disorders and Agoraphobia Treatment Center in Bala Cynwyd, Pennsylvania.

Lay on the lavender. A few drops of lavender oil added to your body lotion can be a source of anxiety-preventing aromatherapy all day long. For a more dramatic effect, add a drop of the oil to a dab of your favorite salve, then rub it into your temples or solar plexus as a reminder to relax and breathe deeply.

Breathe from the bottom. When you're worrying about a deadline or how the dinner party will go, you take quick, shallow breaths high up in your chest, which signals your brain to release anxiety-producing chemicals. "Breathing slowly and fully from your lower abdomen is the best way to calm your body and mind," says Joan Borysenko, Ph.D., director of Mind/Body Health Sciences in Boulder, Colorado. Keep your shoulders still and expand your lungs fully so your belly bulges out, then exhale slowly. Your heart rate will slow, and your anxiety will fade.

Stay in the present. Mindfulness—the practice of being fully absorbed in what you're doing, while you're doing it—anchors you in the present, slowing your breathing and quieting your mind, says Dr. Borysenko. For instance, try eating an orange mindfully: Peel it slowly and deliberately. Notice its nubby feel, garish color, and tangy scent. Savor the sweet-sour juice in your mouth. Linger there, in the moment. If any thoughts—say, of your com-

HOLLER FOR HELP

Get Your Life in Line

If chronic anxiety is seriously limiting the way you live your life, seek help from a mental health professional. You may need a prescription medication such as alprazolam (Xanax) to block the fight-or-flight response and calm your mind and body, as well as short-term cognitive therapy to give you a different way to think about things that happen.

Whether you regularly listen to NPR's Dr. Dan Gottleib or to Dr. Laura, you may want to turn off the docs every once in a while and either slip in a Brahms CD or turn the dial to a classical station. According to one study, 30 minutes of classical music can be as calming as 10 milligrams of Valium.

ing day—intrude, gently turn your attention back to the orange. When you practice mindfulness in everything you do, you're less likely to be led astray by worries.

Hold the joe. A Duke University study revealed that even low to moderate doses of caffeine can cause difficulty concentrating, nervousness, trembling, insomnia, irritability, and disorientation. Caffeine can add to the physical symptoms of anxiety and make it worse, says Dr. Welsh. So switch to decaf, and see if you don't feel less anxious. Dr. Welsh suggests cutting back on sugar, too, because it has a similar effect on anxiety.

Shift mental gears. If panic rises when you're in the midst of a crowd, concentrate on something else: Wiggle your toes in your shoes. Read a nearby sign. Fumble for your keys. Ask someone for directions. Focusing on concrete, familiar objects and activities keeps your anxiety from commandeering your thoughts—and building to all-out panic. Heidi Weinhold, N.D., a naturopathic physician in Pittsburgh, also suggests whispering "soft belly." Saying the words will shift your focus, and they will remind you to take a deep breath, which will instantly diffuse the fight-or-flight hormones, she says.

Go ga-ga over GABA. Gamma-amino butyric acid (GABA) is the calming chemical in your brain that regulates all of your feel-good hormones. Hyla Cass, M.D., assistant clinical professor of psychiatry at the University of California, Los Angeles, School of Medicine, says that supplementing with GABA (available at health food stores) reduces overall tension. She suggests taking 250 milligrams twice daily after meals. As always, however, you should consult your doctor before trying it, and avoid GABA altogether if you take anti-anxiety or antidepressant medications.

Sip some oatstraw. Sipped as a tea, the herb oatstraw (which you can find at a health food store) is both calming and energizing and is "awesome" if you're trying to cut back on caffeine, says Dr. Weinhold. Another plus: Oatstraw is packed with B vitamins, which soothe jangled nerves. Buy the herb in tea bags or add 20 to 60 drops of tincture to a glass of water and take it up to four times a day.

Calm your heart with passionflower. This herb is tailor-made for hyped-up people with thumping hearts, says Dr. Weinhold. Add 20 to 40 drops of passionflower extract (available at health food stores) to a glass of water and drink four or five glasses a day. Don't use it if you're pregnant, though.

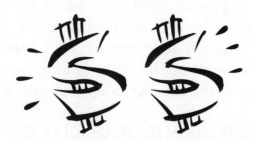

Arthritis

Fight the Force of Friction

Are your hinges so creaky in the morning that you feel like the Tin Woodman without his trusty oilcan? Do your fingers, knees, and hips get so stiff that even simple activities, such as working in the garden, make you feel like you're doing hard time in the mines?

Mother Nature doesn't mess up very often, but she sure could have done a better job of joint design. By age 40 or 50, many of us begin to notice some joint tightness. It's usually caused by osteoarthritis, the "wear and tear" arthritis that occurs when the spongy cartilage that covers and protects the bones of our joints becomes thinner due to age and daily friction.

WHEN YOUR JOINTS ARE OUT OF JOINT

Without their protective cushioning, bones may start to grind against each other, which can damage the tissue surrounding the joint. The immune system attempts to come to the rescue, but instead, the white blood cells overreact and release inflammatory proteins. These in turn cause swelling, pain, and further damage to the tissue. Joints become stiff and sore, although not all at once and maybe never more than a few.

Osteoarthritis usually announces itself with pain and stiffness, especially in weight-bearing joints such as your hips and knees. Repetitive motion is often the culprit. If you spent your youth hurling a ball, you may be at risk for arthritis in your shoulders. Even relatively young skiers and runners can develop severe knee problems.

> ### Tea Time
>
> #### Get Relief with Ginger
>
> Ginger is a powerful anti-inflammatory herb that can take the edge off arthritis pain, says Grace Ornstein, M.D. To make a healing tea, grate about an inch of fresh ginger and steep it in hot water for 10 minutes, then strain. Drink it once or twice a day.

MOVE WITH EASE

You should call your doctor at the first sign of joint pain. It's always possible that you have rheumatoid arthritis or another kind of joint disease. In most cases, though, your joints are simply wearing out a bit. Don't get panicky and throw a lot of money at the problem right away. In many cases, you can use home remedies to eliminate most—if not all—of your pain.

Watch the clock. Nearly everyone with arthritis takes the occasional pain reliever. It's best to take aspirin and related drugs before noon. Since the pain and inflammation tend to be worst in the late afternoon and evening, you can get a jump on them by starting your treatment in the morning or at midday.

Hide the high heels. Skinny stilettos are murder on your knees—but they're not the only culprits. In fact, high, wide-heeled pumps may predispose you to osteoarthritis of the knee, too. The problem, it seems, isn't the stability of the platform but the height of the heel. Any woman who regularly wears heels higher than 2 inches is twice as likely to develop

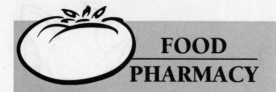

FOOD PHARMACY

Beat Pain with Boron

Raisins, pears, apples, and other fruits, as well as nuts and beans, all contain the trace mineral boron, which can relieve joint pain and stiffness and actually appears to protect against arthritis, says Michael E. Weinblatt, M.D.

arthritis as women who don't, says Michael E. Weinblatt, M.D., co-director of clinical rheumatology at Harvard's Brigham and Women's Hospital in Boston. Heels shift your body weight away from your ankles and onto your hips and the inner part of your knee joints, and arthritis is often the result.

Exercise as much as you can. Exercise is a tricky issue if you have arthritis. You obviously don't want to push yourself too hard when you're hurting. On the other hand, regular exercise lubricates your joints and helps with weight loss. Walking is almost always a good choice. If you have too much knee or ankle pain to walk, ride a stationary bike. "Set the seat high so you don't have to bend your knees as much," says James Herndon, M.D., chair of the department of orthopedic surgery at Brigham and Women's Hospital.

Cut those calories. The next time your bathroom scale sneaks up a hair, don't fret about your fanny—it's your knees that deserve your pity! Each time you gain a single pound of body fat, experts say, it feels like four times that much on your knees. The strain is especially hard on your muscles and tendons—your built-in shock absorbers. The good news is, studies show that if you lose as few as 11 pounds, you can reduce stiffness and pain in your knees by half.

Get action with attraction. Although scientists aren't sure why, studies show that wearing knee wraps embedded with magnets may help you get out of a chair more easily, walk faster and less stiffly, and even sleep better. Attracted to the possibilities? Look for wraps with "unipolar" magnets, then place the positive end of the magnet directly over your sore knee, suggests Martha Hinman, Ph.D., associate professor of physical therapy at the University of Texas Medical Branch in Galveston. You should feel relief within 30 minutes.

Oil your joints. Trout, salmon, and other cold-water fish contain an abundance of omega-3 essential fatty acids, which ease swollen, stiff joints by reducing both inflammation and cartilage destruction, says Dr. Weinblatt. Serve 'em up often.

Pepper the pain. A quick way to ease arthritis pain is to apply a topical cream that contains capsaicin, the hot chemical compound that's found in red pepper. "You get local numbing of nerve endings along with a warming effect," says Kevin R. Stone, M.D., an orthopedic surgeon in San Francisco. Most drugstores carry the cream, which comes in concentrations from 0.025 to 0.075; if you have sensitive skin, try a lower strength first. Follow the label directions and be careful not to get it near your eyes or on any areas of broken skin. Wash your hands after using it.

Add some arnica. To soothe aching joints, add a few drops of

The $2 Deal

Rebuild with Glucosamine

One of the most effective treatments for osteoarthritis is glucosamine sulfate, a supplement produced from shellfish. It combats cartilage-destroying enzymes and halts cartilage loss in the knee and hip. "You start with 500 to 1,000 milligrams three times a day. It takes two to four weeks to get relief from pain—and twice that long to ease functioning in your joint," says Todd Nelson, N.D. Avoid it if you have a seafood allergy.

arnica oil to your favorite healing salve. Try using a warming wintergreen, lavender, or rosemary salve as a base. All three can help increase circulation to the painful area. For every ½ teaspoon of salve, add 3 or 4 drops of arnica oil. Apply to sore joints three or four times per day. Arnica is for external use only, though, and don't use it on broken skin.

Cool it with cabbage. Cabbage leaves have been used for centuries to soothe inflammation. A sturdy, outer leaf is just the right shape to place over a bent knee or an elbow. Blanch a leaf or two, then apply warm or cool to inflamed joints. Wrap it with gauze or an elastic bandage to hold it in place.

Fortify with D. New evidence links low levels of vitamin D to the progression of osteoarthritis, says Lila Wallis, M.D., former president of the American Medical Women's Association and a specialist in women's health based in New York City. One study showed that people with too little vitamin D in their diets were more likely to develop osteoarthritis and three times more likely to have existing arthritis get worse. Your body produces vitamin D when you're exposed to sunlight, but it's also helpful to drink milk that's fortified with the vitamin.

Needle your knees. Research directed by the National Institutes of Health indicates that people with osteoarthritis of the knee who receive acupuncture have less pain and better function than people who receive standard care—even weeks after the treatment. Ask your doctor to recommend a reputable acupuncturist near you.

Get a buzz. Try transcutaneous electrical nerve stimulation

(TENS). A TENS unit is a battery-powered device, smaller than a deck of cards, that you attach to your belt or waistband. It delivers electrical impulses through the skin. Although TENS doesn't offer a cure, Emile Hiesiger, M.D., clinical associate professor in the departments of neurology and radiology at New York University School of Medicine in New York City, notes that it may relieve chronic pain. It increases endorphins—naturally occurring narcotics in the body—that inhibit pain impulses arising from the spinal cord.

Put cold on heat. When an arthritic joint is inflamed, it may be painful, swollen, or even feel hot. Put some ice on that fire. "Ice is very good for inflammation and swelling," says Dr. Herndon. He recommends putting an ice pack on the sore joint for about 20 minutes at a time. Repeat the treatment once an hour, continuing for as long as it seems to help.

Warm the stiffness. When your joints are achy, but there's no swelling, heat works better than cold. It feels good, for one thing, and it promotes the flow of healing nutrients into the joint.

Moist heat seems to work best, so you may want to use a warm compress instead of a heating pad. Soak a small towel in hot water, wring it out, and drape it over your painful joint. When the towel cools, soak it again and reapply it.

HOLLER FOR HELP

Get Prescription Relief

If your joints are so swollen and painfully stiff that you can barely climb out of your car, and you're popping aspirin or ibuprofen tablets as if they were breath mints, it's time for a doctor's visit. Standard treatments for arthritis include the prescription medication celecoxib (Celebrex), a drug that works by blocking the pain-prompting enzyme. Prescription arthritis medications usually have fewer side effects than aspirin or ibuprofen.

Take a hint from the East. The herbs guggul, boswellia, gokshura, and madder are commonly used in India to relieve joint pain, and there's good evidence that they work, says Grace Ornstein, M.D., medical director and scientific advisor for Himalaya USA, a marketer of herbal formulas based in Houston. "They all have anti-inflammatory properties," she says.

These and other anti-inflammatory herbs are available in supplement form in health food stores. Follow the directions on the label, and be sure to let your doctor know you're taking them.

Stop pain with licorice. Licorice root is a friend indeed when your arthritis flares up, because it can counteract the inflammation. "It's a wonderful herb," says Dr. Ornstein.

Licorice root is available in capsules and tablets at health food stores (don't bother with licorice candy, which contains little or no real licorice). Since a substance in licorice called glycyrrhizic acid can cause high blood pressure in some people, look for deglycyrrhizinated licorice (DGL) products, then follow the label directions.

Spice up your menu. The herb turmeric is aromatic and spicy, and research suggests that it's a great inflammation fighter. You can add it to rice, stews, and meat dishes.

Lay off the lattes. If you drink more than four cups of coffee a day, you're doubling your risk of developing arthritis, warns Todd Nelson, N.D., a naturopathic physician in Denver. Caffeine not only alters the mineral balance that's needed to make cartilage, it can also dry up the fluid required to keep cartilage and joints lubricated.

Drink up. Like most people, you probably don't drink enough water, and that could be making your arthritis symptoms worse. Drink at least eight full glasses every day—and don't wait until you're thirsty. By the time you feel thirsty, your body's water levels have already dropped too low.

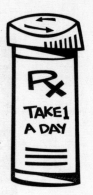

Experiment with drugs. What's the best pill to reach for when you need relief? There's no clear answer, Dr. Herndon says. "I have my favorites, starting with ibuprofen, then aspirin." Other people may do better with naproxen. You'll just have to try different painkillers until you find the one that works best for you. If you're going beyond the guidelines on the label or you have any chronic health problems besides arthritis, consult your doctor first.

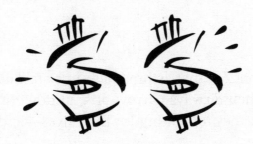

Asthma

Shortcuts to Better Breathing

It's no accident that asthma flare-ups are called attacks. When their airways narrow or shut down, people literally feel as if they're fighting for their lives—and in many cases, they are.

Many people still think of asthma as a childhood disease, yet increasing numbers of adults—more women than men—are developing it. Researchers aren't sure of the exact reason. They suspect that along with the usual triggers (such as pollen, dust, and frigid air) that can inflame airways and cause them to fill with mucus, both increased body weight (which can literally weigh on the chest wall, making it more difficult to breathe) and the surges and drops in hormones associated with menstruation and menopause may play a role.

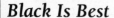

Tea Time

Black Is Best

Afternoon tea is a great relaxer, but it has many other benefits. Regular black tea is a source of theophylline, a bronchial muscle relaxant used to treat asthma. Earl Grey and other great teas can do the trick.

FIGHTING FOR BREATH

Our airways naturally narrow a bit when we're exposed to smoke, pollutants, very cold air, or substances that can harm us if we inhale them. But in people with asthma, perhaps due to a glitch in their genes, this response is exaggerated. Most people can quickly reverse an asthma attack using prescription medication—usually an inhaled bronchodilator—to open the constricted airways. When an attack is more prolonged, however, the inhaler doesn't do much. As airways become more inflamed and often clogged with mucus, it gets harder and harder to breathe. This type of episode is a medical emergency, and you need to get to the nearest hospital emergency room—quickly.

BREATHE EASY

The bottom line? Never fool around with asthma. People can and do die from this disease. While nearly everyone with asthma uses inhalers and other medications, there are drug-free ways to tackle it as well. Here are the best ones to discuss with your doctor.

Put your trust in fish. Tuna, salmon, trout, and other cold-water fish contain loads of omega-3 essential fatty acids (EFAs), which not only inhibit inflammation but may also repair airway

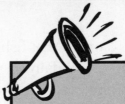

HOLLER FOR HELP

Watch for Warning Signs

Even very mild asthma can flare up as instantly and seriously as severe asthma—and prove just as fatal. Whether you typically have mild, moderate, or severe asthma, if you have wheezing, shortness of breath, or tightness in your chest that doesn't respond to inhaled or oral medications prescribed by your doctor, head to the hospital immediately. Other serious signs include difficulty talking, rapid or shallow breathing, enlarged nostrils, tightly stretched skin on your neck and/or around your ribcage with each breath, and gray or bluish skin around your mouth or under your fingernails.

damage. Eat fish regularly or take 1 to 3 grams of fish oil daily to minimize asthma symptoms. If you don't eat fish often or are sensitive to it, as many people with asthma are, down 1 to 3 tablespoons of flaxseed oil (another source of EFAs) a day. You can find both oils at health food stores and drugstores, but don't use them if you take aspirin, other nonsteroidal anti-inflammatory drugs, or prescription blood thinners.

Cut up some onions. Onions are an old-time remedy for bronchial problems. Researchers have validated this use in recent years after discovering that onions are a rich source of quercetin, an anti-inflammatory compound. Make a pot of onion soup or eat them raw—if you dare—and feel the warmth spreading through your chest and lungs.

Enjoy your daily brew. A few cups of strong coffee can sometimes reduce asthma symptoms. In one survey, 25 people said a jolt of caffeine eased their symptoms, and research at the National Heart, Lung, and Blood Institute seems to back up this observation. Scientists there discovered that regular coffee drinkers with asthma suffer a third fewer symptoms than non-coffee drinkers. Nobody knows exactly why, but it may be because caffeine is a chemical that's similar to the theophylline in tea, which opens bronchial tubes.

Watch for culinary culprits. Asthma is often caused by allergies, and in some cases, the problem is specific foods. Unfortunately, there is no handy list of food allergens—they vary with each individual. If you suspect that foods may be triggering your asthma, talk to your doctor immediately. Then keep a careful record of what you eat, when you eat it, and what kind of symptoms develop afterward. After a few weeks, a pattern may emerge. Take your record to your doctor and ask him to check your suspicions with skin or other allergy tests.

Get a cleaner vacuum. Vacuum cleaners can kick up 2 to 10 times the amount of allergens that normally float around your house. The extra onslaught can persist for up to an hour after you turn off the vac. If you have chronic asthma, look into special vacuums that eliminate this dusty "exhaust." (They're expensive but worth it to ease your symptoms.) You could also wear a dust mask when you vacuum or, better yet, swap housecleaning chores with someone else.

Beat it with borage. The star-shaped flowers of the borage plant are packed with gamma-linolenic acid (GLA), a fatty acid that fights asthma inflammation. Check your health food store for either borage or primrose oil (also packed with GLA) and take 3 grams (3,000 milligrams) daily, suggests Anna Szpindor, M.D., director of Allergy and Asthma Care in Oak Park, Illinois. If you're pollen-sensitive, however, check with your doctor first.

Sleep high. Heading to a dude ranch or rustic retreat anytime soon? Be sure to get dibs on the upper bunk. It's well worth the climb, say researchers in Spain. When you sleep in the bottom bunk, you're showered with dust bunnies and dust mites that fall from the bedding above when the sleeper tosses and turns—and

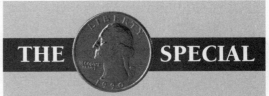

THE SPECIAL

Maximize Magnesium

Studies show that if your diet is deficient in magnesium, your asthma may be more severe. The recommended supplement dose is 800 milligrams of magnesium gluconate (divided into two 400-milligram doses) along with 800 milligrams of calcium citrate a day, says Anna Szpindor, M.D., but check it with your doctor first. This much magnesium may cause diarrhea. If this occurs, reduce the dose, then increase it gradually.

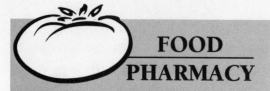

FOOD PHARMACY

Munch an Apple a Day

The skin of organic apples (as well as tomatoes, onions, and the Indian spice turmeric) contains quercetin, a potent bioflavonoid that may help keep your airways clear. Or you can take 500 to 1,000 milligrams of quercetin in capsule form three times a day, along with 100 to 200 milligrams of bromelain, a pineapple-derived enzyme that will boost its absorption. Avoid bromelain if you take blood thinners.

asthma is more likely to flare.

Exercise often. It used to be that if exercise triggered your asthma, you could count on becoming a couch potato. Not anymore. For one thing, doctors now know the couch is home to billions of dust mites, so you can't hang out there. For another, proper exercise helps people with asthma. You need muscle tone, a stronger heart, and increased stamina to fight any disease, and asthma is no exception.

Wheeze less by walking. The best aerobic exercise for most people is walking. You need to walk fast enough so your heart and lungs work hard and you work up a sweat. Obviously, if you have asthma, hard breathing can be stressful, but a consistent, steady walking program will increase your stamina. If you pick up the pace gradually over time, you'll eventually be able to handle some real huffing and puffing. Most doctors advise using an inhaled bronchodilator before doing any strenuous exercise.

Enjoy natural licorice. "An asthmatic person's breath is a thousand times more acidic than it should be," says Richard N. Firshein, D.O., medical director of the Firshein Center for Comprehensive Medicine in New York City. "One theory is that acid backwash in the mouth (from heartburn) inflames the lung tissues and constricts the airways."

To limit both the backwash and the constriction, check your health food store for deglycyrrhizinated (DGL) licorice root, which helps reduce stomach acid. Either sip DGL extract (add about 40 drops of tincture to a cup of hot water) or chew a 200- to 500-milligram DGL wafer before meals, suggests Todd Nelson, N.D., a naturopathic physician in Denver.

Unload your stress. Emotional stress doesn't cause asthma, but it can aggravate it, says Jack Routes, M.D., associate professor of medicine and immunology at the University of Colorado Health Sciences Center in Denver. To reduce anxiety and perhaps improve your breathing, take 20 minutes a day to write nonstop (don't edit yourself, just get it out) about what's stressing you. Studies show that after about four months, you may be breathing easier—which is less stressful by itself!

Breathe more slowly. If you're a wheezer, experts say you're also an overbreather. That is, you breathe heavily or rapidly or inhale through your mouth—any one of which can promote irritation and inflammation of the airways. To slow your breathing, Dr. Firshein suggests using your heart rate as a guide. For every seven heartbeats, breathe in once through your nose. For the next nine beats, breathe out through your mouth with your lips pursed until your air is gone.

Kick your symptoms. It turns out that karate isn't just an

Inhaling steam can unclog tight airways. Fill a teapot with water, bring it to a boil, and remove it from the stove. Place a towel over your head to trap the steam, lean over the teapot (but not so close that you burn your face), and breathe deeply. Or turn on a hot shower and sit in the steamy bathroom for 10 to 15 minutes.

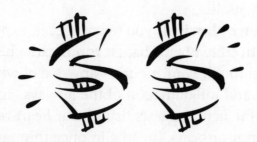

excellent way to ward off bad guys—it's also a solid defense against asthma attacks. "The exclamation that accompanies the forceful kicks forces you to exhale quickly and deeply so you draw in a deep breath before you continue," says Dr. Firshein. And deep, full-lunged breathing (also required when you're walking, running, or swimming) opens airways.

Keep the air clean. Because asthma is often triggered by airborne allergens, make your bedroom an allergy-free zone. It's easy: Simply keep the door and windows shut at all times. Never allow your beloved terrier or tabby to enter. Remove all carpet and throw rugs. Get rid of dust-collecting knickknacks. And use an air cleaner with a HEPA filter (a high-efficiency particulate air filter, which can trap nearly 100 percent of all airborne particles).

Use a peak flow meter. This little gadget costs only a few dollars at the drugstore, and it can save your life. The meter gauges how much air you're able to push out of your lungs, and it may help you predict when an asthma attack is sneaking up on you. Ask your doctor which readings may signal the need to take action, then blow into it twice a day and compare your readings against your "personal best" number.

Athlete's Foot

Foil That Fungus

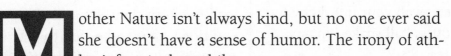

Mother Nature isn't always kind, but no one ever said she doesn't have a sense of humor. The irony of athlete's foot is that while it's rarely serious, it sure feels (and looks) like it could be. To make things worse, it itches most when your feet are swaddled in shoes— the very time when you can't scratch 'em!

The nasty fungus known as *Tinea pedis* that's behind athlete's foot thrives in the warmth and dampness created by the sauna inside airtight shoes or snug socks. It usually settles in the moist area between your fourth and fifth piggies and feeds off dead skin cells. And once the webs of your toes become cracked

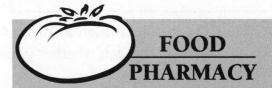

FOOD PHARMACY

Gobble Those Berries!

Strawberries and blueberries are packed with vitamin C, which will help fight your athlete's foot infection from the inside. When fruit's out of season, and if you don't have kidney or stomach problems, take 1,000 milligrams of supplemental vitamin C twice a day, suggests Mike Cronin, N.D.

and red, they itch like the devil.

Because tinea is a fungus—an invader, if you will—it tends to gain a foothold in folks with weakened immune systems and those who have recently used antibiotics. Those drugs kill off all bacteria, including the beneficial types that keep fungi in check, explains Mike Cronin, N.D., a naturopathic physician in Scottsdale, Arizona. People with diabetes are also at increased risk because they tend to have more sugar—a yummy feast for fungi—in their systems. But you don't have to be sick to get athlete's foot. Fungal infections thrive in alkaline environments, so if your diet is high in sugar, yeast, and other alkaline foods, you can get the itch whether you're sick or not.

TREATS FOR YOUR FEET

If the fungus has spread to your arches, or your feet are fiery red, swollen, and covered with blisters, contact your doctor—pronto. If you're on the ball, and you catch the infection in the early stages of itching, you can always fight back with an over-the-counter antifungal agent. But why spend the money if you don't have to? In most cases, you can tackle athlete's foot with simple, homemade cures—and your symptoms should clear up within a week. Here's what to try.

Soak those piggies. Place your feet in a basin of warm water spiked with 2 to 3 teaspoons of tea tree oil and soak for 15 minutes twice daily. This oil, from the Australian malaluca tree, is one of nature's best antifungals.

Or start with a gentler herb.
Since tea tree oil may sting when applied topically, Dr. Cronin suggests first trying one of the gentler antifungal herbs, such as goldenseal, chamomile, or calendula. You can even look for over-the-counter antifungal creams that pack all three for more healing punch.

Zap it with zinc. Not only will zinc increase immunity (and thereby quash fungi), it will also help broken skin heal faster, says Jeanette Jacknin, M.D., a dermatologist in Scottsdale, Arizona. She suggests taking 30 milligrams of supplemental zinc daily, with food, for as long as the fungus persists.

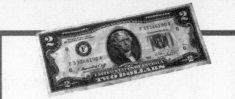

The $2 Deal
Sour Is Sweet

Fungi hate acids, and apple cider vinegar is one of the best acid soaks there is, says Lisa Murray-Doran, N.D., a naturopathic physician in Whitby, Ontario. Here's what to do: Simply fill a basin with equal parts vinegar and warm, soothing water, then soak your feet for 10 minutes daily. Dry each toe and the area between your toes thoroughly when you're done.

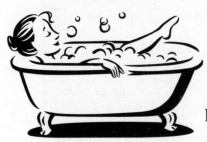

Be a clean machine. Dodge this grungy fungus by meticulously cleaning under your toenails and between your toes during your daily bath or shower.

Dry 'em well. If you're prone to athlete's foot, dry each toe separately, then use a paper towel between them to absorb every drop of moisture. Or use a blow dryer set on low. It'll feel good!

Catch some air. Let those tootsies hang out in the fresh air and sunshine if you're not going anywhere. Just don't walk barefoot around the house. Not only will you track foot powder all over your rugs, but you'll plant contagious little fungus seedlings wherever you go. You don't want to be known as Johnny Fungusseed, do you?

Spoon up some yogurt. *Lactobacillus acidophilus*, which is found in some yogurts, is one of the "good" bacteria that your body needs to keep fungi in check, says Dr. Jacknin. Check yogurt labels to find a brand that contains live cultures (sorry, but frozen yogurt and yogurt-dipped raisins or nuts don't have them), then make a point of including it in your breakfast or lunch menu. Or check at a health food store for acidophilus powder or capsules and take 1 teaspoon of powder or two capsules on an empty stomach twice a day.

Lay on some licorice. Licorice contains a whopping total of 25 fungicidal substances, says Dr. Jacknin. Too bad munching on licorice whips won't do the trick. What you need to do is add 6 teaspoons of powdered licorice to a cup of boiling water and simmer for 20 minutes. Strain out any residue and apply the clear tea to your inflamed toes three times a day.

Take time for thyme. A traditional remedy for athlete's foot is soaking your feet in hot water to which you've added a few

Mama Mia!

Garlic is such a potent topical antifungal that Daniel DeLapp, N.D., a naturopathic physician and instructor in dermatology at the National College of Naturopathic Medicine in Portland, Oregon, suggests placing a clove of raw, peeled garlic between all your toes every night for a week. (Apply a film of olive oil first.) Put on cotton socks before going to bed, then wash and dry your feet each morning. Although you may need to sleep in the guest room, this treatment should stop the itch in its tracks.

drops of oil of thyme to relieve the itching and burning. Then dust your feet with a mixture of myrrh and goldenseal powder in any proportion and put on a pair of heavy cotton socks. Repeat daily for several days.

Count on cotton. While you're treating your athlete's foot, avoid wearing panty hose and stick to socks made of 100 percent cotton. Wash and dry your feet twice daily, then slip into a fresh pair of all-cotton socks sprinkled with antifungal powder.

Give up on cornstarch. This popular ingredient has replaced talc in many powdered anti-sweat products, but it can actually encourage fungus growth, warns Dr. Cronin. You're better off using a medicated antifungal powder or a foot spray that combines calendula and witch hazel, an astringent herb that reduces moisture.

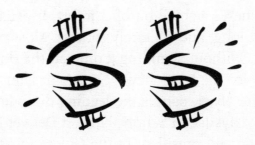

Back Pain

Put Your Aches behind You

There aren't many good things to say about back pain, but here's a small bit of comfort: It usually doesn't last very long, and it's rarely serious. Most people recover in a few weeks without spending a dime at the doctor's office.

Okay, now for the lousy news: Sooner or later, just about everyone gets it. "Back pain is the leading disability for folks under age 45," says Jacob Schorr, N.D., a Denver-based naturopathic physician and president of the Colorado Association of Naturopathic Doctors. "And it isn't just the freight lifters among us who are getting nailed."

Sure, you can injure your back on the job or in a car crash, but by far the most frequent cause isn't anything catastrophic—it's everyday weakness and inflexibility in the muscles that support the back.

STRESS PLUS WEAKNESS EQUALS PAIN

The weaker your muscles (especially those in your upper back, hips, and hamstrings—the muscles at the backs of your thighs), the more apt you are to hurt your back. A sudden, uncharacteristic movement—such as swinging a golf club—strains the stiff muscles, tendons, and ligaments, damaging tissue and causing swelling and intense aching. Your muscles may even seize in spasms to protect your back from further movement and additional injury.

Sometimes you don't even have to do anything to strain your back. Simply living under the burden of chronic emotional stress can create muscle tension, says John Sarno, M.D., professor of clinical rehabilitation medicine at New York University School of Medicine in New York City. That tension in turn can block blood flow to the muscles and create more spasms and pain. "The more pain, the more stress," he says. "It becomes a vicious cycle."

FAST FIX
Get in the Swim

Swimming is one of the fastest ways to take the kinks out of aching back muscles. For one thing, merely submerging yourself in warm water will help reduce muscle tension. More important, the water supports your weight, which allows you to exercise without putting additional strain on your back.

EASE THE ACHE

Don't twiddle your thumbs waiting for Father Time to cure your aching back—you can nudge him along. In fact, you should, because if you treat a back problem in the acute phase, you may reduce the likelihood of long-term pain and disability.

If you stand a lot, as a surgeon or supermarket clerk does, shift your weight from hip to hip to avoid back pain.

Back pain that's severe or doesn't start getting better within a week or two should always be checked by a doctor. For garden-variety aches, though, here's what you need to do.

Move and keep moving. "The worst thing anyone with an achy back can do is to sit still," says Carol Hartigan, M.D., assistant clinical professor of physical medicine and rehabilitation at Harvard Medical School. In fact, resting for more than a day or two reduces muscle flexibility and strength and can lead to further disability. On the other hand, movement keeps blood flowing into the site, waste products flowing out of it, and muscle spasms to a minimum. "Let your pain be your guide," says Dr. Hartigan. "You may not want to move your piano, but it's really okay to lift a bag of groceries. My advice is to do everyday activities as you can tolerate them."

Do the ball stretch. The more you work your back muscles, says Dr. Hartigan, the faster you can return to normal activities. Grab an oversize exercise ball and give this mini-workout a try. First, lie face down across the ball with your hands and feet on the floor. Lift one arm and then the other as high as you can, raising your torso from the ball. Pause for a count of 10, then return both hands to the floor. Next, place both hands behind your head and lift your torso as high as you can. Hold for 5 counts, then release. Repeat as many times as is comfortable.

Stretch and flex. Even if your

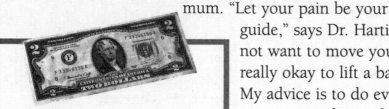

The $2 Deal

Baby It with Bromelain

This anti-inflammatory enzyme, derived from the pineapple plant, may be especially helpful for relieving pain related to inflammation. "I like to use formulas that include bromelain, papain, and trypsin—all enzymes that help calm down the chemical pathways that cause pain," says Tanya Baldwin, N.D., a naturopathic physician in Los Gatos, California. As long as you're not taking blood thinners, check at a health food store for supplements, then follow the label directions.

back pain has you lying on the floor, you can stretch your arms and legs, elongating the tissues in your back and drawing healing blood and oxygen to the area, says Art Brownstein, M.D., clinical instructor of medicine at the University of Hawaii at Manoa. Just remember to stay relaxed, cushion your back with a pad, and use slow, gentle movements as you extend your arms over your head and stretch your legs along the floor. Hold each stretch for about a minute, then relax.

Put cold to work. "Ice is a great analgesic and is preferable to aspirin or other nonsteroidal anti-inflammatory drugs like ibuprofen, which, in large doses, can cause stomach upset," says Dr. Hartigan. Simply fill a paper or Styrofoam cup with water and freeze it, then peel away the rim to expose the ice surface. Grasping the cup, lie on your side, then apply the ice directly to the painful area in a circular motion. Limit the massage to about 5 minutes, and don't place the ice directly on the bony portion of your spine.

Whip up some willow bark. It's a natural source of aspirin-like salicylates, which ease pain. Unlike aspirin or ibuprofen, though, it won't irritate your stomach while it's easing your back pain, notes Glen Rothfeld, M.D., clinical assistant professor of medicine at Tufts University School of

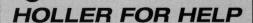

HOLLER FOR HELP

More Than Back Pain

Consult a doctor if you have back pain that persists without abating for more than three days; if it's accompanied by fever, pain at night or when resting, or bowel or bladder changes; or if you are weak or can't stand on your tip-toes, which may indicate nerve damage. If you have back pain as well as a history of cancer or diabetes, you should see a doctor immediately to check for a tumor or nerve damage. Start with your primary care physician, who can refer you to a specialist, such as an orthopedist, if necessary.

Medicine in Boston. To make a tea, pick up some willow bark from a health food store, steep 2 teaspoons in a cup of boiling water, and strain. You can also take capsules or apply willow bark ointment directly to your back. Don't use it in any form, however, if you take aspirin; the double dose of salicylates may be too much for your system.

Relax with an herbal mix. Scour your health food store for herbal pain formulas that contain cramp bark, black cohosh, and oatstraw in capsule form, suggests Dr. Schorr. These herbs are all excellent antispasmodics and muscle relaxants. If valerian, which is a sedative, is also among the ingredients, the capsules will make a great nightcap for a bad back. Follow the dosage directions on the label. Skip the valerian if you're taking other medications, though.

Lie down and say "Ahh!" According to studies from the Group Health Cooperative in Seattle, weekly massages can cut the need for pain medication for back spasms and tight muscles in half.

As a general rule, a muscle spasm should relax when the therapist massages it. If it persists, you probably have some inflammation, too, and mas-

Get a Leg Up

Have you ever wondered why traditional pubs have foot railings that run the length of the bar? It's because bar owners want you to stand there—and buy drinks—as long as you can. Standing with one foot raised greatly reduces pressure on back muscles, so it's a good position when your back is hurting. When you're standing for more than a few minutes, look for any raised surface—a curb, a chair rung, or anything else that's at least a few inches above the ground—that you can use to keep one foot higher than the other.

sage may not be the best therapy for you, notes Beth Mueller, a massage therapist in Appleton, Wisconsin. You'll need at least four massage treatments to smooth out spasms.

Salute your inner soldier. Keep your shoulders back, chest out, stomach in, chin up! That's good posture as well as a good drill for a new army recruit. Correct posture means that your body is aligned so it puts less strain on your lower back.

Sit smart. Keep your feet flat on the floor if you sit at a desk all day. Your arms should be positioned so your elbows form right angles. Set your computer monitor at eye level. Your chair seat should be deep enough to support your hips, but the front edge should not touch the backs of your knees. The chair back should have an angle of about 10 degrees and cradle the small of your back comfortably. If it doesn't, add a wedge-shaped cushion or lumbar pad there.

Here's some back-happy news: An old-fashioned, straight-backed chair is better for your back than many of those high-tech, ergonomic extravaganzas that cost hundreds—or thousands—of dollars. Or you can try a kneeler chair to see if it relieves your back pain, says Emile Hiesiger, M.D., clinical associate professor in the departments of neurology and radiology at New York University School of Medicine.

Take a load off your shoulders. When you carry a shoulder bag, you tend to tense your shoulder to keep the bag from slipping off. This scrunched-up posture causes all kinds of muscle strain and related pain, according to Amy

> The best sleeping position for people with back pain is to lie on their sides with a pillow between their knees. If you're comfortable only when you sleep on your back, at least put a pillow under your knees to reduce the arch in your back and relieve some of the strain.

Klein, D.C., a New York chiropractor who always asks to see what kinds of handbags her back pain clients carry. Check out purses by designers such as Liz Claiborne and Calvin Klein, who are heeding the message with new lines of short-handled carryalls. When you can't sling a bag over your shoulder, you'll be more inclined to switch the weight from hand to hand.

Apply instant heat. Tiger Balm is a familiar remedy from ancient Chinese medicine. Rubbed into the skin, this potent salve creates heat to warm tight muscles and a tingling sensation to divert your attention from the pain.

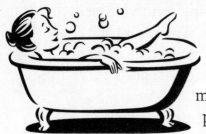

Fill the tub with thyme. Ease your aching back by tossing a handful of dried thyme into the tub as you run hot water for a bath. Soak for 10 to 15 minutes, letting the aromatic oils in this herb take your aches and pains down the drain.

Stop aches with arnica. Arnica gel is an excellent first-aid ointment for muscle or joint pain. For inflamed and irritated nerves, add several drops of St. John's wort oil and apply frequently. Note that arnica is for external use only. Do not use on broken skin.

Ease pain with Epsom. A traditional Epsom salts bath can help ease spasms and relieve pain. Add 2 cups of the salts to a hot bath, sink down, and feel the relief. Afterward, place an ice pack on your back.

Knock down swelling. Studies have shown that aspirin, ibuprofen, and similar drugs often work as well for back pain as more powerful prescription drugs. They help in two ways: They're analgesics, which means they work directly on pain, and they have anti-inflammatory effects, which reduce swelling. Acetaminophen is fine for pain, but it has little or no effect on inflammation.

Bad Breath

Knock Out Oral Odor

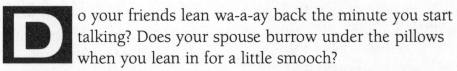

Do your friends lean wa-a-ay back the minute you start talking? Does your spouse burrow under the pillows when you lean in for a little smooch?

If you answered "Yes!" to either of these questions, blame halitosis, the polite term for dragon breath. Bad breath is certainly better than no breath at all, and, truth be told, no one's breath is minty-fresh all the time. But if you have the impression that people are thinking "roadkill" every time you open your mouth, it's time to take a few steps to freshen things up a bit.

Bad breath is almost always caused by odor-causing bacteria in the mouth. Morning breath can be a real killer because while you're sleeping, your saliva production factory is offline. The environment in your mouth shifts from slightly

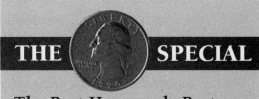

THE SPECIAL

The Best Homemade Paste

To make an effective toothpaste, add a few drops of hydrogen peroxide to baking soda. It won't taste good while you brush, but afterward, your mouth will be wonderfully fresh.

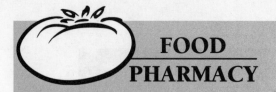

FOOD PHARMACY

Clobber It with Chlorophyll

Vegetables and fruits are not only valuable sources of vitamins and antioxidants, they also contain chlorophyll, a natural deodorant that sweetens your breath. Eat five to nine servings a day for a healthy body and healthy breath.

While you're at it, throw in some sour foods, such as pickles and lemons. They will jump-start the flow of saliva, helping to flush away those nasty halitosis bacteria in your mouth.

acidic to slightly alkaline, bacteria really take off, and you wake up a few hours later with real buzzard breath.

You should definitely talk to your doctor if your breath is always bad. All sorts of conditions, including digestive problems, can cause it. In most cases, though, you can fight the fumes with a few simple strategies.

Get those bristles moving. Are you brushing twice a day with a soft brush? The bedtime brushing is important so plaque doesn't form during the night (when you have less saliva). Massage your gums with the brush, too, and floss before you brush. Flossing every day helps remove plaque—and bacteria—from between your teeth. The American Dental Association also recommends professional cleaning at least annually, and some dentists suggest twice a year.

Rake your tongue. Most bad breath comes from the wet, boggy areas in the back of your mouth, where bacteria breed a sulfurous-smelling plaque on your tongue, according to George Preti, Ph.D., of the Monell Chemical Senses Center in Philadelphia. Before brushing, reach into your mouth as far as you can without gagging and scrape away the plaque, he suggests. Most drugstores carry plastic tongue scrapers, or you can simply use your toothbrush.

Munch an apple. It will not only keep the doctor away, it will also keep bad breath at bay. In fact, an apple is a great remedy for garlic breath. In a healthy mouth, garlic odor usually goes away after a while, but you'll speed up the process if you dilute the pungent aroma by eating an apple, then brushing your teeth.

Swish, swish, swish. Use an antiseptic mouthwash that kills bacteria. Other mouthwashes just mask odor with a minty solution, but some can be quite pleasant and long-lasting. Try making your own odor-masking mouthwash with whole or powdered cloves steeped in hot water.

Try a myrrhvalous mouthwash. Add 1 teaspoon of tincture of myrrh to ¼ cup of water, then swish and spit. It instantly freshens breath—and it tastes good, too. (Tinctures are potent liquid plant extracts; you can find them at many health food stores.)

Chug plenty of H$_2$0. Keeping yourself well hydrated is a good health practice in general, but it's especially important to help keep bad breath at bay. Drink those eight glasses a day to help keep saliva production going and reduce bacteria buildup.

Love those leaves! Some Native American traditions call for using spearmint or bergamot leaf as a quick and easy digestive aid and breath freshener. Chew a leaf or two slowly. Then make a cup of mild mint tea by steeping three leaves in a cup of boiling water for

HOLLER FOR HELP

When Bad Breath Means Bad Health

Bad breath is usually a result of poor dental hygiene, a poor diet, or a sinus or gum infection, but it can also signal something as serious as kidney failure, liver disease, or diabetes. Visit your doctor if you have persistent bad breath that you can't clear up with simple home care.

10 minutes. Strain out the leaves, let the tea cool, and use it as a gargle, rinse, or spray. Also, carry a sandwich bag or pouch of mint or parsley leaves so you can chew on them periodically throughout the day.

Refresh and brighten. Here's a cleansing and refreshing mixture that clears up bad breath while brightening the teeth. You can use this tooth powder daily or alternate it with a commercial brand. In a small dish, mix 1 tablespoon baking soda, ½ teaspoon sea salt or kosher salt, ½ teaspoon powdered allspice, and ½ teaspoon ground sage. Sprinkle onto your toothbrush and brush, or stir 1 teaspoon into a cup of warm water and gargle.

Feel fresh with fennel. Chewing fennel seeds after meals will help freshen breath and promote healthy digestion.

Pepper away mouth germs. Red pepper (cayenne) not only kills germs, it leaves your breath spicy fresh as well. Just dilute 5 to 10 drops each of cayenne tincture and myrrh tincture in half a glass of warm water and use it to rinse your mouth.

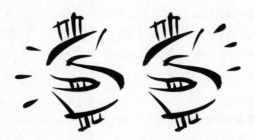

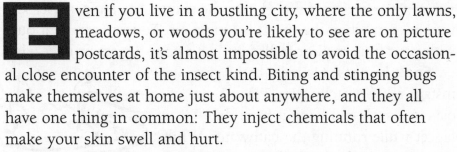

Bites and Stings

Vanquish the Venom

Even if you live in a bustling city, where the only lawns, meadows, or woods you're likely to see are on picture postcards, it's almost impossible to avoid the occasional close encounter of the insect kind. Biting and stinging bugs make themselves at home just about anywhere, and they all have one thing in common: They inject chemicals that often make your skin swell and hurt.

With a few dangerous exceptions (the black widow comes to mind), most bites and stings are only minor nuisances. See a doctor if you get bad hives or other serious reactions. Otherwise, try these quick tips for nearly instant relief.

Freeze the bite. As with other types of inflammation, some well-applied ice can freeze a painful insect sting in its tracks. Ice also soothes the itchiness of mosquito bites.

Wrap some ice cubes in a washcloth or small towel to make a cold pack, then hold it against the affected area for about 20

HOLLER FOR HELP

A Dangerous Reaction

If you have any sign of body swelling or difficulty breathing after a sting, call 911 or get to an emergency room immediately. Stings can cause a life-threatening reaction, called anaphylaxis, in some people. If you know you're allergic, your doctor will probably prescribe an epinephrine self-injector so you can take fast action if you're bitten or stung.

minutes. Remove it for at least 20 minutes, then continue applying it in this way until you're feeling better.

Cool it down. Soak a washcloth in cool water, wring it out, and drape it over the bite, suggests Laura Pimentel, M.D., chair of emergency medicine at Mercy Medical Center in Baltimore. "A cool compress is soothing and will help reduce itching," she says.

Take away the sting. If the insect left a stinger embedded in your skin, your best bet is to remove it as quickly as possible. Otherwise, it will continue to irritate the skin; a bee stinger releases venom even when the insect is long gone. You can scrape it out with your fingernail or pull it out with your fingers or tweezers.

Soak in oats. Oatmeal baths give instant relief to itchy skin. Place 1 cup of oats in a sock and hang it from the faucet while running the bathwater. While you're soaking, squeeze the sock and let the milky water cascade over the bites. Very hot water can sometimes exacerbate the itch, so take your soak in warm water only.

Make a venom vacuum. The next time you get a bite or sting, mix a little baking soda with water and smear a generous layer of the paste on the sore spot. It helps pull venom out of the skin, explains Heidi Weinhold, N.D., a naturopathic physician in Pittsburgh. Don't have baking soda? Apply a dab of mud.

Soil almost always contains a little clay, which also helps draw out the venom and reduce pain and swelling.

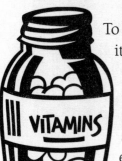

Prepare to repair. To help your skin repair itself, be sure to get plenty of vitamins C and E, two nutrients that are critical for skin health. You'll get enough of both— along with other important vitamins and minerals— just by taking a daily multivitamin.

Think prevention. Natural mosquito repellents are effective only if you use them frequently and there aren't too many of the little blood suckers around. Some doctors think that the best kinds are products that contain neem, lemongrass, or citronella oils. Test an area of your skin first to be sure the repellent doesn't irritate you, then spray or dab it directly on your skin, following the package directions. Studies show that neem oil (from an Indian tree) provides significant protection from malaria-carrying mosquitoes for up to 12 hours; another study found that lemongrass and citronella oils are highly effective against most species of mosquitoes.

Keep your shoes on. Bees often hover just above the ground, gathering pollen from clover and ground flowers, so they can be hard to see. Don't go barefoot across that tempting lawn in bee season— you could step on a bee and get seriously stung.

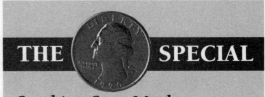

THE SPECIAL

Soothing Sage Mash

You can make a great poultice using sage and vinegar. Just run a rolling pin over a handful of freshly picked sage leaves to bruise them. Put the leaves in a pan, cover with apple cider vinegar, and simmer on low until they soften. Remove the leaves, carefully wrap them in a washcloth, and place it on stings and swellings for instant relief.

Black Eyes

Help for Hard Knocks

If you like old movies, you've probably seen some unfortunate character holding a steak to his injured eye after a run-in with a bully or a barn door. While no one really uses steaks to soothe black eyes (have you checked the price of beef lately?), the idea wasn't so far-fetched. Black eyes hurt, and putting something cool on it probably felt pretty good.

A hard knock can break blood vessels beneath the skin, causing swelling and a lot of tenderness. It takes a week or two for a black eye to heal completely, and in the meantime, chemical changes in the skin give it its astonishing range of hues.

BANISH THE BLACK-AND-BLUE

Since shiners always look terrible, you can't go by appearance alone in deciding whether you're seriously injured. If you have bleeding, pain in the eyeball (as opposed to the surrounding area), or vision changes (double vision, for example) after the injury, get to a doctor right away. Otherwise, you can speed healing without spending a bundle on fancy ointments.

Start with cold. Nothing is better for a black eye than

applying ice right away. Cold causes blood vessels to constrict, or
narrow, which reduces internal
bleeding, swelling, and those
unsightly color changes, says
Priscilla Natanson, N.D., a naturopathic physician in Plantation,
Florida. Cold also numbs the area
and helps ease the throbbing.

Make an ice pack by wrapping
some ice cubes in a washcloth or
small towel, then gently hold it
against the area for 15 to 20 minutes every few hours during the 24
hours following the injury, Dr.
Natanson advises.

Then use heat. You don't want
to apply heat to a black eye right
away because it may increase bleeding under the skin. From
24 to 48 hours after the injury, though, a warm compress is just
the thing. The heat promotes circulation and helps flush pain-
causing substances from the area. Soak a washcloth in warm
water, wring it out, and apply it for a few minutes as often as
necessary to reduce discomfort.

Run the hot-cold cycle. You can also try a technique called
contrast hydrotherapy, in which you alternate warm and cold
compresses. It's a wonderful treatment for a black eye, says Dr.
Natanson. The combination of heat and cold helps the body
flush and clean the tissues and will help your eye heal more
quickly.

Start by applying a warm compress for about 3 minutes.
Switch to cold for 30 seconds, then go back to heat. Repeat the
process two or three times, always ending with the cold applica-

FAST FIX
Terrific Tannins

One of the quickest ways to soothe
a black eye is with a tea bag. Black
and green teas contain tannins,
chemical compounds that help
reduce swelling. After brewing a
cup of tea, let the tea bag cool for a
few minutes, then squeeze out the
excess moisture. Lie back,
close your eyes, and
hold the tea bag against
the injured area for 10
minutes or so.

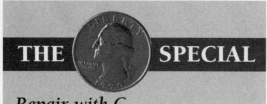
Repair with C

Vitamin C does more than relieve the sniffles. When you have a black eye, it helps strengthen and repair tiny blood vessels called capillaries. As long as you don't have stomach or kidney problems, think about trying 2,000 to 3,000 milligrams of vitamin C daily until the black eye is gone. Take it in divided doses at different times of the day to prevent diarrhea or stomach upset.

tion. Use this technique three times a day until your eye is completely healed.

Heal with comfrey. The herb comfrey is among the best treatments for minor wounds and bruises, and it's perfect for a black eye, says Dr. Natanson. If you're using fresh leaves, mash them into a paste and apply it directly to the bruise. If you're using the dried form, crush the leaves between your fingers and add just enough water to moisten. Wrap the powder in a piece of cheesecloth, then hold it on the area. Apply either form of the herb for about 20 minutes twice a day. Comfrey is available at health food stores.

Forget the white pills. Even though it's a great remedy for pain, aspirin reduces the ability of blood to clot normally, which could result in even more bruising in the days following the injury. A better choice is acetaminophen, which has the same painkilling properties as aspirin but is less likely to cause additional bleeding or bruising.

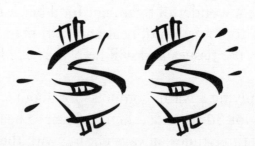

Blisters

No More Trouble with Bubbles

You have to give your skin credit: It's not only weather resistant, germ repellent, and self-healing, it also knows how to protect itself. When you exert too much pressure—by spending all day on your knees scrubbing floors, for example, or wearing tight shoes without socks—the skin responds to potentially damaging friction by forming a blister, a protective, fluid-filled pad.

Most blisters go away on their own, usually within a few days to a week, but that doesn't mean you can ignore them. Blisters can easily become infected—and when that happens, they hurt like the dickens!

HURRY THE HEALING

Your doctor will charge a bundle to open and drain a blister. You might need the help—but probably not. Except when they get infected, there's no reason to pop blisters to drain out the fluid, says Lisa Arnold, N.D., a naturopathic physician in Orleans, Massachusetts. Here are some easy, inexpensive steps to prevent infection and help blisters heal more quickly.

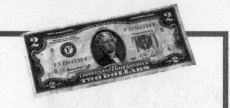

The $2 Deal

Comfort from Calendula

To reduce blister tenderness and help speed healing, apply a salve that contains the herb calendula along with skin-protecting vitamins A and E. "Calendula is really helpful for skin problems," says Lisa Arnold, N.D.

You can apply the salve, available at health food stores, once a day. Or buy dried calendula, crumble it between your fingers, and add enough water to make a paste. Cover the blister with the paste and leave it on for about 20 minutes, then rinse it off.

Catch 'em quick. Before a blister appears, you'll usually notice a hot spot—a red, tender area on your skin. Acting quickly at this stage may prevent a blister from forming.

If you've had a burn, for example, quickly apply ice to the area and keep it there for about 20 minutes. If the hot spot is caused by friction, cushion the area with moleskin, gauze, or another type of padding.

Wash away the germs. The best way to keep infection-causing germs out of blisters is to clean them (and the surrounding skin) once or twice a day. Wash the area well with soap and water, then dry it thoroughly. Too much moisture will soften the blister and make it more likely to break open before it's ready.

No worries with "wort." The herb St. John's wort is great for killing germs and easing pain. Use an alcohol-based tincture, available at health food stores, to moisten a square of gauze, then apply it to the blister after you've washed it.

Lay on some yarrow. Big blisters sometimes take a long time to heal. You can speed things along by applying yarrow, an herb that naturally (and safely) draws out the fluid. "It's an astringent herb that will help dry it out," says Dr. Arnold.

If you're using fresh or dried yarrow (available at health food stores), chop or crumble it as finely as you can, then add enough water to make a paste. Apply the paste to the blister and cover it with an adhesive or gauze bandage. Replace the dressing once a day until the blister is gone.

Count on clover. Red clover oil is a great choice for healing blisters. You can put the oil directly on the sore, then cover it with a bandage to promote healing. Repeat the treatment once a day until the blister's gone.

The oil is available in most health food stores, but be sure the product you buy is made for topical use. What you don't want is an essential oil, which is too concentrated to apply directly to your skin.

Let it breathe. Even though it's good to protect a blister with a bandage, you want to expose it to the air for at least 20 minutes a day. A little air circulation will help protect the area from infection-causing bacteria, which thrive in dark, moist places.

Tone up with tannins. These compounds, which occur in many plants and trees, can strengthen the skin. To prevent blisters, soak your hands or feet in a strong, tannin-rich infusion of black tea, oak bark, or pine twigs. To make it, simply soak a handful of the tea, bark, or twigs in a basin of freshly boiled water. When the water cools, strain the solution, then soak your hands or feet for 10 to 15 minutes. One caveat: If you have diabetes, talk to your doctor before soaking your feet.

Lace tight. When putting on running or other sports shoes, be

FAST FIX
A Spicy Solution

You probably have two of the strongest antiseptic herbs in your kitchen right now. "Rosemary and thyme can really help if you're worried about infection," says Lisa Arnold, N.D. Add a tablespoon of each herb to a cup of hot water and steep for about 10 minutes. Let the liquid cool to room temperature, pour some on a cloth, and hold it against your blister for about 20 minutes. You can repeat the treatment once or twice a day until the blister is gone.

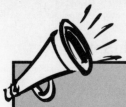

HOLLER FOR HELP

Watch for Red

The only time blisters are really dangerous is when they get infected. If the pain is getting worse, or if you notice the area is swelling or turning red, it's worth taking the time to apply an over-the-counter triple antibiotic ointment a few times a day. If that doesn't help, you're going to have to see a doctor to be sure the infection doesn't continue to spread.

sure to lace them up properly, so your feet are held firmly in place. Otherwise, they'll rub around against the insides of the shoes and create blisters.

Fight the friction. Blisters on the feet are most likely to develop if your feet are either too sweaty or too dry. If your socks are often soggy, the origin of your blister problem may be that sweaty skin. Try sprinkling a little cornstarch into your socks before you put them on, and dust some between your toes, too.

If the skin on your feet is very dry, smooth a thin film of petroleum jelly over them before you pull on your socks and sneakers.

Take care of your hands. Wear gloves when you work with household or construction tools. Likewise, wear gardening gloves when you're raking or pruning.

Lighten up. A golf club, squash racket, or tennis racket is a blister machine, so loosen your fingers and change your grip as often as you can while playing.

Get tough. If you are about to embark on a home improvement project or other activity that will be a shock to your soft hands, get them ready. Rub denatured alcohol on your hands three times a day for several weeks before doing the manual labor, recommends Andrew Weil, M.D., director of the Program in Integrative Medicine at the University of Arizona in Tucson.

Bloating

Drain the Tank Naturally

The human body is naturally awash in water, but that doesn't mean that more is necessarily better. At certain times of the month, or after pigging out on chips, pickles, or other salty foods, women can accumulate so much extra fluid that it makes their skin puffy. They may actually need to use soap to help slip off a ring.

Bloating is a problem mainly for women because the increase in estrogen right before menstruation encourages water to accumulate in the spaces between the cells, making tissues swell and skin plump up. In fact, some women gain a whopping 10 pounds of water weight in the week prior to their periods, when higher estrogen levels spur the body to retain sodium, which in turn makes tissues hold onto more water. Estrogen replace-

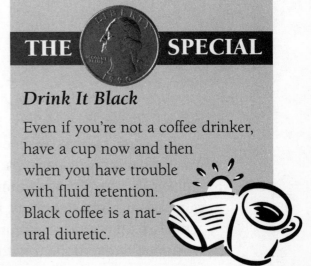

THE SPECIAL

Drink It Black

Even if you're not a coffee drinker, have a cup now and then when you have trouble with fluid retention. Black coffee is a natural diuretic.

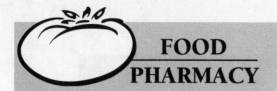

FOOD PHARMACY

Eat "Lawn Salad"

Avid weed whackers may consider it a nuisance, but bloaters should think of it as a plus—the lowly dandelion, that is. The fresh, young leaves of the dandelion plant (which the French call *pissenlit*, or "urinate in bed") act as a natural diuretic. In fact, in head-to-head tests, dandelion leaf tea was shown to be as effective as the prescription diuretic furosemide (Lasix).

If you have fluid retention due to heart problems, talk to your doctor about slowly adding dandelion to your diet and decreasing your dosage of diuretic drugs. Do not do it on your own. And don't use dandelion if you're taking potassium supplements.

ment drugs used to treat menopausal discomforts such as hot flashes can cause bloating.

There are other reasons for water retention as well, such as the aforementioned salty foods. "Proper fluid regulation requires a balance of salt and of potassium gleaned from fruits and vegetables," explains Michael DiPalma, N.D., a naturopathic physician in Newtown, Pennsylvania. Bloating can also be due to steroid medications, blood pressure drugs, and inflammatory reactions to everything from insect bites to sunburn to bread. Belly bloating, in particular, can be an allergic reaction to foods (especially the gluten in wheat) or a result of lactose intolerance—a lack of the lactase enzyme that breaks down the milk sugar (lactose) in dairy foods. The lactose ferments and forms a gas, which puffs the belly.

BEAT THE BLOAT

The conventional treatment for bloating related to simple water retention is water pills, or diuretics. These drugs help the kidneys excrete excess sodium and water in the tissues, but they can also flush out important minerals, such as potassium, which actually battles fluid retention. For occasional bloating—such as when you've overdone it with the tortilla chips or you're about to menstruate—try these more natural ways to siphon off the fluid.

Prune water weight with potassium. You can beat bloating (and retain ample potassium) by sipping potassium-rich teas. Parsley is a good choice, as is cleavers, a nineteenth-century herb once known as bedstraw because it was used to stuff beds. "It's a common weed that acts as a diuretic and clears waste and excess fluid," explains Judith Boice, N.D., a naturopathic physician in Portland, Oregon. Just be sure to have only one cup of either of these teas a day—too much can drain important minerals from your body.

Slim down with silk. Next time you're shucking corn, don't chuck the silk—instead, dry it and save it to make cornsilk tea, a time-honored folk remedy that will help your kidneys flush out fluids. Because cornsilk is rich in potassium, it will also help balance the sodium in your system that may be making you hold water. For the tea, steep 1 tablespoon of dried silk (also called stamens, which you can buy at a health food store if you don't have corn on hand) in 1 cup of boiling water for 5 minutes. You should see an effect within an hour or two, and you can continue to drink up to three cups a day for four days.

Add more water. That's right: Although it may seem counterintuitive, drinking ample water—at least eight glasses daily—is crucial for combating fluid retention, espe-

HOLLER FOR HELP

Trouble in the Water

Don't assume that bloating is normal. In some cases, it's a sign of underlying liver, heart, or kidney conditions, so you'll want to talk to your doctor. Likewise, talk to your physician if simply pressing on your skin leaves a dent. It's a sign of edema, a type of very serious fluid retention that can block blood flow.

cially fluid that pools in your belly after eating. "Food allergies can irritate the digestive tract and cause the body to retain more fluid to try and dilute the irritating substances," says Dr. Boice. "Drinking water helps the kidneys flush it all out."

Prowl the produce aisle. That's where you'll find literally piles of potassium-rich foods that send puffiness packing. Among the best are sunflower seeds, dates, figs, oranges, peaches, bananas, tomatoes, and all the leafy greens—even the tops of celery stalks are rich in this precious mineral!

Read the label. While you're shopping, check the labels on prepared and processed food with an eagle eye. Sodium, which promotes fluid retention, hides in everything from cereal and cheese to colas. Your goal is to keep sodium intake to 1,000 to 2,000 milligrams a day, but that can be tough. Just 2 ounces of American cheese packs 800 milligrams, and 3 cups of microwave popcorn contains 500 milligrams.

Try B$_6$. "Bloating can occur if you're deficient in vitamin B$_6$, which helps your body metabolize hormones—including the hormones that cause premenstrual bloat," says Dr. Boice. "That's why I recommend that women regularly take a B-complex supplement—to balance out the B$_6$." Avoid individual vitamin B$_6$ supplements.

Do the dairy thing. All dairy foods, especially milk, are loaded with calcium. A study of more than 400 women found that getting 1,200 milligrams of calcium daily reduced bloating and other premenstrual symptoms by half.

Kick back. If your ankles swell, it means that fluid, including lymphatic fluid, is pooling in your legs. Sitting with your legs raised will allow the fluid to be moved more easily by your circulatory system. If ankle swelling is a chronic problem, check with your doctor—and keep a footstool handy.

Wrap up with yarrow. Make a strong infusion of yarrow and peppermint by steeping 2 tablespoons of each in 1 pint of water for 15 minutes, then strain and chill. Meanwhile, prepare several lengths of gauze, muslin, or cheesecloth. When the infusion is thoroughly chilled, saturate the cloths, wrap them around your lower legs, and relax—with your legs elevated—for 20 minutes or so. This will leave your legs refreshed and help discourage fluid retention.

Sip a bloat-free tea. To enhance lymphatic flow, combine equal parts of the following herbs: hawthorn, horse chestnut, ginkgo, cleavers, and dandelion leaf. Steep 2 tablespoons of the mixture in 1 quart of boiling water for 15 minutes, let cool, and drink throughout the day. Some caveats: Dandelion is rich in potassium and should not be taken with potassium tablets, and people taking blood-thinning medications should consult their physicians before using ginkgo.

Feel better with melons. The Chinese use cucumbers and watermelons and other melons to reduce fluid retention. These foods contain cucurbocitrin, which is said to increase the natural leakiness of tiny blood vessels, or capillaries, in the kidneys. This means that more water escapes into the kidneys for elimination.

Tea Time

Sip the Stalk

When you steam asparagus, save the water, let it cool, and gulp it down (it'll taste vaguely of asparagus, but mostly like water). "Asparagus drippings make a great diuretic," says Michael DiPalma, N.D. Other excellent diuretic foods include artichokes and watercress.

Body Odor

Stop the Stink

We've all had occasions when no matter how frequently or ferociously we've scrubbed, we smell more foul than fresh, and the lingering odor has turned our favorite sweaters into instant castoffs. The culprits are bacteria that thrive on skin. When they devour the fatty sweat produced by the apocrine glands in the underarms, scalp, and genitals, the result is a very pungent smell.

KEEP ODOR AT BAY

Strong body odor can sometimes be a sign of a serious medical condition or skin infection. That's why you should call your doctor if an unusual odor permeates your skin despite your best attempts to get rid of it. In most cases, though, you can take care of body odor without chipping in for a new Lexus for your doctor's kids. Here are some tips.

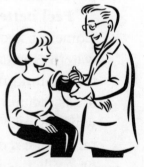

Sweeten your diet. Some body odor is caused by what you eat; the famous smells of garlic and onions can come right through your pores. But there's no need to boycott these favorites. Just neutralize their potent aromas by also eating parsley and other green leafy vegetables with chlorophyll, a natural deodorant. (That's the origin of the parsley-as-garnish tradition.) If you keep it up, you'll begin to notice the difference in just a few days.

Change deodorants periodically. After years of use, your usual deodorant may no longer work as well as it used to. It may have been altered by the manufacturer, your own body chemistry may be changing, or you may simply have developed a tolerance for the brand. Try another—change is good! You'll be using a deodorant every day for years, so why have bored armpits? If you get a rash from one deodorant, try another designed for sensitive skin. You may also want to look for a plain deodorant rather than an antiperspirant, since the latter contains aluminum chloride, which can be a skin irritant.

Clean up your digestion. "Just as old garbage can stink up your whole house, the odor from decaying matter in your intestines can radiate throughout your body," says Daniel DeLapp, N.D., a naturopathic physician and instructor of dermatology at the National College of Naturopathic Medicine in Portland, Oregon. For starters, he recommends cutting back on red meat, which can sometimes create a stink. "Protein is harder to break down in the gut," says Dr. DeLapp, "and the more food left hanging around, the more chance for smelly bacterial by-products to hang around, too."

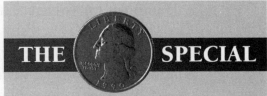

THE SPECIAL

Slap on Soda

That lowly box of baking soda you use to keep your fridge moisture-free and smelling sweet can do the same for your feet and underarms, says Nelson Lee Novick, M.D., associate clinical professor of dermatology at Mount Sinai School of Medicine in New York City. Pat it under your arms and on the soles of your feet at least twice daily.

Load up on yogurt. The best way to control odor-causing "bad" bacteria in your gut is to fill it with "good" bacteria. You can accomplish this by eating yogurt that contains live, active cultures of *Lactobacillus acidophilus* (check the label; frozen yogurt and yogurt-covered snacks don't have live cultures) or downing acidophilus capsules, which you can find at health food stores.

Munch your veggies. Raw veggies and fruits provide roughage that helps escort smelly waste through—and out of—your intestinal tract. Cooked foods, on the other hand, are slower to move through your intestines. Plus, says Dr. DeLapp, "when you cook foods, you change the oxidation, which can prompt more odor during digestion."

Splash it on. Splashing some rubbing alcohol under your arms may reduce the bacteria population. For a persistent odor problem, try using alcohol in place of deodorant—but not after shaving or if you have any nicks or cuts in your skin. That would sting like crazy!

Carve that jack-o'-lantern. Pumpkins provide a good, concentrated source of the mineral zinc, a deficiency of which can prompt body odor. If you're not keen on the seeds, you can take 30 milligrams of supplemental zinc daily to help reduce body and foot odor—but not without your doctor's guidance. If taken continu-

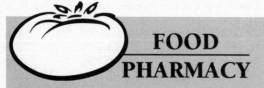

FOOD PHARMACY

Freshen Up with Juice

"Using a juicer is a great way to get a range of chlorophyll-rich foods such as kale, chard, and other dark green vegetables all in one shot," explains Jennifer Reid, N.D. Chlorophyll can restore the pH balance of blood that's too acidic—and therefore too friendly to bad bacteria—due to a diet heavy on meat and other proteins.

ously, zinc can deplete copper and other minerals, and it could be toxic. "In fact, I wouldn't exceed 15 milligrams a day without guidance from a health-care practitioner," warns Jennifer Reid, N.D., a naturopathic physician at the Columbia River Natural Medicine Clinic in Troutdale, Oregon.

Try odor-killing herbs. That tangy-smelling sage you use to season poultry stuffing contains compounds that can tame wetness, plus oils that fight bacteria. Pine-scented rosemary is another natural antibacterial herb. Mix 1 tablespoon of each with 1 cup of baking soda and sprinkle on any odor-causing body part.

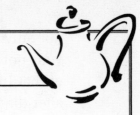

Tea Time

Sip Some Sage

Sage tea can help curb sweat gland activity and may be especially helpful when your perspiration is stress induced. Simply steep 2 teaspoons of dried sage in 1 cup of boiling water for 10 minutes, then savor in small doses—but only during tense situations. Regularly ingesting sage may cause dizziness, hot flashes, and other problems. Don't drink sage tea if you're pregnant or nursing.

Wear odor-fighting fibers. Polyester and most synthetic fabrics keep odors close to your body. Cotton, silk, and some of the new wicking fabrics designed for athletes allow moisture to circulate, so it won't cling to your body or clothing. Check at a sporting goods supply or camping store for lightweight, wicking underwear.

Cut back on coffee. You probably already know that odorous oils in garlic, onions, fish, and exotic spices can linger in your body, but coffee and tea are also bad news because they increase the activity of the sweat glands. Try eliminating these offenders and see if that foul odor fades.

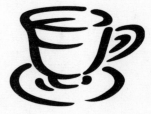

Feel fresh with fennel. It makes a sweet postmeal drink, especially if you've had garlic, onions, or other smelly foods that not only cause bad breath but may also make odor pour from your pores. In fact, fennel is such an excellent natural deodorizer that Indian restaurants often offer fennel seeds instead of after-dinner mints.

Rub on the "magic mineral." If you're going through deodorants and antiperspirants like there's no tomorrow, consider trading your stick for a stone—a crystal deodorant stone, that is. Not only will one stone last much longer than a standard stick, it may be much kinder to your system. The aluminum chloride in antiperspirants completely plugs up the sweat glands, whereas crystal stones contain alunogenite, a natural astringent that may only partially block the glands.

Love that lemon! Giving your body a steady stream of water—no fewer than eight glasses a day—is one of the best ways to flush out toxins and eliminate the stink. But Jeanette Jacknin, M.D., a dermatologist in Scottsdale, Arizona, offers a twist on the standard advice. Each evening, add a squeeze of fresh lemon juice and 1 teaspoon of chlorophyll (available at health food stores) to your glass, she suggests. Both will help eliminate odor-causing bacteria from your gut.

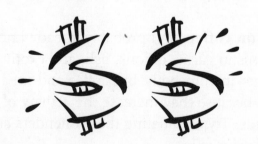

Breast Pain

Ease the Monthly Aches

Women today are almost desperate for more regularity in their lives. Soccer practice that ends when it's supposed to. Weekend chores that get done on time. Friends who show up for dinner at the appointed hour. In today's high-octane world, a little predictability just makes things easier.

In many women's lives, unfortunately, one of the few things that happen like clockwork is breast pain during their monthly menstrual cycles. "After ovulation, the breasts get ready for a possible pregnancy," explains Jana Nalbandian, N.D., a naturopathic physician and faculty member at Bastyr University near Seattle. "There's increased circulation to the mammary glands, which causes fluid retention and possibly some discomfort."

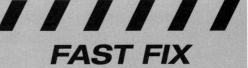

FAST FIX
A Heavenly Compress

When your breasts are aching, you can get quick relief by draping them with a bath towel that's been soaked in hot water and wrung out, says Jana Nalbandian, N.D. Heat promotes circulation and can help flush away excess fluid, she explains.

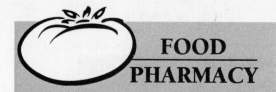

FOOD PHARMACY

Spoon Up Some Yogurt

The beneficial organisms in yogurt slightly decrease the time that stools—and the estrogen they contain—stay in your intestine, and eliminating excess estrogen from the body can help reduce monthly breast pain. Check the label to be sure the yogurt contains live cultures of *Lactobacillus acidophilus*, the helpful form of bacteria.

BABY YOUR BREASTS

Most women just live with breast pain because they figure they can't do anything about it. Nothing could be further from the truth. You should certainly check with your doctor just to be on the safe side, but there are many simple strategies that are just as effective as anything you'll find in a high-priced specialist's office.

Lighten up. Some dark-colored foods may aggravate monthly breast pain. The worst offenders seem to be chocolate, black tea, cola, and coffee, so try avoiding these foods in the week or so prior to your period.

Take a poke at pain. The herb pokeroot is a favorite among herbalists for relieving breast pain. Health food stores carry pokeroot tincture and oil. Put either on a cotton ball and rub it all over your breasts for relief. The herb is for external use only.

Count on cabbage and clay. Long before there were doctors or corner drugstores, herbalists treated breast pain with a poultice made from green clay (available at health food stores) and cabbage. The mixture appears to soften breast tissue and reduce monthly breast lumps and discomfort. Combine 4 parts shredded cabbage with 1 part clay, mix well, and apply it to your breasts at bedtime. Cover the poultice with a moist cloth, then wrap a layer of gauze bandage around your body or wear a loose-fitting, soft cotton bra to hold it in place. Your breasts will probably feel a whole lot better in the morning.

Toss a salad. Dandelion greens have a pleasant, slightly bitter taste, and they contain compounds that reduce fluid retention. As long as you don't use pesticides on your lawn and you pick the leaves before the flowers bloom, you'll have the fixings for a fresh-tasting, wholesome salad that keeps breast pain at bay. Mix 'em up with spinach, which also helps reduce excess fluid. Go easy on the dandelion if you take diuretics or potassium supplements, though.

Prime your body with primrose. Evening primrose is a traditional remedy for breast pain, and there's some evidence that it works. It's rich in omega-6 fatty acids, which inhibit the body's production of inflammation-causing prostaglandins, natural chemicals that cause pain. Dr. Nalbandian advises women to take 1,500 milligrams of evening primrose oil in capsule form twice a day.

One problem with evening primrose oil supplements is that they're expensive. Some less costly supplements include borage oil, flaxseed oil, and black currant oil, all of which also contain beneficial omega-6 fatty acids.

Shop for color. Fruits and vegetables with bright red, yellow, or orange hues are loaded with carotenoids, plant pigments that appear to prevent breast pain in some women. Add as many to your diet as you can.

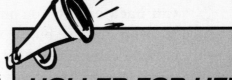

HOLLER FOR HELP

Monthly Trouble Signs

If you have regular breast pain, stay in touch with your doctor and report any changes in your monthly symptoms. You'll definitely want to make an appointment if the pain is severe or getting worse, affects only one breast, or is accompanied by signs of infection, such as redness, nipple discharge, a fever, or general aches.

Cut back on fat. You already know that dietary fat is loaded with calories, but there's another reason to cut back. Red meat, rich desserts, fast-food burgers, and other foods high in fat stimulate estrogen production, and high levels of estrogen can promote monthly breast pain, says Dr. Nalbandian.

Tame pain with herbal tea. Chasteberry, or vitex, helps normalize hormone levels that, when unbalanced, can contribute to breast swelling and discomfort. To make chasteberry tea, add 1 teaspoon of dried berries to 1 cup of boiling water, steep for 15 minutes, and strain. Drink a cup twice a day.

Shake the salt habit. When your breasts are tender and sore, any swelling can make them hurt even more. To reduce fluid retention, cut down on salt. Don't just set aside the saltshaker, though—read food labels, too. Many packaged foods contain high amounts of sodium.

Count on castor oil. Castor oil packs are a soothing anti-inflammatory. To make one, saturate a clean cloth with castor oil and place it on your breasts, covering them completely. Cover with plastic wrap (castor oil stains clothing), then with a hot water bottle or a heating pad set on low. Leave everything in place for 1 hour. Repeat three or four times a week.

Ease it with E. A number of scientific studies have shown that vitamin E supplements can help ease breast pain. The recommended dose is 400 to 800 IU daily. Be sure to get supplements that contain d-alpha tocopherols, which are thought to be more effective than other forms of vitamin E.

Wear a sports bra. Even if you're not an athlete, a sports bra is an important piece of equipment if your breasts are tender and sensitive. It will keep them in place so they don't rub against each other or your clothing. Also, avoid underwire bras, which can impede circulation.

Bronchitis

Banish the Barking

If your voice is so crackly and you're coughing so hard that you sound like a circus seal, you probably have bronchitis, a temporary inflammation of the mucous membranes of the bronchi, the main, branching airway passages of the lungs.

Acute bronchitis—which usually lasts about a week—typically follows a cold, when the virus travels from your nose to your air passages. Most cases of acute bronchitis, like most colds, disappear on their own after several miserable days. Your doctor may prescribe an inhaler (the kind that's used for asthma) to help open your bronchial tubes and clear out mucus. But there are many gentle, less expensive ways to accomplish the same thing. Ask your doctor if the following strategies wouldn't do the job just as well.

Steam out secretions. Warm steam soothes the lining of the bronchial tubes and loosens secretions. To make your own steam machine, first boil a pot of water. Carefully fill a bowl with the water, then put a towel over your head and the bowl to make a "tent" to trap the steam. Lean over the bowl (but not

If you're coming down with a cold, whip up a batch of chicken soup—or, better yet, get a loved one to do it. Chicken contains the amino acid cysteine, which is chemically similar to the bronchitis drug acetylcysteine. Plus, new research suggests that chicken soup helps block the production of neutrophils, white blood cells that contribute to upper respiratory symptoms.

close enough to burn your face) and inhale deeply through your nose. You can add a bit of eucalyptus or sage oil to the water to give the steam added medicinal punch. Don't try to use an electric vaporizer this way, though; its concentrated stream of steam is dangerous when used near the face.

Fight back with flax. A flaxseed poultice retains heat for a long time and is ideal for soothing an irritating, spastic cough. Add ½ cup of ground flaxseed to ¾ cup of boiling water, then simmer and stir until it makes a thick paste. Spread the paste on a piece of cheesecloth and apply it as hot as you can tolerate it (without burning) to your chest. For deep penetration, try adding 5 or 6 drops of an oil such as thyme or eucalyptus to the poultice. Leave it on for 1 to 2 hours.

Keep the water glass full. You need lots of fluids to keep your lungs healthily hydrated and working at their best, so drink at least eight glasses of water a day.

Dump the dairy. When you were a kid, you may have been given ice cream to soothe a tickle in your throat, but when it comes to bronchitis, it's a no-no. "You want to lay off foods that produce phlegm and those that cause inflammation," says David Zeiger, D.O., a family physician in Chicago. This means skipping not only dairy foods but also wheat, soy, sugar, margarine, peanut butter, preserved meats, and processed foods. What's left? Fish, legumes, and green vegetables—all of which are rich in magnesium, which helps relax the smooth muscles of your bronchial tubes so you can breathe easier.

Gobble garlic. One of garlic's key components—the volatile oil allicin—helps relax the bronchi so more air can pass through them. Garlic also stimulates the immune system and reduces phlegm.

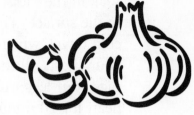

Clear congestion with a fennel chest rub. Just combine 10 drops each of fennel oil, thyme oil, and eucalyptus oil with 4 ounces of sunflower oil, then massage the mixture gently onto your chest.

Sip a soothing tea. Soak 2 heaping tablespoons of marshmallow root in 1 quart of cold water overnight. Strain, then heat 1 cup of the tea to a boil. Add ½ teaspoon each of licorice root and thyme, cover, and steep for 15 minutes. Drink three or four cups a day. One caveat: Avoid licorice root if you have high blood pressure or kidney disease.

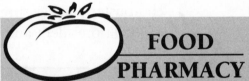

Run hot and cold. You can short-circuit bronchitis by flushing out mucus with hot-and-cold wraps. Here's how: Immerse a towel in water and wring it out, then heat it in the microwave for 5 to 10 minutes. Next, lay a wool blanket over your chest and cover

FOOD PHARMACY

Magic Mushroom

Studies indicate that the reishi mushroom—a reddish-orange fungus that grows on the bark of withered Japanese plum trees—may be highly effective for treating bronchitis. In fact, in one study, people with bronchitis who took reishi extracts had a 60 to 90 percent improvement in their symptoms. The typical adult dosage for acute bronchitis is 30 drops of reishi extract (available at health food stores) added to a glass of water every 2 to 3 hours while symptoms last.

it with a sheet. Place the steamy towel on top of the sheet and cover it with another blanket. Let your chest soak in the moist heat for 5 minutes to bring the blood to the surface. Then repeat the process with a very cold towel, which will shunt blood away from your chest. All the while, have someone massage your legs, rubbing vigorously toward your heart for 10 minutes. The heat and cold, combined with the rubbing, create a kind of pump to flush out phlegm and draw white blood cells into circulation to kill off the virus behind your bronchitis.

Break up congestion. To get mucus flowing, try this broncho-buster cracker spread suggested by James A. Duke, Ph.D., president and CEO of Duke's Herbal Vineyard in Fulton, Maryland, and a former specialist in medicinal plants for the USDA. Mix small amounts of garlic, ginger, mustard, turmeric, chopped chile peppers, and horseradish into a paste. Spread very thinly on crackers and nibble gingerly, one tiny bite at a time. The ingredients will make everything run, promises Dr. Duke—your eyes, your nose, and even the thick mucus clogging your bronchial tubes.

Cook up a curry. Indian curries contain turmeric, which is a great source of quercetin, a bioflavonoid-antihistamine combo that can calm reactivity in the airways. Or simply supplement with three 200- to 300-milligram capsules of quercetin (available at health food stores) a day— one before breakfast, lunch, and dinner—for as long as your symptoms last, suggests Michael DiPalma, N.D., a naturopathic physician in Newtown, Pennsylvania.

Breathe better with onion. Like garlic, onions contain the volatile oil allicin, which can open your airways by relaxing your bronchi. Coat a cast-iron skillet with olive oil and add a handful of chopped onions, a teaspoon of apple cider vinegar, and a pinch of cornstarch. Cook over low heat to make a paste. Let the paste cool and place it on a cloth. Lay the cloth on your bare chest and cover it with plastic wrap, add another cloth, and top everything with a heating pad set on low. "The onion will be absorbed into your body," says Dr. DiPalma. "You'll know, because you'll have the onion breath to prove it."

Take echinacea. In one study, people who took echinacea twice a day for eight weeks reduced the duration of respiratory tract infections by half—possibly because the herb boosts the body's infec-

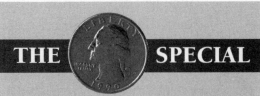

THE SPECIAL

Powerful Mustard Plaster

One of the oldest and most popular remedies for chest congestion is a hot mustard plaster, which helps break up stubborn mucus in the lungs by bringing heat to the area, according to naturopathic physician Elizabeth Burch, N.D., of iVillage's health Web site. The powder of black mustard seeds releases potent oil when mixed with water. Mix 1 part mustard powder with 10 parts flour and enough tepid water to make a paste, then spread a thin layer onto a cloth. Coat your skin with some olive oil and place a layer of cloth on your chest before applying the plaster, mustard side out. Leave it on for 10 minutes or less. To prevent blisters, remove it when your skin begins to redden.

tion-fighting cells so they attack the virus with a vengeance. You can find tinctures at a health food store. "Drink 1 to 1½ teaspoons of echinacea tincture added to a shot glass of warm water two or three times daily for the duration of your symptoms," suggests Dr. Zeiger. Disregard the slight numbness you may feel in your mouth from the herb, he says; it will quickly pass. But don't use echinacea if you have an autoimmune disease such as lupus, rheumatoid arthritis, or multiple sclerosis, or if you are pregnant or nursing.

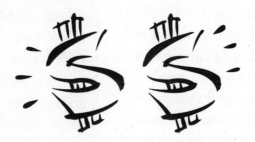

Soak away discomfort. Climb into a steaming tub laced with 2 drops each of eucalyptus, thyme, and rosemary oils, plus a cup or so of Epsom salts. The steam will increase the flow of nasal mucus; the molecules from the oils will dilate your small airways, easing your breathing; and the Epsom salts will provide bronchi-relaxing magnesium that's absorbed through the skin.

Bruises

Super Skin Savers

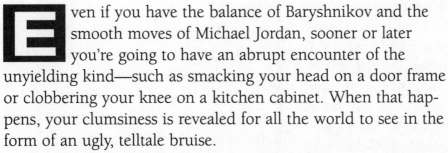

Even if you have the balance of Baryshnikov and the smooth moves of Michael Jordan, sooner or later you're going to have an abrupt encounter of the unyielding kind—such as smacking your head on a door frame or clobbering your knee on a kitchen cabinet. When that happens, your clumsiness is revealed for all the world to see in the form of an ugly, telltale bruise.

Any hard impact can damage tiny blood vessels, called capillaries, beneath your skin. Broken capillaries bleed, but you don't see blood because it's under the surface. What you do see is the dark "stain," which can range in color from slightly yellow to eggplant purple. Apart from being an unsightly mess, a bruise hurts because the same impact that damages blood vessels also injures skin and muscle.

FADE AWAY

Most bruises aren't a big deal. Daily, your body slowly cleans up the damage by removing fluids and damaged cells. While you're healing, of course, the pain and tenderness can be a real

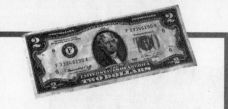

The $2 Deal

Bromelain Is Best

A natural substance found in the pineapple plant, bromelain helps your body break down and remove the chemical spill that causes bruises. Fresh pineapple doesn't contain enough of the enzyme to be helpful, so it's better to take it in supplement form. The recommended dose is 400 milligrams two or three times a day on an empty stomach. Don't take bromelain if you're taking prescription blood thinners.

nuisance—and you'll have to answer those endless questions about how you got that ugly blotch. There's no secret strategy for making bruises disappear like magic, but there are ways to help them heal more quickly. Here's how to do it.

RICE to the rescue. The oldest treatment for bruises, and still the most effective, goes by the initials RICE: rest, ice, compression, and elevation. Performing these steps in sequence will minimize discomfort and help bruises heal much more quickly.

• **Rest** means just what it says. When you've bruised an area, give it some downtime in order to let the damaged tissues start healing.

• **Ice** the area immediately after the injury. Apply an ice pack for about 20 minutes every few hours for the first day or two. Cold reduces the bleeding under the skin that causes pain and discoloration.

• **Compress** the area by wrapping it with an elastic bandage. You want the wrap to be snug, but not so tight that it cuts off circulation. You'll know you're stretching it tight enough if you can see light through the bandage while you're applying it. The pressure restricts blood flow and helps prevent swelling.

• **Elevate** the bruised area above the level of your heart as often as you can. This allows excess fluid to drain away from the bruise and back into circulation.

Use heat and cold. After a few days of RICE, switch to a technique called contrast hydrotherapy, in which you alternate between hot and cold compresses. "This creates an artificial pumping action that brings more nutrients to the area and pumps out waste products," explains Sean Sapunar, N.D., a naturopathic physician and clinical faculty member at the Bastyr Center for Natural Health near Seattle. The alternating temperatures cause blood vessels to expand and contract.

Here's how it works: Soak some washcloths in hot tap water and others in cold. Apply a warm compress to the area for 3 minutes, then switch to cold for 30 seconds. Several times a day, repeat the cycle three times, always ending with the cold compress.

Cure it with castor. A traditional and powerful way to treat bruises is to apply a castor oil pack. "Castor oil has excellent anti-inflammatory properties, and it penetrates the skin very well," says Dr. Sapunar. Spread castor oil over the bruise, then wrap the area with plastic wrap. Place a heating pad (set on low) or a washcloth soaked in hot water on top of the wrap. Leave it in place for about 20 minutes, then wash off the oil. You can repeat the treatment several times a day until the bruise is gone.

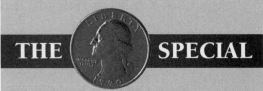

THE SPECIAL

Strengthen Capillaries with C

Your body uses vitamin C to repair damaged capillaries. When you have a bruise, you've injured dozens or even hundreds of them, so you need as much of this important nutrient as you can get. While the bruise is healing, eat plenty of fruit (especially citrus fruit) and vegetables, which are loaded with vitamin C. As long as you don't have kidney or stomach problems, it's also helpful to take 2,000 to 3,000 milligrams of vitamin C supplements for a day or two. Since large amounts of vitamin C can cause diarrhea or upset stomach, it's a good idea to take smaller amounts several times a day. Taking it with food also helps.

Fix it with fish oil. It sounds like something your grandmother would recommend—and, as usual, she'd be right on the money. Fish oil is rich in omega-3 fatty acids, natural substances that make your body less prone to inflammation. As long as you're not taking aspirin or prescription blood thinners, take a tablespoon or two of fish oil daily until the bruise is gone, says Dr. Sapunar. "You can get similar benefits by eating fish and flaxseed, but it takes a little longer," he adds.

Get to the root of it. Ginger tea is an effective treatment for bruises because it reduces inflammation and dilates, or widens, blood vessels. Wider blood vessels allow more blood to circulate, which removes pain-causing compounds and brings in more healing nutrients. You can make ginger tea by steeping 1 tablespoon of powdered ginger in a cup of boiling water for 5 to 10 minutes. Drink the tea at least three times a day until the bruise is gone.

Pump up your nutrients. Your body's need for nutrients increases dramatically when you have a bruise. Important bruise beaters include zinc, vitamin A, and selenium. You'll get plenty of these and other healing vitamins and minerals by taking a multivitamin every day until the bruise fades.

FOOD PHARMACY

Give Bruises the Blues

Remember the girl who turned into a giant blueberry in the film *Willy Wonka and the Chocolate Factory*? It wasn't a pretty sight, but the good news is that she probably never bruised again. Blueberries are loaded with vitamin C and chemical compounds called bioflavonoids, which are essential for blood vessel repair. "I advise people to eat a half-cup of blueberries a day," says Sean Sapunar, N.D. The nutrients in the berries will help bruises heal and make your blood vessels stronger and better able to resist future damage.

Knock it out with nuts. Brazil nuts are loaded with selenium, the nutrient that's essential for skin health. Eat about a cup daily while the bruise is healing.

Pop some arnica. A major bruise buster, arnica gel is available at health food stores. If you'd rather not use a gel, you can take arnica in homeopathic form, following the package directions.

Try the salt strategy. Here's a chance to use that box of Epsom salts that's been sitting in the back of your bathroom cabinet all these years. Add a cup or two of the salts to a warm bath (or a smaller amount to a basin), then soak the area for about 20 minutes. "The magnesium in the salts is very soothing for bumps and bruises," says Dr. Sapunar.

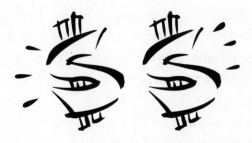

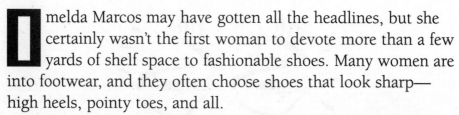

Bunions

Step Away from Foot Pain

Imelda Marcos may have gotten all the headlines, but she certainly wasn't the first woman to devote more than a few yards of shelf space to fashionable shoes. Many women are into footwear, and they often choose shoes that look sharp—high heels, pointy toes, and all.

Unfortunately, buying shoes for style instead of comfort can literally change the ways your foot bones grow. Can you feel a knobby bump at the base of your big toe? If you can, that's a bunion, and it means your shoes are forcing your bones to grow in some pretty unnatural ways. Bunions really hurt when you squeeze them into tight-fitting shoes—and they can make your feet feel tired and achy at the end of a long day.

BUNION BUSTERS

Short of surgery, there's no way to get rid of bunions once they form. Before you consider foot surgery, though—and the mortgage-size payment that comes with it—you'll want to explore some gentler ways to reduce pain and keep bunions from getting worse. Here are a few that may help.

Can it with cola. Love an ice-cold soda? Your aching feet will, too. Before you pop the tab, place the can sideways on the floor, slip off your shoes, put your sore foot on the can, and roll it back and forth for several minutes. The cold will help reduce inflammation, and the motion will give your foot a good massage.

Heat it up. On your tongue, the fiery capsaicin in red pepper makes you want to guzzle a gallon of water. But when you apply capsaicin cream (available in drugstores) to a painful bunion, you'll feel sweet relief. Capsaicin relieves pain by gradually decreasing the concentration of something called substance P, which transmits pain signals to the brain. The cream stings, so be careful not to get it in your eyes or on any area of broken skin, and wash your hands well after using it.

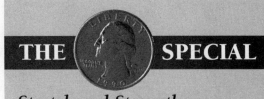

THE SPECIAL

Stretch and Strengthen
They can be your best friends when you're fighting bunion pain, because they'll make your toes strong and flexible. Sit with your feet together and loop a thick rubber band around both big toes. Move your feet as far apart as they'll go, hold the stretch for 5 seconds, then relax. Repeat the exercise 10 times at least once a day.

Cream it. "One of the best painkillers for bunions I've found is called Fortex," says John Hahn, N.D., D.P.M., a naturopathic physician and podiatrist in Bend, Oregon. "It packs aspirin-like salicylate in a peanut-oil base, and it can penetrate the skin and quell inflammation rather quickly." Check for Fortex at a health food store and smooth the cream on your bunion several times daily, if you can.

Pass on the pressure. Surround your burgeoning bunion with over-the-counter doughnut-shaped moleskin or a gel-filled

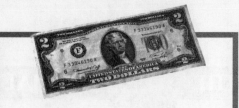

The $2 Deal

A Soothing Herbal Blend

The next time your bunions are barking, stop off at a health food store and get the ingredients for a soothing herbal rub. A time-tested formula consists of 6 parts oak bark, 3 parts marshmallow root, 3 parts mullein, 2 parts wormwood, 1 part lobelia, 1 part skullcap, 6 parts comfrey root, and 3 parts walnut bark. Put the herbs in a double boiler, add olive oil to cover, and cook for 1 to 2 hours. Strain out the herbs and throw them away. Add an equal amount of melted beeswax to the oil and store the mixture in an ointment jar with a tight-fitting lid. Apply it daily whenever your feet hurt, advises Rowan Hamilton, Dip.Phyt., professor of botanical medicine at Bastyr University near Seattle. "You'll probably notice good results within a few days," he says.

pad to reduce pressure and friction from shoes. Check your drugstore or supermarket for protective pads impregnated with anti-inflammatory medicines. They'll deliver first aid to your bunion as they cushion it.

Straighten 'em out. If your big toe is starting to drift and a bunion is sprouting, a sponge-rubber toe spacer, which you can find at any drugstore, can keep it from angling outward and relieve the pressure while you're wearing shoes. Start with a small spacer and gradually use wider ones until your toe feels comfortable.

Head to the shore. Your feet may appreciate a trip to the seashore as much as you do. Walking barefoot in the sand is a great way to strengthen your feet and make them less sensitive to bunion pain.

Rub out pain. Massage is excellent for reducing bunion pain, and you'll get even better results when you combine it with a soothing bath. The next time you're in the tub, lather your hands with soap. Slip your fingers between the toes of one foot and gently reach around to massage the bottom of your foot. Bend your wrist while you rub so your foot moves in every direction. Then do the same thing with your other foot. You may be a little sore the first few times you do it, but after that, your bunions should start feeling a lot better, says Mark Hoch, M.D., president of the American Holistic Medical Association.

Buy some new shoes. The main cause of bunion pain, and the one thing that always makes it worse, is wearing shoes that don't fit. Shoving your foot into a poorly fitting shoe literally changes the shape of your foot, says Cherise Dyal, M.D., an orthopedic surgeon in Wayne, New Jersey, and chair of the Public Education Committee of the American Orthopedic Foot and Ankle Society.

FAST FIX
Comforting Comfrey

A comfrey footbath soothes painful bunions fast. The herb contains chemical compounds that reduce skin discomfort and help sore areas heal. To make a footbath, steep an ounce of dried comfrey leaves (available at health food stores) in a few cups of simmering water for 10 minutes. Add enough cool water to make the temperature comfortable, pour the water into a basin, and soak your feet for 20 minutes or so. If you can't find comfrey, it's okay to substitute Epsom salts, says Rowan Hamilton, Dip.Phyt.

Always have your feet measured when you buy new shoes, she advises. Avoid narrow styles with pointy toes. You want shoes that are wide enough for your feet to slip into comfortably, preferably with a flat or low heel.

Burns

Put Out the Fire

You probably remember the old Saturday morning cartoons that featured Yosemite Sam. The pistol-packin' bandolero would say things like, "Now, get that flea-bitten carcass off'n my real estate!"—just before Bugs Bunny tricked him into a crackling campfire.

That's life in toon town. In real life, though, there's nothing funny about burns. They're among the most painful injuries you're ever likely to get. Even a small burn damages nerves as well as the surface layers of skin, and the exposed raw tissue can take a long time to heal. Worse, it's extremely vulnerable to infection.

The darned thing about burns is that they happen so fast. Unlike other types of injuries—a knife cut, for example—with burns, there's virtually no time to react and save yourself from danger. By the time sensations of heat have traveled from your skin to your brain, the damage has been done.

CHILL THE PAIN

You need immediate medical attention for serious burns or for any burn that's bigger than 2 to 3 inches around. Minor burns, however, are easy enough to treat at home. Here are some suggestions for cooling the pain and helping them heal more quickly.

Get the water flowing. It's almost instinctive to throw water on something that's burning, and that's the perfect response when you've touched something that's too hot to handle, says Lisa Arnold, N.D., a naturopathic physician in Orleans, Massachusetts. "Cold water is the best thing," she says.

As soon as possible, flood the area with cold running water for about 10 minutes. This will stop the pain and help prevent swelling. If the pain persists, repeat the cold-water treatment for 15 minutes each hour. "The cold constricts the blood vessels, and taking it away opens them up again," she explains. This creates a pumping action that improves circulation and helps the burn heal more quickly.

Improvise if you need to. If the closest cool liquid happens to be milk or even a soft drink, well, any port in a storm. "You have to work with what you've got," Dr.

HOLLER FOR HELP

Don't Mess with Bad Burns

You can treat minor, first-degree burns at home. Second-, third-, or fourth-degree burns, which penetrate progressively deeper into the skin, always need a doctor's care—and can be life-threatening in some cases. Get to an emergency room if the burn covers a large area of skin, looks infected, or appears charred or white. Even a small burn that doesn't heal within 10 days or looks infected needs medical attention.

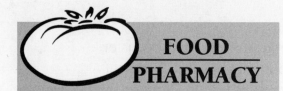

Crunch Some Seedy Soothers

Pumpkin seeds are loaded with zinc, an essential mineral that helps all wounds, including burns, heal more quickly, says Jeanette Jacknin, M.D.

Arnold says. The more quickly you cool the injury, the sooner you'll stop the damage.

Leave the ice in the freezer. Even though you want to cool a burn as quickly as possible, ice will probably make things worse. It will make the area too cold, and sometimes it sticks to the skin.

Forget about butter. "Putting butter or any oily substance on a burn is the worst thing you can do, because it will seal in the heat," says Jennifer Reid, N.D., a naturopathic physician at the Columbia River Natural Medicine Clinic in Troutdale, Oregon. "After heat singes your skin, it continues to cook the tissues, so you want to try to cool the burn immediately. For that to happen, the heat has to be able to escape."

Love that aloe! To hasten healing and guard against infection, you can't do much better than the thick juice inside the leaves of the aloe plant—even if you head to the hospital. "Aloe's so effective that it's included in a product developed for burn victims to reduce the need for skin grafting," says Dr. Reid. Simply cut a notch in a leaf, squeeze until the juice appears, and apply it directly to the burn. The cooling liquid will ease pain, keep skin from blistering, stave off infection, and speed wound healing by helping fresh skin cells grow.

Ease it with oregano. You love oregano on your pizza, and your scorched skin will love it, too. Oil of oregano contains vitamins A and C as well as minerals, including calcium, phosphorus, iron, and magnesium. When rubbed on the skin, it aids in healing minor burns.

Get comfort with comfrey. The leaves and roots of the comfrey plant contain the healing agent allantoin, which stimulates healthy tissue growth. To make a cooling, cell-growth-encouraging poultice, simply mash 1 cup of fresh leaves or soak 1 cup of dried leaves (you can find both at health food stores) in enough water to cover them. Then wrap the mash in a thin cloth and apply it to the burn as needed.

Apply plantain. If the blisters on your burn burst, dab the area with plantain tea. This antibacterial Native American plant contains the healing agent allantoin and is sometimes called nature's Bactine because it's good for healing all kinds of wounds, says Michael DiPalma, N.D., a naturopathic physician in Newtown, Pennsylvania. Brew a tea (you can find packaged plantain tea at a health food store), let it cool, and apply the liquid to your burn.

Soothe it with St. John's. You may know this herb for its role in easing mild depression, but it also helps heal minor burns quickly and with minimal scarring, says Jeanette Jacknin, M.D., a dermatologist in Scottsdale, Arizona. Apply the extract (available at health food stores) directly to the burn several times a day.

Use an herbal mix. Even the best herbs for burns can be made a little better by using them in combination. Dr. Arnold advises picking up a cream or ointment that contains several skin-friendly herbs, such as comfrey, calendula, and goldenseal, at a health food store. Apply it

The $2 Deal

Clean with Calendula

This herb is an anti-inflammatory, astringent (cleanser), and antiseptic (germ killer) all rolled into one. Plus, it helps repair tissues and prevent scarring. "Some physicians advise applying calendula cream directly to a burn," says Jennifer Reid, N.D. "I prefer to add several drops of calendula tincture to a cup of water, dip a cloth in the mixture, and dab the cloth onto the wound a day or two after the burn occurred, so it won't sting the tissues." You can find both calendula cream and tincture at health food stores.

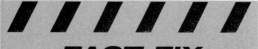

FAST FIX
Bring On the Toothpaste

To quickly ease minor burns, apply some toothpaste. Most toothpastes contain menthol, which has a cooling effect on the skin, explains Lisa Arnold, N.D.

according to the package directions.

Keep it clean. One reason that burns are so dangerous is that they strip away the protective outer layers of skin—and there are plenty of germs that will jump right in. To prevent infection, wash the area with soap and water a few times a day. Cover it with a bandage if you think it's likely to get dirty, and be sure to change the bandage at least twice a day. Just remember to wash gently: Overzealous scrubbing can easily damage burned skin.

Raise it high. "Elevating the burned area, if it's on a part of the body that can be elevated, is definitely good," Dr. Arnold says. You want the area to be higher than the level of your heart so fluids that accumulate there will drain back toward the body as the normal flow of blood and other fluids mops up the damage.

If you can, keep the area elevated for about 20 minutes, Dr. Arnold advises. For larger burns, elevate it several times during the first 24 hours.

Spread on extra protection. To prevent infection, apply a thin layer of triple antibiotic ointment every time you wash the burn and change the bandage.

Bursitis

Ease Those Aching Joints

Have you ever heard of housemaid's knee, miner's elbow, or weaver's bottom? They sound like they could be characters in Shakespeare's comedy *A Midsummer Night's Dream*. In fact, they're whimsical names for bursitis, a condition that's about as far from comedic as you can get.

Bursitis occurs when small, fluid-filled sacs called bursae, which normally help joints move smoothly, get inflamed and swollen. Your body has more than 150 bursae, so you can imagine the painful possibilities. The most common sites for bursitis are joints that undergo heavy wear and tear, such as the shoulder, hip, and knee.

BE GENTLE TO YOUR JOINTS

If you notice that one or more of your joints hurts like the dickens, check with your doctor. Bursitis is rarely serious, but sometimes other conditions, such as arthritis, cause similar symptoms. An x-ray will show what's causing your pain. In most cases, though,

Bursitis

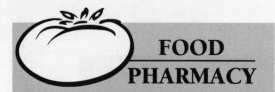

you won't have to fork over a pile of cash for expensive pain-relieving drugs. Here are a few simple tips to reduce pain and prevent additional injury.

Stop the swelling. If your joint feels hot and swollen, the first thing you should do is get some ice on it. Applying cold constricts blood vessels and reduces the flow of fluid and inflammatory chemicals to the painful area.

Apply a cold pack or ice cubes wrapped in a small towel or a washcloth to the area for about 20 minutes. Repeat the treatment every hour or two until the pain goes away.

Raise your arm. Or elevate your leg or whatever else hurts. Raising the area higher than the level of your heart causes gravity to help pull out fluids and reduce swelling.

Wrap it up. Snugly wrapping the injured area with an elastic bandage will also reduce swelling. Don't make the bandage so tight that it cuts off circulation, though. If you can just barely slip a finger under the edge, it's tight enough.

Add some heat. Pain that lingers after a day or two often responds well to a heat treatment. Soak a small towel in hot water, wring it out, and place it on the area that's hurting. You can also use a heating pad set on low.

Swap heat and cold. This traditional healing method uses alternating hot and cold treatments to improve circulation in an injured part of your body. It brings in more nutrients while flushing out toxins and waste products, says Phoebe Yin, N.D., a naturopathic physician and faculty member at Bastyr University near Seattle.

First, soak a small towel in hot water, wring it out, and place it on the sore spot for about 3 minutes. Then soak a towel in cold water and apply it for 30 seconds. Repeat the cycle two or three times, always ending with the cold.

Pound pain with peppers. Call it chile pepper, call it cayenne, call it capsaicin. Just call it—this ointment is really hot stuff! Smooth it over your sore joint, and you'll begin to feel relief. The heat from the chemical capsaicin brings more blood circulation to your sore bursa, and with it, more healing nutrients. You can buy capsaicin cream over the counter at your local drugstore or health food store. The best products contain 0.025 to 0.075 percent capsaicin. Use it up to three times a day, but be careful—keep it away from your eyes and any areas of broken skin.

Get relief from the garden. Two common garden plants, chickweed and comfrey, are used traditionally to relieve swelling and pain. Pick a handful of chickweed and one or two large comfrey leaves. Blanch them both in hot water and apply, using the chickweed as the first layer and holding it in place with the comfrey leaves.

Put bromelain to work. This enzyme from the pineapple plant is one of nature's anti-inflammatories. To relieve bursitis, take 200 milligrams in capsule form daily on an empty stomach. Avoid bromelain if you're taking

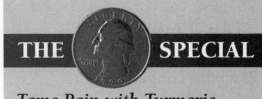

THE 〔coin〕 SPECIAL

Tame Pain with Turmeric

This pungent spice contains chemical compounds that can relieve an inflamed, irritated joint. If you're not a big fan of spicy foods, you can take supplements that contain curcumin, the active ingredient in turmeric. They're available at health food stores; follow the label directions.

blood-thinning medications or are sensitive to pineapple.

Count on castor. A castor oil pack is an old-time pain treatment that's never out of style. First, smear some castor oil over the area that hurts. Put some plastic wrap on top of the oil, then cover the whole thing with a heating pad set on low.

The heat will push the oil's healing components into the aching joint. Since this is a heat-based treatment, though, don't use it if you have swelling or inflammation.

Get in shape. Resistance training, or exercising with weights, will help build strong muscles. And the stronger the muscles around your joints, the better they can protect you from the kinds of injuries that cause bursitis. If you've already been treated for bursitis, have your doctor prescribe an exercise program to prevent further complications.

Hey, relax. When you're doing repetitive tasks that can lead to bursitis, take frequent breaks. Stretching and moving around, even for just a few minutes each hour, can make a real difference.

Get extra C. Vitamin C is critical for repairing injured joints. You could take supplements, but a tastier solution is to add some crunch to your next salad. "Green and red peppers are good sources of vitamin C," says Dr. Yin. Not a pepper fan? Then load up on oranges—but don't peel them too carefully. "There's a lot of vitamin C in the white part next to the peel," she says.

Pop a morning multi. The multivitamin you take every day with breakfast is especially important when you're coping with bursitis. "There are a lot of nutrients that are important for connective tissue health," says Dr. Yin. A multivitamin provides them all.

Oil your joints. The omega-3 essential fatty acids found in fish are important for good health, especially when your body is coping with inflammation. Until your joints are better, plan on eating two or three servings of fish a week. The oils will help tame inflammation and help you recover more quickly.

If you're not a fish fan, you can get healthy amounts of omega-3's by eating ground flaxseed. Every day, add a tablespoon or two of seeds to cereal, smoothies, yogurt, or salads.

Flood your tissues. "Your joints and bursae have a lot of water in them," says Dr. Yin, "so hydration is very important for joint health." Plan on drinking eight glasses of water throughout the day, every day.

Analyze your life. Sometimes the best way to fight bursitis is to do some creative thinking. Pay close attention to what you do as you go about your daily life. Are repetitive motions putting your arms or legs in awkward or strained positions? Do you spend long periods of time with a knee or elbow pressed against the floor or a chair?

"Things that put pressure on a joint or tendon or restrict blood flow might cause problems down the road," says Dr. Yin, so try to eliminate them from your daily routine.

Calluses and Corns

Tackle the Tough Spots

Mother Nature must be a shoemaker at heart. If you walk barefoot a lot, you'll naturally develop calluses, thick layers of dead skin that act like the soles on a good pair of shoes. The tough skin covers the sensitive layers underneath and protects you from whatever's underfoot.

People who work hard with their hands usually form calluses that protect them from nicks and cuts. And as anyone who has ever tried to play a guitar can tell you, learning's a painful process until you develop good calluses on your fingertips. Calluses, however, sometimes have painful nerves and bursal sacs beneath them that can cause symptoms ranging from shooting pain to aches.

CALLUS COMFORT

If a callus hurts so much you can hardly stand it, or if it's starting to ache or bleed, call your doctor. Otherwise, you can probably take care of calluses with simple home care. Here are some things to try.

Do the ol' soft shoe. Stiff leather shoes look great, but they don't feel so good when you have corns (small calluses on the toes), says Pamela Taylor, N.D., a naturopathic physician in Moline, Illinois. The only way to get rid of corns is to get rid of friction. That means wearing shoes made from cloth or soft leather for a few weeks, she advises. Sandals are also a good choice as long as the straps don't rub against the tender areas.

Soften tough skin. Treat yourself to one of the many creams and lotions made to soften calluses; they have ingredients such as peppermint and apple-kiwi. Also try a moisturizer, such as vitamin E oil, cocoa butter, or lanolin, to make calluses softer and less painful.

Go barefootin' at the beach.

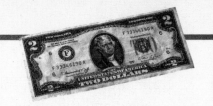

The $2 Deal

Oil Away Aches

Herbal oils are nearly perfect for corns and other calluses. Any oil softens the skin, but herb-infused oils stimulate circulation and help keep your feet healthy and ache-free, says Pamela Taylor, N.D. She recommends the following blend of oils, which you can find at health food stores. Add 2 drops each of peppermint oil and carrot seed oil to an ounce of calendula oil, then mix in 5 drops each of lavender oil and geranium oil. Store the mixture in a small bottle and massage it into your feet once a day—more often when your corns are aching.

Those gray, gritty pumice stones we use to sand down calluses are made of volcanic rock. While few of us have access to volcano slopes, sand on the beach acts like a pumice stone—only better! If you live near a beach, walk in the sand as often as you can. Your feet will feel fabulous.

Bring out the salts. The next time

you take a bath, treat your feet to a moisturizing salt rub. Moisten a handful of Epsom salts with a small amount of almond or olive oil, then scrub your feet until the salt's dissolved and the oil has softened your skin.

Soften with citrus. Rubbing half a lemon on your feet, elbows, and heels will give you softer, smoother skin.

File, don't cut. Corns are just dead skin, so you'd think they'd be easy to cut away. Don't try it, though: There's a good chance that you'll damage healthy tissue and wind up with a painful sore—or even a nasty infection. "It's much safer to use a nail file or a pumice stone to file the corn down," says Dr. Taylor.

Don't file it down all the way at one time; instead, remove just a little bit of skin each day. Most of the corn will be gone in a week or two, and you'll be less likely to hurt yourself in the meantime. People with diabetes should be especially careful when filing corns.

Soften before scraping. Corns are a lot easier to remove if you soften the skin before using a file or pumice stone. First, soak your foot in warm water for 5 to 10 minutes. Once the skin is soft, gently abrade the toughened area to remove a few layers of skin, then leave it alone for the rest of the day. Repeat the soak-and-scrape routine once a day until the corn is gone.

Enjoy a rubdown. A foot mas-

FAST FIX
A Touch of the Tropics

To soften a callus, apply a piece of pineapple rind and cover it with adhesive bandages overnight, suggests James A. Duke, Ph.D., president and CEO of Duke's Herbal Vineyard in Fulton, Maryland, and a former specialist in medicinal plants for the USDA. An enzyme in the rind does the trick.

sage is a super soother when your corns are a-poppin'. But don't put a lot of pressure directly on the corns—it hurts! Instead, work around them. Massage your entire foot, starting at the tips of your toes and working backward to your heel. If your foot is particularly tender, you may want to use a massage technique called effleurage: long, stroking movements with just a little bit of pressure.

Redistribute the load. Use orthotic inserts in your shoes to transfer pressure away from callused areas and absorb shock. These may help if you have calluses because of an abnormal gait, flat feet, high arches, or very bony feet. Inserts are available in most drugstores, but it's a good idea to ask a podiatrist about orthotics that can be specially made for you.

Size counts. Twenty years ago, clerks in shoe stores routinely measured your feet to ensure a good fit. These days, you're lucky if you can even find someone to help you find the size you think you need.

"Find a store where the clerks measure both of your feet," says Dr. Taylor. "They should check the fit at both the heel and the toe. After that, wear the shoes and walk around to make sure they're truly comfortable."

THE SPECIAL

A Soothing Soak

Periodically soak your feet in a pan of water to which you've added a teaspoon of baking soda or soap. As the callused skin loosens, gently rub it away a bit at a time with a pumice stone or emery board. Follow up with lotion or cream to soften your feet. This remedy is not appropriate for people with diabetes, who may have poor circulation in their feet and thus may injure their skin.

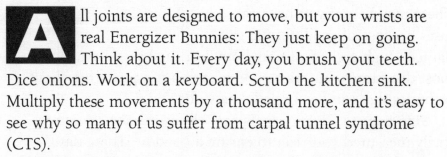

Carpal Tunnel Syndrome

Take Away Wrist Woes

All joints are designed to move, but your wrists are real Energizer Bunnies: They just keep on going. Think about it. Every day, you brush your teeth. Dice onions. Work on a keyboard. Scrub the kitchen sink. Multiply these movements by a thousand more, and it's easy to see why so many of us suffer from carpal tunnel syndrome (CTS).

Carpal tunnel syndrome has nothing at all to do with muscle soreness and everything to do with nerves. There's a nerve in the wrist that passes through a narrow channel called the carpal tunnel. Even under normal circumstances, there's barely enough room in there for the nerve to move freely. If anything happens to make the tunnel smaller—swelling caused by too much typing, for example—the nerve gets a little mashed. That's what causes the tingling, numbness, and/or pain that are the telltale signs of CTS.

UNDO THE PINCH

In extreme cases of CTS, surgery may be needed, but it rarely goes that far. You can probably reduce painful nerve pressure with some simple home approaches—without having to pay for a high-priced operating suite. Here are a few things to try.

Back off for a while. Don't make the mistake of ignoring tingling or other symptoms in your hands or wrists. Stop what you're doing immediately. It may be that a few days' rest will reduce the internal swelling, though it's more likely that you'll have to give your hands a few weeks off—and perhaps longer. It's worth doing because inflammation and swelling in the wrist can cause permanent nerve damage if they're stopped early enough. If the tingling continues, check with your doctor.

Immobilize your wrist. One of the best remedies for carpal tunnel pain is to wear a splint that holds your wrist straight while you work. It keeps your wrist from flexing and putting unnecessary pressure on the nerve, explains Kevin Conner, N.D., a naturopathic physician and faculty member at Bastyr University near Seattle. "Have it fitted by a doctor or physical therapist," he adds. Over-the-counter splints rarely fit correctly. A splint that's too loose won't work very well, and one that's too tight could cause circulation problems.

Splint while you sleep. Don't use your splint only when you're working. It's also important to wear it while

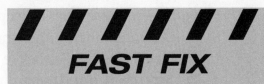

FAST FIX
Flood Away Pain

A fast way to ease carpal tunnel flare-ups is to flood your wrists with cold water, says Kevin Conner, N.D. Go to the kitchen or bathroom sink, turn on the cold water tap, and let the water flow over your wrists for 5 to 10 minutes. "It's the quickest, easiest way I know to reduce pain and inflammation," says Dr. Conner.

you sleep. Most people sleep with their wrists bent at an angle at least some of the time, and this can aggravate carpal tunnel problems even while they're snoozing.

Stretch it out. It's hard to reverse CTS once you have it, so doctors stress the preventive approach. Before working with your hands—typing, operating a cash register, or working in the yard, for example—take a few minutes to warm up with some gentle stretching.

For example, extend your arm in front of you with your palm facing down. Slowly raise your hand so your wrist flexes upward. Keep going until you feel a good stretch, then bend your hand down for another stretch. Do this at least a dozen times, up and down, and repeat it several times a day.

Drain excess fluids. CTS tends to get a lot worse if you're retaining more water than you should, says Dr. Conner. It makes sense, because all that water has to go somewhere, and some of it ends up in tissues in your wrist. The more the tissues swell, the more likely you are to experience carpal tunnel pain. This is why women often develop symptoms during pregnancy or even at the bloating stage of their menstrual cycles.

There are a number of herbal treatments for easing water retention—dandelion and parsley are two of the main ones—but don't use them without checking with a doctor. Water retention is a sign

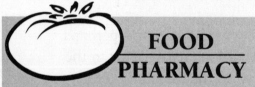

FOOD PHARMACY

Have a Wrist-Friendly Salad

Mix your favorite salad fixin's with hard-boiled eggs for vitamin A, red peppers for vitamin C, and sliced almonds for vitamin E. All these nutrients are excellent anti-inflammatories and may help reduce the swelling in your tendons that's causing your pain, says Andrew Lucking, N.D.

that something's wrong with your body's natural balance, and you'll want to correct the underlying problem rather than merely treat the symptom.

Put your thumb to work. Gentle self-manipulation of the bones and soft tissues of the wrist can shift the fluids responsible for swelling, releasing the trapped nerve. As an added benefit, it can keep your forearm agile. Here's what to do: Gently press your thumb into the soft bottom side of your wrist, 1 to 2 inches back from the crease, then slide it back and forth over one tendon at a time as well as up and down your wrist.

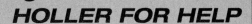

HOLLER FOR HELP

Save That Nerve

Any problem affecting the nerves is potentially serious, so you'll want to see a doctor as soon as you notice carpal tunnel symptoms, especially numbness, tingling, or pain in your fingers or wrist that doesn't go away within a few days. Without quick treatment, compression of the nerve within the carpal tunnel may cause permanent damage.

Repeat several times throughout the day or as often as you feel you need to.

Cast off pain with castor oil. "A compress made from castor bean oil is a great way to get an anti-inflammatory to the source of the pain," says Andrew Lucking, N.D., a naturopathic physician in Minneapolis. Soak a cloth with castor oil (available in health food stores), heat it in the microwave until it's warm but not hot, and place it on your wrist. Cover the compress with plastic wrap and leave it in place for several hours.

Try the feel-good burn. Capsaicin—the compound that makes red pepper so fiery—also reduces inflammation by blocking the release of pain-causing substances. You can pick up a commercial pain-relief salve that contains capsaicin at any drugstore, or simply make your own by mixing

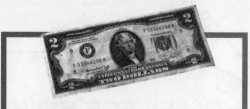

The $2 Deal

Restore Flexibility with EFAs

Flaxseed is a rich source of omega-3 essential fatty acids (EFAs), which have anti-inflammatory properties. Drizzle 1 tablespoon of flaxseed oil (available in health food stores) on your salad daily, and your wrist woes may be over within two weeks. Don't take flaxseed oil if you're taking aspirin or prescription blood thinners.

1/2 to 1 teaspoon of powdered red pepper into 1/4 cup of skin lotion. Rub no more than 1 teaspoon of the mixture on the sore area, being careful not to get it on any areas of broken skin or near your eyes. Wash your hands thoroughly afterward.

Resist the rests. Whether they're filled with gel, foam, or buckwheat, the wrist rests you use with your keyboard to reduce pressure on your wrists may actually double the pressure inside your carpal tunnel—and increase the likelihood of developing CTS. Instead, position your keyboard on an adjustable platform so the space bar is higher than the function keys. When you're not typing, rest your hands on the arms of your chair or in your lap—anywhere but on your keyboard or mouse pad, which will cause your wrist to bend upward and increase the pressure inside that trouble-prone tunnel.

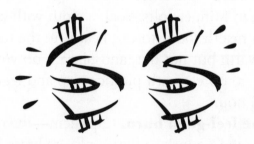

Cataracts

Keep Your Vision Sharp

I f it's true that the eyes are windows of the soul, then the view must get a little cloudy in our later years. With advancing age, proteins in the lenses of the eyes naturally discolor and lose some of their natural transparency. In some cases, the eyes get so filmy that incoming light is blurred or even blocked. This condition, known as cataracts, is among the leading causes of vision loss in older adults.

The good news is that cataracts progress slowly over time and are usually detected during routine eye examinations. The better news is that most cataracts are almost completely curable. Modern laser surgery that removes the cloudy lens, which is replaced with a clear implant, is now safe and effective, says Alex Eaton, M.D., an ophthalmologist and retina specialist in Fort Myers, Florida.

The very best news, though, is that you may not ever have to think about surgery if you take steps to prevent cataracts from forming in the first place. Here's what you need to do.

Make the produce aisle your second home. All of those fruits and vegetables are loaded with antioxidants, chemical compounds that block the eye-damaging effects of toxic oxygen molecules in the body—molecules that play a leading role in causing cataracts, says Dr. Eaton.

Go for the green. Kale; spinach; and collard, mustard, and turnip greens are loaded with lutein and zeaxanthin, two compounds that are important for eye health. Two Harvard University studies—one of 36,000 men, the other of 50,000 women—found that those who ate foods richest in these compounds had about a 20 percent lower chance of needing cataract surgery than those who didn't eat such foods.

Have some tea with your onions. One study showed that drinking several cups of tea a day was associated with lower risk of cataracts. Tea is rich in quercetin, an antioxidant that's essential for eye health. Onions are even better, because the body absorbs twice as much quercetin from them as from tea. And quercetin survives heat, so you can enjoy your onions cooked as well as raw.

Shade your eyes. Sun exposure triples the risk of cataracts—and it's

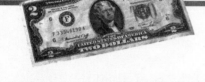

The $2 Deal

Bilberry Protects Peepers

A close relative of the blueberry, bilberries may help to prevent cataracts, or at least slow their growth. This shrubby plant is high in bioflavonoids, nutrients that enhance the action of vitamin C. Because the lens of the eye naturally contains so much vitamin C, some scientists believe a deficiency can lead to cataracts. You can find bilberry in tincture form; the usual dose is 1 to 2 milliliters twice a day. Don't use bilberry or supplemental vitamin C without your doctor's okay.

so easy to avoid. Simply wear a brimmed hat and good sunglasses every time you're out in the sun. And keep in mind that reflected light—from water, snow, or pavement—is often even more damaging than direct sunlight.

Put out those butts. Cigarette smoking increases the risk of developing age-related cataracts, and an article in the *Journal of the American Medical Association* suggests that quitting reduces that risk. Men who had quit smoking had a 23 percent reduced risk of cataracts and a 28 percent reduced risk of cataract extraction than men who currently smoked. If quitting has been a losing battle so far, ask your doctor for advice. There are many new and effective ways to help you quit, and the sooner you do it, the better off you'll be.

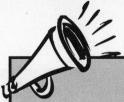

HOLLER FOR HELP

Be Vigilant about Vision

In the early stages of cataracts, you can pretty much carry on as usual, since they have only a minor effect on your vision. You may find you're becoming more sensitive to light and glare and that your sight is gradually blurring. You may also discover that you need a new eyeglass prescription more often than usual. See your doctor as soon as you notice any vision changes—especially if you are seeing double, you see halos around street lights, or your vision is actually dimming. This could indicate a more serious problem, such as a detaching retina, which needs emergency treatment.

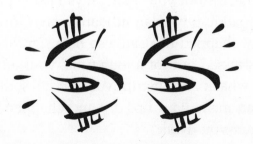

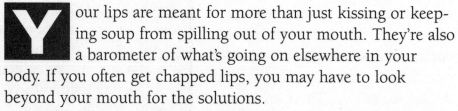

Chapped Lips

Caress Your Kisser

Your lips are meant for more than just kissing or keeping soup from spilling out of your mouth. They're also a barometer of what's going on elsewhere in your body. If you often get chapped lips, you may have to look beyond your mouth for the solutions.

Chapped lips usually indicate nothing more serious than too much exposure to sun or wind. Chapping is especially a problem in winter, because indoor heat sucks a lot of moisture out of the air. But if your lips stay chapped for weeks at a time, or if they get better for a while, then get chapped again, you should probably see your doctor. "You may not be absorbing all the nutrients you need from your diet," says Priscilla Natanson, N.D., a naturopathic physician in Plantation, Florida.

Continually chapped lips can also be a sign of chronic stress. When you're stressed out for a long time, your adrenal glands can get out of whack and disrupt your body's sodium balance. This in turn can make your lips dry and chapped, no matter how much water you drink.

PUCKER POWER

The skin on your lips is shed and replaced more rapidly than other tissues, says Dr. Natanson. If you aren't getting enough key nutrients in your diet, for example, the problem may start to show up on your lips before you notice other symptoms. Also, dry lips may be a signal that your body isn't retaining fluids as well as it should.

So don't think of chapped lips as just a nuisance. At the very least, a lack of proper TLC can result in deep, painful cracks that are agonizingly slow to heal. Lip balm should always be the first line of defense for parched lips, but if yours still seem rough enough to scour pots, consider these additional tips.

Top off your tank. Sometimes chapped lips are simply a signal that your body's water tank is low. Try drinking several large glasses of water daily to give your lips the moisture they're craving.

Cook up some veggies. Eating more green vegetables is a great way to keep your lips in the pink. They're rich in zinc, essential fatty acids, and riboflavin—everything your lips need to retain moisture and stay healthy, says Dr. Natanson.

Pump moisture into the air. An indoor humid-

FAST FIX
Buy Natural Balms

Herbal lip balms that contain marigold or calendula are better than synthetic goop from the cosmetics counter because they contain natural compounds that promote healing, says John Hibbs, N.D., a naturopathic physician and professor at Bastyr University near Seattle. Other lip-healing ingredients to look for in balms include lanolin, olive oil, and echinacea.

ifier is a great way to keep your lips supple and healthy. It's especially important to use a humidifier during cold weather because heating systems, especially oil heat, draw moisture out of the air.

Screen the sun. Too much sun does more than just dry your lips; it can give them a ferocious burn, says Dr. Natanson. She recommends using a lip balm with the highest sun protection factor (SPF) you can find. Be sure it's waterproof, and use it as often as the directions on the package recommend.

Bag the balm. "I'm not real keen on using petroleum-based products," says Dr. Natanson. Rather than covering your lips with an oil slick, she recommends using protective products that contain beeswax or other natural forms of oil.

Lay off the licking. If you find that your lips get severely chapped during stressful times—when visiting your in-laws at Thanksgiving, for example—you could be licking them more than usual, says Dr. Natanson. "Licking your lips actually dries them out," she says. Her advice: Chew gum or suck on lozenges when you're nervous.

Toss the smokes. Need another reason to quit smoking? Smoking dries your lips and makes them more prone to chap-

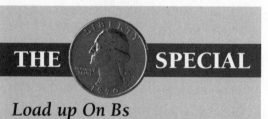

THE SPECIAL

Load up On Bs

Chapped lips or cuts at the corners of the mouth are classic signs of a B vitamin deficiency, says John Hibbs, N.D. "B vitamins are required for cell division and reproduction," he explains. "When the tissues in the corner of the mouth are weak from lack of B vitamins, cracks or splits appear." A good multivitamin that includes all of the B vitamins should put your lips back in working order.

ping. And we hear it's bad for your lungs, too.

Try some new makeup. Some women get chapped lips when they use foundation makeup or lipstick. In fact, almost any cosmetic ingredient that comes near the mouth can cause reactions in some people, says Dr. Natanson. If chapping is a frequent problem, try using different kinds of makeup until you find the brands that agree with you.

Switch mouthwashes. Or try a new toothpaste. As with makeup, these products may contain ingredients that cause chapping. A simple step such as changing brands may make a big difference.

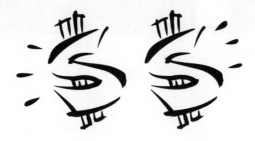

Chronic Fatigue Syndrome

Put Some Spring in Your Step

It used to be called the yuppie flu because it seemed to afflict so many people struggling to balance high-powered careers and parenthood. Before that, doctors just called it being dog-tired. These days, it's better known as chronic fatigue syndrome (CFS), a baffling set of symptoms that can make you feel as though all your energy went right down the drain.

CFS usually begins with cold or flu-like symptoms, along with an intermittent low-grade fever, muscle and joint pain, memory loss, and insomnia. Then there's the chronic, disabling fatigue that can last for at least six months—and sometimes years. A 1990s study from the Centers for Disease Control and Prevention showed that CFS may be more widespread than previously thought, and a Harvard Medical School study showed its prevalence may be even more than double previous estimates.

FIGHT THE FATIGUE

Chronic fatigue is probably triggered by an infection, but there isn't a definitive treatment. It's essential to see your doctor, because the symptoms of CFS are nearly the same as those caused by many other problems, some of them quite serious. If you've already been diagnosed with CFS, however, the following tips will help put your energy back on the fast track.

Eat better than ever. "Good nutrition may be the single most important strategy for whipping CFS," says Ralph Ofcarcik, Ph.D., a nutritionist and guest education manager at the Red Mountain Health Resort in Ivins, Utah. Until you're feeling better, forget the junk food and sodas. "Since the immune system is functioning at less than an optimum level, it makes good sense to focus on nutrient-dense, unprocessed foods," he says.

In other words, load up on fruits, vegetables, legumes, and whole grains, and go easy on red meat and other fatty foods.

Feel your oats. Oats, specifically the "straw," are rich in minerals and can help restore a compromised nervous system. Make a cold infusion by soaking 2 tablespoons of oatstraw in 1 quart of cold water overnight. Strain and drink

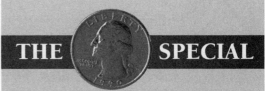

THE SPECIAL

Take Your Morning Multi

In addition to eating a nutritious diet rich in fresh fruits and vegetables, it's essential to take a multivitamin/mineral supplement, preferably one that contains extra magnesium, says Ralph Ofcarcik, Ph.D. People with chronic fatigue who take these simple steps often feel a lot better, he explains.

HOLLER FOR HELP

CFS Pretenders

Chronic fatigue syndrome is worrisome enough by itself, but there are a number of other medical conditions that mimic its symptoms. See your doctor if you have a history of ongoing fatigue. It's possible that you have a thyroid condition or any one of a dozen different diseases.

throughout the day.

Fight back with an herbal blend. Combining tonic, relaxing, and restorative herbs may help ease fatigue and improve immune function over time. Measure out equal parts of lavender, lemon balm, licorice root, skullcap, wood betony, and vervain. Add 1 heaping teaspoon of the mixture to 1 cup of hot water and steep for 20 minutes. Strain out the herbs and drink two cups a day. If you have high blood pressure, though, don't use licorice root.

Fish for primrose. According to one study, 85 percent of a group of people with CFS reported some improvement after 15 weeks of taking a combination of evening primrose oil and fish-oil supplements. As long as you're not taking heart medications, start with 1,500 milligrams twice a day.

Get some shuteye. Everyone needs a good's night rest, but with CFS, it's a real priority. Establish a regular sleep routine and sleep for 7 to 9 hours a night. Ask your doctor for help if you're having serious problems sleeping.

Simplify, simplify. This may be the time to delegate housekeeping or line up more baby-sitters. If you have a spouse and children, work out a plan to share the chores. If you can afford to hire help, spend money on that and cut back on things that matter less.

Save your strength. For example, invest in a

wheeled suitcase or duffel bag and buy a lightweight folding cart that you can toss in the backseat and use for groceries or even as a briefcase. Have groceries and other supplies delivered whenever possible so you can conserve your strength.

Turn off the ringer. Screen phone calls with an answering machine and answer only when you feel up to it. Constant interruptions add stress and make you feel defeated. Establish a habit of returning calls when you aren't busy or feeling exhausted.

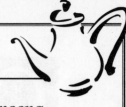

Tea Time

Get Zip with Ginseng

To boost your energy, bring about 5 cups of water to a simmer, then add 1 teaspoon of ground ginseng root. Cover, remove from the heat, and steep for about 30 minutes. Then add 1 teaspoon of dried borage leaves and 1 teaspoon of dried mint leaves and steep for another 15 to 20 minutes. Finally, add 10 to 20 drops of ginkgo tincture. Strain out the herbs, sweeten to taste, and sip up to three cups a day. Ginseng can raise your blood pressure, so avoid it if you're taking blood pressure medication.

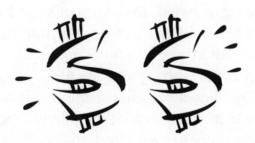

Colds

Stop the Sniffles

If you can't figure out why modern science hasn't found a cure for the common cold, consider the numbers. A cold is actually 1 of about 200 mild viral infections of the upper respiratory tract. Even if doctors figured out how to cure one of them, what about the other 199?

The trouble is, over-the-counter drugs just don't do much—and cost a bundle besides. Antihistamines, for instance, will dry up a runny nose from allergies, but they won't affect the dripping and sneezing of a cold. Decongestants can leave you jittery. Aspirin and acetaminophen can suppress your immune system. And those all-in-one nighttime remedies? They come with a shot glass for good reason: The "knockout" ingredient is alcohol. It may help your head hit the pillow, but it won't do a thing to fight infection.

FEEL BETTER FAST

Other than curling up in bed, what's the alternative? Try some of these natural remedies. Some of them—if taken at the first sneeze—can cut your sick time by more than half.

Steam out infection. Steam kills cold germs on contact if water temperatures are 110°F or more. Herbs such as eucalyptus add a penetrating scent and have disinfectant properties. Put some fresh leaves in a bowl, pour boiling water over them, and drape a towel over your head and the bowl to make a "tent." Lower your face over the bowl (carefully—you can scald yourself if the steam is too hot) and breathe in. You can also add a few drops of oregano oil to the water. It's nice—a bit like diluted Vicks.

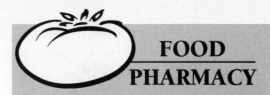

FOOD PHARMACY

Mushrooms for Immunity

Smoky-tasting shiitake mushrooms amp up production of interferon, a protein that girds the body to defend against viral invaders, while reishi mushrooms may help ease respiratory tract inflammation. Either add these 'shrooms to your therapeutic chicken soup or look for them combined in extract form and follow the directions on the label, advises John Hahn, N.D., D.P.M., a naturopathic physician and podiatrist in Bend, Oregon.

Stay lubricated. When you're in artificially controlled environments with really dry air, such as offices and airplanes, your nasal membranes dry out, and tiny cracks that invite viruses may form in your nasal passages. The best defense? Drink plenty of liquids and use saline nasal spray often to hydrate the tender membranes.

Make a chest rub. Using a poultice when you have a cold is a good way to make yourself rest. Make your own chest rub by adding 3 or 4 drops of herbal oil (try eucalyptus, lavender, or thyme) to 1 tablespoon of olive oil. Apply the mixture liberally to your chest, cover with a clean cloth, and settle into a comfy chair with a cozy afghan and a good book.

Make a Bloody Mary. You can use booze or not, as you prefer. To the tomato juice, add some lemon, a celery stalk, and horseradish, then drink it quickly. Tomato juice is full of vitamin C, but it's the horseradish that really does the trick. Its powerful fumes will loosen congestion, making your cold more bearable.

Mine some zinc. Research indicates that zinc may cut the duration of colds by about two days by acting as a physical barrier to prevent viruses from entering the cells that line the nose and throat. All you have to do is spritz an over-the-counter zinc nasal spray (which you can find in drugstores) in each nostril four times a day within 48 hours of the first inkling of a cold. With zinc lozenges, you have to act even more quickly—within 24 hours of your first symptom. "Look for zinc gluconate tablets that aren't flavored with citric acid, tartaric acid, or sorbitol," advises David Zeiger, D.O., a family physician in Chicago. When these ingredients mix with saliva, they cancel out zinc's benefits.

> A cup of hot tea with honey usually feels great when you have a cold. You can try different types, such as red pepper tea, that are meant to loosen up mucus. Lemon and honey, added to weak tea or even plain hot water, also ease head pain and help break up congestion.

Echinacea is excellent. Studies have shown that the herb echinacea shortens the duration of colds from nine to six days and makes them less severe—possibly because the polysaccharides it contains boost the body's infection-fighting cells. The best way to take echinacea is as a tincture (an alcohol-based extract, which is available at health food stores) so it bypasses digestion and flows directly into your bloodstream.

At the first hint of a cold, Dr. Zeiger recommends taking 30 drops of tincture every 2 hours. After a week, go to 20 drops three times a day, for a total of 10 days. Use the herb only during your cold (with continued use, it loses effectiveness), and never use it if you have an autoimmune disease such as lupus, rheumatoid arthritis, or multiple sclerosis, or if you are pregnant or nursing.

Breathe easy with olive. Research shows that leuropein, the active ingredient in olive leaf extract, has powerful healing properties that may beat bacteria, viruses, fungi, and even parasites. The recommended dose is a 300-milligram capsule three times a day for no more than two days. After that, gradually reduce your intake, suggests Jennifer Reid, N.D., a naturopathic physician at the Columbia River Natural Medicine Clinic in Troutdale, Oregon. Check with your doctor first, and never take olive leaf in any dosage for more than seven days.

Slurp some soup. Why did the chicken cross the road? Perhaps to get into the soup pot. Nobody knows exactly why chicken soup works, but it does help relieve cold symptoms. Most doctors believe that the steam from the hot soup promotes drainage and thus makes you feel better. There must be some-

Tea Time

Pungent Protection

Garlic has long been used for its potent healing effects, and it does double duty as a cold preventive because it keeps other people at a distance! Surprisingly, garlic tea doesn't taste as bad as you'd think. Chop two medium cloves and simmer in 1 cup of water for 10 to 15 minutes. Add two to three slices of fresh ginger to improve the taste and increase the warming action of the garlic. Honey and lemon are optional. Drink two to four cups per day. People who take blood-thinning medications should steer clear of garlic unless given the green light by their physicians.

thing to it; it's been in use as a remedy since the twelfth century.

Pony up for horseradish. This powerful herb contains allyl isothiocyanate, which stimulates the nerve endings in your nose and makes it run like a faucet. Plus, horseradish has antiviral properties. "I suggest patients take a teaspoon of freshly grated root or a half-teaspoon of horseradish extract three times a day," says Michael DiPalma, N.D., a naturopathic physician in Newtown, Pennsylvania. The extract is available in health food stores.

Soothe your cough with elm. If you're coughing so much that your chest and back ache, try slippery elm tea. This time-honored expectorant will help break up the sticky mucus that may be clogging your bronchial tubes, says Dr. Reid. Look for it at health food stores and follow the directions on the label.

Fight the bug with astragalus. This Chinese herb stimulates the release of interferon in the body and thereby boosts your immune system. Unlike echinacea, you can take astragalus (available at health food stores) every day during cold and flu season to bolster your resistance. A typical regimen is eight 400- to 500-milligram capsules or 15 to 30 drops of extract daily.

Wash often. Hardy cold viruses can live for hours on door-knobs, faucet handles, books, money—all the things we touch

Snooze with Booze

Try a hot toddy as a cold rescue. Before hundreds of cold remedies became available at drugstores, certain home remedies were probably a lot more fun to take. And if you took enough, you absolutely felt better, because pretty soon you didn't notice the symptoms anymore. There are many variations on the hot toddy, which apparently originated in Scotland. Start with juice, honey, or tea and add the liquor of your choice.

every day. Frequent hand washing is the single best way to avoid catching a cold or spreading your own. Unfortunately, the habit is in decline. Researchers from the American Society of Microbiology and the Centers for Disease Control and Prevention watched 8,000 people in restrooms in several cities. Only 67 percent stopped at the sink. In a related survey, only 40 percent of women reported washing their hands after sneezing or coughing, and men were even worse—just 22 percent. (They were also asked if they washed their hands after changing a diaper or petting an animal—and believe us, you don't want to know their answers.)

Toss the germs. Bacteria and viruses live on cloth towels and sponges for hours, so use paper towels, tissues, and napkins when someone in the house has a cold.

Mist away throat pain. Here's a blast of natural relief for a sore throat. First, buy yourself a new plant mister. Then make a triple-strength tea by adding 3 teaspoons each of dried slippery elm, echinacea, and licorice to 3 cups of water. Bring it to a full boil, then reduce the heat and simmer for 10 to 15 minutes. Strain out the herbs, cool, and

The $2 Deal

Decongest with Licorice

The steam from licorice tea speeds the flow of mucus from your nose, and the licorice itself stimulates production of interferon, a protein that helps the body defend against viral invaders, brings mucus up from the lungs, and soothes a scratchy throat. Check your health food store for packaged licorice tea and follow the label directions. Don't use this remedy if you have high blood pressure.

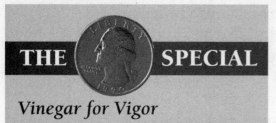
Vinegar for Vigor

Appalachian healers make a cold remedy from common household ingredients: Mix a dash of red pepper and a pinch of salt into 1 ounce of apple cider vinegar and drink it three or four times a day. Another remedy some folks use for colds is 1 tablespoon each of honey and lemon juice. Add them to a cup of hot water or tea and sip it three times a day.

pour the brew into your new spray bottle. Open your mouth, stick out your tongue, and spray the back of your throat as needed during the day. Ahhhh, relief! Don't use licorice, though, if you have high blood pressure or kidney disease.

Decline dairy. When you have a cold, stick to juices, water, and hot beverages. Avoid milk and milk products, because moo juice promotes mucus formation. If you do indulge in dairy during a cold, you'll not only get a milk moustache, you'll also get more congestion.

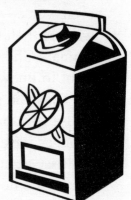

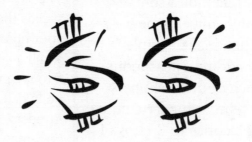

Cold Sores

Quick Tips for Pain-Free Lips

Pain isn't always proportionate to size, as anyone who's ever had a cold sore knows. Those pesky little blisters on or near the lips are hardly bigger than a pencil eraser, but they can feel as though someone's digging into your lip with a hot poker.

Despite the name, cold sores—also known as fever blisters—don't have anything to do with colds or fevers. They're caused by a virus called herpes simplex type 1. (A close relative, herpes simplex type 2, is responsible for genital sores.) Millions of Americans are infected with the virus but never have symptoms. Others aren't so lucky.

The cold sore virus survives in the body forever, although it spends most of its life in dormancy. Periodically, it "wakes up," trav-

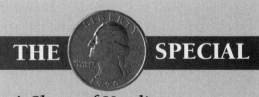

THE SPECIAL

A Sheen of Vaseline

Applying petroleum jelly is an easy way to soften the skin surrounding cold sores to prevent cracks or bleeding. Smooth a generous layer on the area once or twice a day and keep applying it until the cold sore is gone.

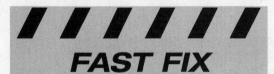

FAST FIX
Ice It Up

It's often possible to stop cold sores in their tracks by applying ice at the earliest sign. Most people experience a slight tingling sensation days before cold sores erupt, and that's the time to apply an ice cube to the area. Keep it there for about 30 minutes and repeat the treatment throughout the day. "If you catch it early enough, it could abort the whole outbreak," says John Hibbs, N.D.

els up nerves to the skin, and erupts in a painful, fluid-filled blister. The blister goes away in about a week, but that doesn't mean the virus is gone. It's just back in hiding, where it will stay dormant until the next time conditions are right for it to appear.

HEALING HELPERS

Most people don't get cold sores often enough to worry much about them. If you're one of the exceptions—maybe you get sores every month, for example, or they're unusually large or painful—your doctor may write a prescription for acyclovir (Zovirax), which can shorten the duration of outbreaks if taken within a day or two after symptoms appear. There are also topical creams available, such as Abreva.

Whether or not you decide to use medication, you'll certainly want to take steps to eliminate the sores as quickly as possible—and help keep them from coming back. You don't have to buy a lot of fancy medicines to do it. Here's what doctors advise.

Dab on lemon balm. Studies show that lemon balm, also known as melissa, helps cold sores heal faster with less crusting. "Lemon balm contains at least four antiviral compounds," explains Jeanette Jacknin, M.D., a dermatologist in Scottsdale, Arizona, "so it's considered by some to be a first-choice herbal treatment." The key is to apply it at the first inkling of an outbreak. Make a tea by steeping 2 to 4 teaspoons of dried lemon balm leaves in a cup of hot water for 10 minutes or so, then apply the cooled solution directly to the sore. Or look for a commercial lip balm that contains lemon balm and slather it on your sore.

Excellent extracts. At the first indication of a blister outbreak, scan the shelves of your local health food store for extracts of calendula, tea tree oil, slippery elm, and myrrh; they're all either excellent astringents or inflammation and infection fighters. Add several drops of each to a cup of hot water, let it cool, and dab the solution directly onto your cold sore for instant pain relief.

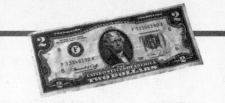

The $2 Deal

Lick the Pain with Licorice

Don't head to the candy aisle; instead, go to a health food store for natural licorice root extract. It contains chemical compounds that inhibit the activity of the virus and can help cold sores heal more quickly, says John Hibbs, N.D. As soon as a sore appears, dab it with the molasses-like extract four to six times a day.

Go for the gold standard. Goldenseal is another antiviral herb that can treat cold sores. Add 1/4 teaspoon of extract (available at health food stores) to your echinacea drink three times a day.

Put your trust in E. Studies show that if you apply vitamin E oil (from either a bottle or a capsule) directly to a cold sore, you may speed your recovery and relieve the pain—possibly within a single day.

Sip echinacea. Echinacea isn't just a plain old cold fighter; it battles cold sores, too, perhaps by boosting the antiviral immune fighters in mucous membranes. Mix 1/4 teaspoon of extract (available at health food stores) in water or juice and drink it three times a day for as long as your symptoms last, suggests Dr. Jacknin. Don't take echinacea if you have an autoimmune disease such as rheuma-toid arthritis, lupus, or multiple sclerosis, or if you are pregnant or nursing.

Zap sores with zinc. The same white ointment that lifeguards use on their noses to protect against sunburn may heal cold sores in 5 days instead of the usual 10. The catch, according to research, is that you have to apply zinc oxide four times a day—and perhaps every hour—starting within 24 hours of the first hint of an outbreak. You can find the ointment at drugstores.

Buy the right balm. The herbal balms sold in health food stores reduce cold sore pain and keep the skin moisturized as the blisters dry and crust. In addition, some balms help combat the virus directly. "Marigold and calendula balms are healing and have antiviral properties," says John Hibbs, N.D., a naturo-pathic physician and professor at Bastyr University near Seattle.

Oil 'em. Both lavender and St. John's wort oils, available in health food stores, inhibit the activity of herpes simplex, says Dr. Hibbs. Once or twice a day, use a cotton swab to dab a small amount of oil on the sore. Be careful not to get the oil in your mouth, though. Even in tiny amounts, these oils should not be taken internally.

Ax the arginine. The cold sore virus can't thrive without an amino acid called arginine, so as soon as you feel a cold sore coming on, avoid arginine-rich foods, such as chocolate.

Flood the pain. Even if you don't drink a lot of water most of the time, you really want to tank up when you have a cold sore. The more fluid you have in your body, the easier it is for immune cells to get where they're needed to start the healing process, says Dr.

Hibbs. He recommends drinking 8 to 12 glasses of water a day until the sore is gone.

Load up on lysine. Like arginine, lysine is a naturally occurring amino acid. Unlike arginine, it inhibits the effects of the herpes simplex virus. "Take 3,000 to 4,000 milligrams of lysine daily during outbreaks," says Dr. Hibbs.

Put your feet up. The herpes simplex virus tends to awaken during times of stress, probably because tension and anxiety make the immune system work less efficiently. It's impossible, of course, to eliminate all the stress from your life, but keeping it at manageable levels reduces the risk of getting cold sores. Even if you already have an outbreak, reducing stress can prevent one sore from triggering another.

Everyone controls stress in different ways. Daily exercise is a great stress reducer. Relaxation techniques, such as meditation and deep breathing, can help, as can setting aside time to do things you enjoy, such as going to the movies or spending time with friends.

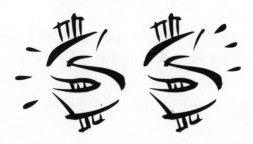

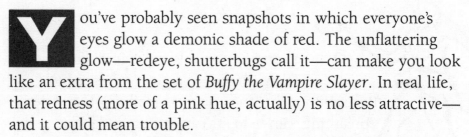

Conjunctivitis

Get the Pink Out

You've probably seen snapshots in which everyone's eyes glow a demonic shade of red. The unflattering glow—redeye, shutterbugs call it—can make you look like an extra from the set of *Buffy the Vampire Slayer*. In real life, that redness (more of a pink hue, actually) is no less attractive—and it could mean trouble.

A condition called conjunctivitis, better known as pinkeye, occurs when the conjunctiva—the protective membrane covering the insides of your eyelids and the exposed whites of your eyes—gets infected.

If your eyes are itching, burning, and discharging some sticky goop, chances are good that you have pinkeye. It usually begins in one eye and quickly spreads to the other. It can be caused by bacteria or an allergy, but it's most commonly the result of a virus.

EASE THE IRRITATION

While pinkeye is quite contagious, it's usually not very serious. Once in a great while, however, a case of conjunctivitis can do some real damage. If your pinkeye doesn't clear up within a week, or if you have a fever or changes in vision along with it, call your doctor. Otherwise, here's how to soothe the garden-variety types that trouble most of us.

Shut your eyes and chill. Ice-cold compresses can soothe your eyes. Simply place a damp washcloth that's been chilled in the freezer or a cool, wet paper towel over your closed eyes for about 20 minutes. Stop for 30 to 60 minutes, then do it again. Apply cold as often as you feel the need.

Relax with a berry good compress. Strawberry tea helps soothe inflamed eyes and fight infection. Steep 1 teaspoon of leaves in 1 cup of hot water for 10 minutes, strain, and cool. Use the solution in a compress or put it in an eye cup and rinse your eyes with it once or twice daily.

Stay on the dry side. Until your eyes have cleared up, don't go swimming! Not only can you spread conjunctivitis germs to others in the pool, but the chlorinated water can increase the irritation.

Hands off. While your eyes are infected, avoid shaking hands; use disposable tissues that you discard yourself; and be sure to disinfect doorknobs, countertops, and telephones. Also, don't share towels or pillows.

The Chamomile Cure

To make a soothing eyewash from chamomile, steep 2 to 3 teaspoons of herb in 1 pint of boiling water (or use a tea bag) for 10 minutes. Let cool and strain through a sterile cloth. Use an eye cup to rinse your eye with the solution two or three times daily until the problem is resolved. People with ragweed allergies may be sensitive to chamomile.

Conjunctivitis

Unload your mascara. Get rid of any mascara, eyeliner, or eye shadow that you've used since you developed pinkeye. They're harboring germs. Then, when your peepers are no longer pink, treat yourself to some new cosmetics.

Get out your glasses. Don't wear contacts while you have pinkeye. Your eyes will feel worse with them in, since the lenses hold the germs against your eyeball.

Put on some shades. Wear sunglasses to protect your eyes from glare and irritation. You'll look cool, and you'll feel less self-conscious about your inflamed eyes and mascara-free lashes.

Get all weepy. Check your local drugstore for artificial tears and other soothing eye remedies. According to the American Academy of Family Physicians, these lubricating eyedrops are especially helpful if your pinkeye is due to allergies, but they can also help reduce swelling of the conjunctiva.

Stop allergy attacks. If your conjunctivitis is allergy related, ask your doctor if you should take an over-the-counter antihistamine such as diphenhydramine (Benadryl), which can help reduce itching, swelling, and discomfort. If a drug doesn't do the job, ask if prescription antihistamine eyedrops are right for you.

Constipation

Get Up and Go!

Sometimes constipation, like beauty, exists only in the eye of the beholder. Most of us grow up thinking that a daily bowel movement is necessary for good health, but everyone experiences constipation in different ways. For someone who's accustomed to having a bowel movement every day, a reduction to three or four a week could be a sign of constipation. For others, having three bowel movements a week is normal, but having fewer than that is a problem.

Since there's so much individual variation, doctors offer this advice: If there's been any change in your usual bathroom habits, get professional advice. There are literally hundreds of things that can cause constipation. Sometimes it's a side effect of medications. Lack of exercise can cause it, or drinking too little water, or not eating enough fiber. The list goes on and on.

START THINGS MOVING AGAIN

Fortunately, you don't have to put up with constipation—and you definitely shouldn't fork over your hard-earned cash for

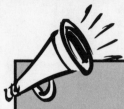

over-the-counter laxatives. There are a lot of less expensive—and safer—treatments to try first. Here are the best.

Fill 'er up. All experts agree that the simplest way to wake up your colon is to drink water—lots and lots of it. "Try to down 10 glasses (a total of 80 ounces) within 24 hours," recommends Gary Gitnick, M.D., chief of the division of digestive diseases at the University of California, Los Angeles, School of Medicine. Need to get things moving right now? Drink a large glass of water every 10 minutes for 1 hour to soften your stools and spur elimination.

Praise the plants. The best diet for beating constipation is the same one that doctors recommend for preventing heart disease, cancer, and dozens of other serious health problems: a lot of plant foods and very little, if any, junk food.

In other words, eat as though processed foods had never been invented. "You want a diet that's high in fiber and complex carbohydrates," says Rob Dramov, N.D., a naturopathic physician in Tigard, Oregon. That means lots of fruits and vegetables, whole grains, and legumes every day, as well as high-fiber cereals such as oatmeal and oat bran.

Have another slice of pie. Just make sure it's rhubarb—one of the yummiest natural laxatives around. Rhubarb stimulates mucus production in the large intestine to ease elimination, which typically occurs within 6 to 10 hours. You can eat it stewed or try this lip-smacking smoothie: Juice 3 cups of raw rhubarb stalks and 1 cup of fresh or frozen strawberries. Add 1/4 cup of water and 1/4 cup of honey, then sip and go!

Heed the call. If you're reluctant to use a public restroom no matter how urgent the need, you're setting yourself up for trouble. Resisting the urge to have a bowel movement—whether you're at a restaurant or at home—can make it difficult to go later on. In fact, delaying bowel movements can make your large intestine lazy, Dr. Dramov says. Essentially, you're teaching your body to resist its natural urges. You'll be a lot more regular if you go as soon as possible when you feel the need.

Rub in regularity. To encourage movement in sluggish bowels, try a simple belly-button rub. Use your favorite massage oil and lightly massage your stomach with the tips of your fingers, starting at your belly button and moving in small clockwise circles. Gradually expand the circles until you're massaging your entire abdomen. If you do this for 10 to 15 minutes every morning, you may find that your daily routine will be a bit more regular.

Move often. Any kind of physical activity—walking, lifting weights, riding a bicycle—helps the intestine work more efficiently. In fact, it's not uncommon for people who have been constipated for years to get completely better once they start exercising for 20 to 30 minutes daily.

Regulate with supplements. The mineral magnesium helps soften stools and make bowel movements easier, says Dr. Dramov. Talk to your doctor about starting the day with 500 milligrams of supplemental magnesium. Another option: As long as you don't have stomach or kidney problems, take 1,000 to 2,000 milligrams of vitamin C a day, split into two or three doses. Relatively high doses of this vitamin often soften stools, he explains. If either supplement causes diarrhea, though, reduce the dose.

Dig some dandelions. To make a dandy drink that'll relieve constipation, puree some young dandelion leaves in a blender with water, then pour the juice into a glass. Drink up to three glasses of this tonic daily. Just be sure your dandelion comes from a lawn that hasn't been blasted with chemicals. And don't use dandelion if you're taking diuretics or potassium tablets.

Mind your medicines. Constipation is among the most common side effects of medications. Antacids are common culprits, as are pain medications. It's worth making a list of all the drugs you're taking to review with your pharmacist. If it turns out that one of them may be responsible for your constipation, your doctor shouldn't have any trouble finding an acceptable alternative.

Multiply by three. In hospitals, prunes, bran, and applesauce are frequently mixed together and offered to patients to get things going. To make your own cocktail, mix 4 to 6 chopped prunes with 1 tablespoon of bran and

½ cup of applesauce. Try it just before bed.

Give psyllium a try. Check a health food store or drugstore for powdered laxatives that contain psyllium seeds. Once a day, add 2 tablespoons to a large glass of water or juice and drink it immediately, before it thickens. To avoid intestinal blockage, be sure to drink lots of water throughout the day—at least six extra glasses—while you're taking psyllium. And don't use it within 2 hours of taking any other supplements or medications, since it could delay their absorption into the bloodstream.

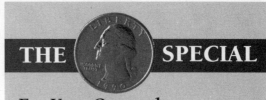

THE SPECIAL

Eat Your Oatmeal

A certain type of gummy fiber called mucilage soaks up water, softening stools and making them easier to pass. Oatmeal has lots of mucilage, which is the reason it's often recommended as an excellent breakfast choice to jump-start your system. Just don't top your bowl with bananas, which can be binding.

Pop some prunes. Ounce for ounce, prunes are packed with more fiber than almost any other fruit or vegetable—including dried beans. What's more, they contain dihydroxyphenyl isatin, a natural laxative. Down a glass of prune juice before bed to encourage a morning movement, then nibble on dried prunes (or figs and raisins, which also contain isatin) during the day. For a tasty, high-fiber dessert, try baked apples stuffed with prunes, figs, or raisins.

Say yes to yoga. Perform this yoga exercise, and you'll have a bowel movement within 10 minutes, promises Jeff Migdow, M.D., a holistic medical practitioner at the Kripalu Center for Yoga and Health in Lenox, Massachusetts. First, stand with your hands at your sides, inhale deeply through your nose, exhale through your mouth, and lift your arms over your head while inhaling deeply again through your nose. Next, exhale while lowering

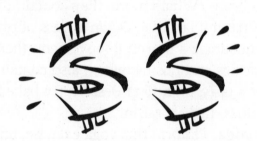
yourself into a squat, with your hands on your knees and your head lowered. As you finish the exhalation, still squatting, pump your abdomen in and out 20 times. Stand up and repeat the sequence three times.

Kick back after meals. It's the best way to encourage your digestive tract to shift into gear. If you're the type who likes to eat and run, you're diverting blood to other parts of your body and leaving your intestine short-changed. "The old adage 'rest and digest' is just as true today as it ever was," says Dr. Dramov.

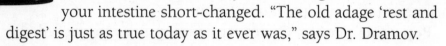

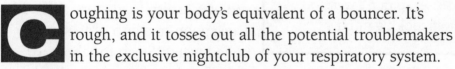

Coughs

Halt Annoying Hacking

oughing is your body's equivalent of a bouncer. It's rough, and it tosses out all the potential troublemakers in the exclusive nightclub of your respiratory system.

Unfortunately, there are a lot of troublemakers out there: dust, pollen, viruses, and smoke from your grandfather's cigar, to name just a few. Coughing does its job pretty well, and for the most part, you want to encourage it. But you also want to soothe the irritated tissues in your throat and airways until the cough goes away naturally, as well as boost your immune system so that any germs disappear as quickly as possible.

SLIP, SLIDE, AND SLEEP

A simple cough responds to simple solutions. Here's what may help.

The poultice that pleases. Traditional healers swear by herbal oil poultices for easing coughs. To make one, add a few drops of thyme or eucalyptus oil to a teaspoon of olive oil. Rub the mixture on your chest and the outside of your throat, then cover the area with an old towel or a piece of flannel so you

HOLLER FOR HELP

Count the Days

If your cough really hurts, is accompanied by fever, or is getting worse instead of better after a week or so, check in with your doctor. You may have a hard-hitting infection that won't go away until you take antibiotics. Coughing can even be a symptom of heart disease, so don't wait too long before looking into it.

don't stain your clothes. Leave the poultice on for about 20 minutes. The vapors will soothe your irritated airways and reduce the urge to cough.

Hang out with hyssop. A good way to eliminate mucus—and the coughing that goes with it—is to drink hyssop tea. A traditional herb for treating coughs, hyssop makes mucus thinner and easier to cough up, says Priscilla Natanson, N.D., a naturopathic physician in Plantation, Florida. Buy dried hyssop at a health food store and add 1 teaspoon to a cup of freshly boiled water. Steep for about 10 minutes, then strain out the herb. Drink it throughout the day.

Heat some wine. A traditional Belgian remedy for coughs is to combine hot red wine with lemon, cinnamon, and sugar. At the very least, it will put you right to sleep, so you won't know if you're coughing (and probably won't care). Alcohol is a component of many cough medicines, but use it cautiously—too much will weaken the immune response, which you need to fight infection.

Sleep on a slant. When your chest is congested, and you're coughing up a lot of mucus, pile on several pillows or sleep on a foam wedge. Sleeping with your head raised 6 to 8 inches will prevent the mucus from pooling in your bronchial passages, thus promoting more peaceful sleep.

Keep fluids flowing. Any time is the right time to drink lots of fluids, but especially when you've got a cough. Enjoy a cup of hot tea or a tall glass of lemonade with honey—these are also good at loosening mucus.

Take a break for a change. Since most coughs are caused by upper respiratory infections, your first approach should be to help your body heal. The best way to do that—and one that most of us, with our too-busy schedules, don't do often enough—is to kick back and take it easy until you're feeling better, says Dr. Natanson.

Add extra nourishment. Even if you get all of the essential nutrients in your diet, your body needs extra vitamins and minerals when you're fighting an upper respiratory infection. Taking a daily multivitamin is an easy way to ensure that you get all the nutrients you need to heal quickly.

Forget the fruit juices. While vegetable juices are great when you have a cold or the flu, fruit juices can hurt more than they help. They're loaded with sugar, and all that sweetness is just what germs need to flourish. Also, the acids in citrus juices can irritate your throat and make a cough worse. Stick with vegetable juice until you're well again.

Pop extra C. This all-purpose nutrient is

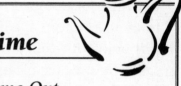

Tea Time

Take Thyme Out

This familiar kitchen spice is great for fighting off a nagging cough. It inhibits bacteria and reduces cough-causing inflammation in your throat and other tissues. Thyme is also an effective expectorant: It makes mucus thinner, so you don't have to cough as hard to get rid of it. You can make thyme tea by steeping 1 teaspoon of dried herb in a cup of hot water for 10 to 15 minutes, then straining out the herb. Or visit a health food store, pick up a bottle of thyme tincture, and take 10 to 20 drops up to four times daily.

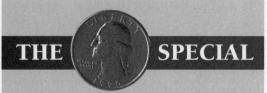

Soothe with Sweet Syrup

Honey mixed with onion juice was widely used for coughs during the Great Depression, when few folks could afford drugstore remedies. To this day, people still use it. Honey or sugar is used to draw the juice from an onion, forming an effective cough syrup. The onion, it's said, stimulates saliva flow, which clears the throat and perhaps reduces inflammation.

Here's what to do: Slice an onion into rings and place them in a deep bowl. Cover them with honey and let stand for 10 to 12 hours. Strain out the onion and take 1 tablespoon of the syrup four or five times a day. Or you can finely chop an onion, mix with ½ cup of granulated sugar, and let stand overnight. Take 1 tablespoon of the resulting syrup every 4 to 5 hours. Never give raw honey to children under one year of age.

essential when you're sick because it strengthens your immune system and can help reduce cold symptoms, including coughs, in a hurry. Unless you have kidney or stomach problems, take 500 milligrams every few hours until you're feeling better. If you start having diarrhea, reduce the dose to a level you can tolerate.

Ask for anise. The herb anise, which has a pleasant licorice flavor and fragrance, is another traditional cough remedy. You can buy anise tea bags at health food stores or raid your spice cabinet and steep a teaspoon of anise in a cup of hot water. It's also fine to use a tincture. The recommended dose for quelling a cough is about 20 drops up to four times daily.

Gulp down some gum weed. Also known as grindelia, this common herb is a top-flight cough remedy. "It's great when you have a dry, raw kind of cough," says Dr. Natanson. She advises taking about 20 drops of grindelia tincture two to four times daily. You can find the tincture at health food stores.

Soften with marshmallow. When mixed with hot water, the

herb marshmallow (which was used to make the candy in the days before high-tech laboratories) forms a slippery liquid that coats and moisturizes a dry, raspy throat. Slippery elm has similar effects. You can buy both herbs in powdered form at most health food stores. Add a tablespoon of either to a cup of hot water and sip it slowly several times a day.

Drink your veggies. Fresh vegetable juice is packed with nutrients that will feed your immune system. The advantage of juices over solid foods when you're sick is that your body is able to absorb the nutrients quickly and easily. Unpack that juicer someone gave you for your birthday five years ago and crank it up. "Green leafy vegetables are the best choices for juicing," says Dr. Natanson. Be sure to use organic veggies so you don't ingest any pesticides.

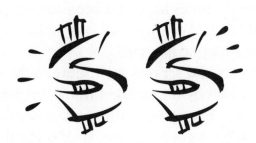

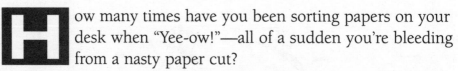

Cuts and Scrapes

Help Healing and Battle the Bugs

How many times have you been sorting papers on your desk when "Yee-ow!"—all of a sudden you're bleeding from a nasty paper cut?

Most of the cuts and scrapes we endure in the course of our busy lives are caused by the smallest things: trimming gnarly tree branches, say, or moving a little too fast with the paring knife. When you get a cut or scrape, your body almost immediately mobilizes specialized cells in your skin and blood vessels. They secrete a host of chemical compounds, including gluelike substances that stop bleeding and seal the cut.

FAST FIRST AID

These small wounds are painful because some parts of your body, especially your fingertips, are jammed with sensitive nerves. Even shallow cuts on your hands or fingers can deliver a surprising amount of pain, and the risk of infection is very real.

Obviously, you need to see a doctor if you're bleeding a lot or have a deep puncture wound. In most cases, though, all you need is some simple first aid. Here's what to do.

Clean and clean again. Hold your wound under running water or pour cool water over it from a cup. Using mild soap—the brand you normally use when you bathe should be just fine—and a soft washcloth, thoroughly clean the edges of the wound and the surrounding area, being careful not to let any soap stray into the open skin. If dirt is embedded in the wound, dip some tweezers in rubbing alcohol, then pick out the particles. Better yet, use a very soft, clean nailbrush to remove any tiny, deeply embedded bits of debris.

Put on some pressure. Once the wound is clean, press a clean cloth or tissue on it for 15 minutes (about how long it takes to stanch the flow of blood), especially if the cut is on your scalp, hand, or foot, where blood vessels are close to the surface. If blood seeps through the cloth, add another layer and reap-

HOLLER FOR HELP

Don't Mess with Infection

Even minor abrasions sometimes become infected. When you change the bandage, look for redness, swelling, pus, or increased tenderness. These are all signs that bacteria are winning the battle, and you may need antibiotics to turn the tide.

Another risk to be wary of is tetanus, especially if there was wood or rusted metal in the injury. Tetanus is a life-threatening condition, so be sure you're protected. If you haven't had a tetanus vaccination in the past 10 years, go to your doctor and get the shot. It stings for only a moment, but it provides long-lasting protection.

Cuts that bleed a lot or continue bleeding for more than a few minutes may be too much for you to handle. If you can see deep inside the cut—if it extends, say, more than $1/4$ inch into the tissue—see a doctor right away.

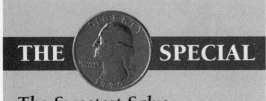
The Sweetest Salve

When crude, undiluted honey was applied to wounds in a recent study, they healed twice as fast as wounds treated with antiseptics. "The thick honey covers the wound and may serve as an antibacterial to keep infection at bay," explains Manfred Kroger, Ph.D., professor emeritus of food science at Pennsylvania State University in University Park. Plus, honey appears to reduce swelling and pain. Just be sure to thoroughly wash your cut, use pasteurized honey (which won't harbor bacteria of its own), and watch for signs of infection, such as red streaks around the wound, a fever, or increased tenderness, cautions Dr. Kroger.

ply the pressure gently but firmly. If the cut is on your arm or leg, you can raise it above the level of your heart to help slow the bleeding. Note: If your cut bleeds in spurts or blood drenches the bandage after 10 minutes of firm, direct pressure, go to the emergency room immediately.

Cover it. Once the injury is clean, cover it with an adhesive bandage. "It should be snug enough to keep out dirt, but not so tight that it prevents circulation," says Sean Sapunar, N.D., a naturopathic physician and clinical faculty member at the Bastyr Center for Natural Health near Seattle.

Do it all again. Even if you wash and cover a wound promptly, bacteria can get inside while it's healing. To prevent infection, it's important to change an adhesive bandage every day. Wash the wound with soap and running water, dry the area with a clean towel, and apply a fresh bandage. Most cuts don't require any more attention than that. "I'd stay away from hydrogen peroxide," says Dr. Sapunar. "It can actually damage the tissue in some cases."

Knock out the germs. Calendula fights a broad range of bugs, including bacteria and fungi. "I like to use it as a poultice to clean out debris," notes Sharol Tilgner, N.D., a naturopathic physician and director of the Wise Acres Herbal Education Center in Eugene, Oregon. To prepare a poultice, saturate a piece of sterile gauze or cloth with calendula extract (available at health food stores), place the soaked material on your injury, and leave it there for about an hour to help soften the skin and make any debris easier to remove. Afterward, pour a drop or two of extract directly onto the wound to keep it germ-free and reduce the chance of scarring.

Put rosemary to work. To reduce the risk of infection, wash the wound with rosemary extract, available at health food stores. This aromatic herb is a mild antiseptic that appears to penetrate the skin and may allow the wound to dry out better than antibiotic creams and ointments, which can smother the skin and may seal in germs.

Yell for yarrow. "Yarrow is my favorite herb for healing minor wounds," says Dr. Tilgner. "It's easily found, and it acts as both an astringent to stem the flow of blood and an anti-inflammatory to calm the pain." Simply rinse some fresh yarrow leaves, chew them into a paste, and spit out the mashed poultice directly onto your wound. The fresher the leaves, the more quickly the bleeding will stop.

Nature's Germ Fighter

If you have a laceration or puncture wound, echinacea, a natural immune booster, will help bring white blood cells to the area to fight infection, says Sharol Tilgner, N.D. "I usually suggest taking two capsules three times a day for a week. Or take one or two droppers of tincture in a cup of water three times while you're healing." Both forms of echinacea are available at health food stores. Don't take the herb if you have an autoimmune disease such as rheumatoid arthritis, lupus, or multiple sclerosis, or if you are pregnant or nursing.

Heal faster with comfrey. The leaves and roots of the comfrey plant contain the healing agent allantoin, which stimulates healthy tissue growth, speeding healing and reducing scar formation. You can find comfrey cream at a health food store, or you can crush 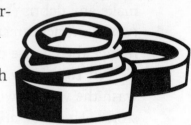 fresh, clean leaves to apply to your wound as needed. Since comfrey encourages scab formation, however, use it only on shallow cuts that you've cleaned thoroughly, warns Dr. Tilgner. Otherwise, you may inadvertently seal in some germs.

Stop scars with gotu kola. This versatile Indian herb contains no fewer than three compounds that simulate collagen, the connective tissue that forms the basis for skin repair and scar reduction. In fact, studies indicate that gotu kola can help prevent keloid scars—those large, bulging scars marked by more tissue growth than is needed to repair the wound. Simply pour a drop or two of extract (available at health food stores) directly onto the wound daily as it heals.

Clobber pain with cloves. Raid your spice rack for whole cloves, which contain the chemical eugenol—an excellent antiseptic and painkiller. Crush the cloves into a powder, then sprinkle it directly onto your wound to speed healing.

Dandruff

Fight the Fallout

It's amusing to think what our interplanetary neighbors (assuming that there are any) would think of life on Earth if they somehow managed to intercept television signals during commercial breaks. They'd naturally assume that we're obsessed with cars, clean floors, and—oh, dear!—the horrors of dandruff.

Shampoo manufacturers have somehow convinced us that dandruff is a serious social faux pas, if not exactly life-threatening. The truth is, we all shed dandruff flakes now and then, especially in winter, when the scalp tends to dry. We're usually not even aware of it. It's only when the flakes multiply that we begin to notice little specks in our hair or on the shoulders of dark jackets or shirts.

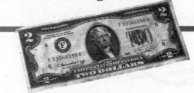

The $2 Deal

Beat It with Bs

The B vitamins, particularly biotin, are essential to a healthy scalp, so make sure you get a multivitamin that contains biotin. Or take a B-complex supplement that includes 300 micrograms of biotin.

HIGH-SPEED TURNOVER

Most dandruff occurs when tiny oil glands at the base of the hair roots run amok. The scalp's skin normally replaces itself once a month, but if you have dandruff, somehow this shedding process is accelerated. Your hair becomes greasy, and those telltale crusty, yellowish flakes sprinkle onto your shoulders. Chances are, they're not your favorite fashion accessories.

More men than women have dandruff, so doctors suspect that the male hormone testosterone may have something to do with it. Other factors that can give you a case of the flakes include family history, food allergies, excessive sweating, alkaline soaps, and yeast infections. And although no one knows exactly what causes dandruff, stress does provoke it, according to Alvin L. Adler, M.D., a dermatologist and instructor at New York Hospital–Weill Cornell Medical Center and Beth Israel Medical Center, both in New York City.

BANISH THE FLAKES

You should see a doctor if you're losing hair, your scalp seems inflamed, or you have itchy, scaly skin on other parts of your body, which may indicate a more serious problem such as psoriasis. In most cases, though, you can control dandruff with a few basic steps—

without spending a fortune on expensive hair-care products. Here are some options.

Get a shampoo with fire power. A good dandruff-fighting shampoo reduces scaling of the scalp and allows medication to penetrate, reports Dr. Adler. Look for shampoos that list coal tar or salicylic acid among the ingredients, he advises. Although there are many over-the-counter dandruff shampoos, the FDA has approved only five active ingredients as safe and effective against dandruff: coal tar, pyrithione zinc, salicylic acid, selenium sulfide, and sulfur. The FDA also recognizes a combination of salicylic acid and sulfur as effective.

Wash your hair daily. This breaks up larger flakes of dandruff, making them less noticeable. It also prevents the buildup of hair spray, gels, and other hair preparations, some of which can look a lot like dandruff as they wear off the hair. Massage the shampoo into your scalp and let it sit for 3 to 5 minutes—longer if your dandruff is severe. Rinse thoroughly to get all the shampoo out.

Steam it out. Steaming the scalp with nutritive herbs is a deep cleansing treatment for dandruff. Mix together equal parts of fresh or dried leaves of rosemary, nettle, and peppermint. (If you use fresh nettle, be sure to wear gloves while preparing the mixture to avoid being stung by the prickly leaves.) Steep 2 tablespoons of dried herb mixture or ½ cup fresh herbs in 2 cups of hot water in a covered container for 10 minutes. Strain the infusion, let it cool slightly, and apply it carefully to your scalp. Cover your hair with a shower cap and wrap your head in a hot, wet towel. Leave the treatment on for 30 minutes, then use an herbal rinse.

Soothe with an herbal rinse. Herbal rinses add sheen to the hair shaft and relieve scalp irritations at the same time. Traditional herbs include rosemary and sage for dark hair,

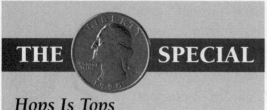
Hops Is Tops

It flavors beer—that's how most of us know about hops. Yet the wild hops plant is found all over the world, and Native Americans use it as a cure for dandruff, among other things. But you don't need to comb the fields and woods for hops—just rinse your hair with beer or add a good squirt of the "suds" to your regular shampoo.

chamomile and marigold for blondes, and cloves for auburn or red hair. Make a strong tea using 4 tablespoons of herb to 1 quart of boiling water. Steep for 15 minutes, then add ¼ cup apple cider vinegar to restore the scalp's normal pH. Use as a final rinse after shampooing.

Tame it with thyme. Another herbal approach to dandruff control is to dab some thyme oil diluted with olive oil (4 drops of thyme oil per teaspoon of olive oil) on your scalp 1 hour before washing your hair. Then, after shampooing, it's thyme for an anti-dandruff rinse. To make it, boil a handful of dried thyme in a quart of water, strain, and cool.

Clear it with yucca. Native American healers use roots of the yucca plant, pounded and whipped with water, to treat dandruff. Yucca roots contain soapy substances called saponins. For a simpler approach, try a ready-made yucca root shampoo, available in some health food stores.

Turn off the power. Whenever you can, let your hair dry naturally rather than blowing it dry. When you must have extra volume for a special occasion, be sure to use a lower setting. That hot wind really dries out the scalp, making you more vulnerable to dandruff.

Brush it out. Using a natural-bristle brush, brush your hair from the scalp outward with steady, firm strokes. This carries excess oil away from your scalp, where it can cause dandruff, to the hair strands, where it gives your hair a healthy shine.

Denture Pain

Soothing Sore Gums

Denture technology has come a long way since George Washington wore his famous artificial teeth. Today, it's almost impossible to distinguish dentures from natural teeth, at least by the way they look. Wearing them, on the other hand, does take some getting used to. If the fit isn't perfect, dentures can feel clumsy or uncomfortable. And even if they fit perfectly, they simply don't feel like real teeth. There's always an adjustment period—and the adjustment, in some cases, can be downright painful.

Your own teeth come properly fitted, and even the best dentist can't compete with Mother Nature. When you get dentures, your dentist will do everything possible to ensure proper fit and minimize pressure points on your gums. For various reasons, however—changes during adjustments, for example, or even changes in your mouth—the way dentures fit can vary over time. You'll know there's a problem if you develop a sore spot somewhere along your gum line. It's similar to the blisters you get when your shoes don't fit well, and the pain increases every time the area is rubbed the wrong way.

TAKE A BITE OUT OF PAIN

Denture pain is incredibly common, but that doesn't mean it's normal. Pain always means that something's wrong. If your dentures start hurting, you need to visit your dentist to have them adjusted. You probably won't have to shell out big bucks for a whole new set, however. Here are a few ways to reduce the pain and help the sore spots heal properly.

Eat softly. New dentures are always uncomfortable at first. "In the first two months, most patients will probably need to have their dentures adjusted two or three times," says David Austin, D.D.S., a dentist in Columbus, Ohio, and a member of the American Academy of Orofacial Pain. During that time, you can keep soreness to a minimum by sticking to foods that are soft and easy to chew, such as pasta or steamed vegetables.

Give your gums a break. Once you get a sore spot on your gums, your best bet is to wear your dentures as little as possible until it heals. Otherwise, they will continue to irritate the area. Most sores heal completely within 10 to 14 days, although you'll probably be able to wear your dentures comfortably before then.

Count on chamomile. Here's a quick (and tasty) way to ease denture-related gum pain. Drop a teaspoon of dried chamomile (available at health food stores) into a cup of hot water, steep for 10 to 20 minutes, and strain.

HOLLER FOR HELP

Hidden Heart Trouble

If you wear dentures, the last thing you would expect is to have a "toothache" in your lower jaw. Don't ignore it—you could be having a heart attack. "I've had two patients call me under those circumstances, and both times it turned out that they were having heart attacks," says David Austin, D.D.S. "If you wear dentures and are having what seems to be tooth pain in your lower jaw, call 911 just to be safe."

When it's cool, take a mouthful of tea, swish it around for 30 seconds or so, and spit it out. Keep rinsing with the tea until it's all gone. You shouldn't use chamomile if you're allergic to ragweed.

Heal faster with gargles. Antibacterial mouthwashes can help gum sores heal more quickly because they prevent bacteria from irritating the open wound. Be sure you choose a brand that's formulated to kill germs, not just freshen breath.

Get plenty of vitamin C. It's an essential nutrient for gum health. If your dentures have rubbed you the wrong way, take 2,000 to 3,000 milligrams of vitamin C daily to help the sore heal more quickly. Don't take this amount of C, however, if you have stomach or kidney problems. And since high doses can cause stomach upset or diarrhea in some people, take it in two or three smaller doses during the day. It also helps to take it with food.

Check your belt size. Have you lost or gained weight recently? If so, you may have found the reason for your denture pain. "The gums can shrink with weight loss or swell if you gain weight," says Dr. Austin. Even small changes in the size and shape of your gums can throw your denture fit out of whack. If

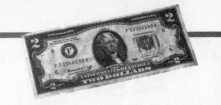

The $2 Deal

Count on Q₁₀

Available in health food stores, drugstores, and supermarkets, coenzyme Q_{10} is a supplemental nutrient that promotes gum healing by increasing the amount of oxygen that's available to tissues in the mouth. Check with your doctor first, but it should be okay to take anywhere from 30 to 200 milligrams daily until the sore spots heal. Keep your mouth properly lubricated by drinking at least eight full glasses of water daily. You don't have to drink it all at once; just sip it throughout the day to keep your tissues moist.

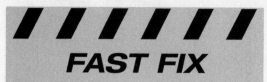
you aren't able to maintain a stable weight, stay in touch with your dentist, who will adjust your dentures to compensate for weight changes.

Brush often. Plaque and tartar, the same nasty substances that promote tooth and gum disease, can adhere to dentures just as easily as they cling to natural teeth. Once plaque and tartar build up, they can push your dentures out of alignment. "Brush your dentures at least twice a day, before you put them in and again after you take them out," Dr. Austin advises. It's a good idea to use a toothbrush that's specially made for dentures and designed to get into all the cracks and crevices.

Feel better with folic acid. This B vitamin is another nutrient that's good for the gums. It helps the body replace cells that were damaged by poorly fitting dentures. If you have a gum sore, take at least 400 micrograms daily until it heals.

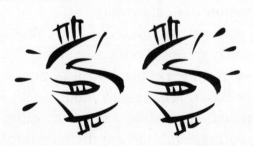

Depression

Nature's Best Mood Boosters

Think depression is just about the blues? Think again. Serious, clinical depression can last for months or even years, and it has a profound impact on physical as well as mental health.

Researchers at Johns Hopkins University found that depressed people were *four* times more likely to have heart attacks than those who said they were not depressed. A study of middle-aged women found that those who had depressive symptoms (sleeping problems, lack of energy, frequent boredom, and crying) and who felt unsupported by their friends and families had low levels of high-density lipoprotein (HDL), the "good" cholesterol that helps prevent heart disease.

WHAT'S BEHIND IT?

Genes, which help determine the levels of various brain chemicals that affect mood, may be partially to blame, but depression is usually a one-two punch. Genes set the stage, and then a stressful event tips your brain chemistry into the abyss. And chronic stress—the kind that arises from constantly trying

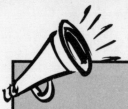

It's important to distinguish between a passing feeling of sadness or the blues and the symptoms of major depression. Untreated depression can lead to suicide, which is the third leading cause of death in teenagers and the fifth leading cause of death in adults ages 25 to 64.

If you have any thoughts of suicide, are depressed for more than two weeks, can't concentrate, feel guilty, can't sleep or sleep too much, or have a noticeable change in weight, get professional help right away. If you have even one thought of suicide, head straight for the nearest emergency room.

to meet too many daily obligations—floods the body with the hormones cortisol and prolactin, which can lower levels of the mood-stabilizing brain chemical serotonin.

There are other causes of depression as well. The spikes and dips in hormones that normally occur during the menstrual cycle (giving rise to the irritability and general moodiness of premenstrual syndrome, or PMS), after giving birth (triggering postpartum depression), and before menopause can affect brain chemistry and dampen your mood. Abnormalities in the thyroid, pituitary, and adrenal glands can do the same.

Even the gloomy days of winter or simply being cooped up in a dark house or windowless office can add to your doldrums, since inadequate exposure to sunlight can inhibit the release of serotonin. This sleepy, moody type of low is called seasonal affective disorder (SAD) and usually lifts during the sunny spring and summer months. If you're underexposed to light in general, however, it can contribute to general depression year-round.

NATURAL MOOD LIFTERS

Depression needs to be diagnosed by a doctor. People with moderate or serious depression need to be under a doctor's care and should seriously consider taking medication if it's recommended; in some cases, antidepressant drugs can be lifesavers. But if your depression is mild, you might not have to start out with antidepressants—or spend the rest of your life (not to mention your bank account) in therapy. At least in the beginning, ask your doctor if you can try some of these gentle (and less expensive) treatments. Just one caveat: If you're already taking prescription antidepressants or have bipolar disorder (also called manic depression), avoid the herbal antidepressants recommended here.

Build up your Bs. Nearly 80 percent of people with depression are deficient in vitamin B_6, says Hyla Cass, M.D., assistant clinical professor of psychiatry at the University of California, Los Angeles, School of Medicine.

Check with your doctor first, but to get B_6 plus the rest of the Bs (all of which your body needs to deliver oxygen to the brain, turn blood sugar into energy, and keep feel-good brain chemicals in cir-

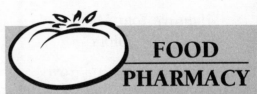

FOOD PHARMACY

Talk Turkey

Don't wait until the holidays to get your dose of tryptophan, an amino acid that's ultimately converted into serotonin in the body. In one study, when women who were depressed feasted on foods such as turkey, chicken, fish, dairy products, soybeans, nuts, and avocados, which are high in tryptophan, their depression eased without the help of medication, reports Hyla Cass, M.D.

When you're eating turkey or another tryptophan-rich food, pair it with a lower-fat carbohydrate, such as whole grain bread, brown rice, or mashed potatoes. Carbohydrates trigger the release of insulin, which allows tryptophan to freely enter your brain so that eventually, serotonin levels rise.

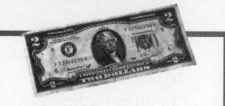

The $2 Deal

*Improve Your Mood
with St. John's*

A slew of studies since the 1970s have shown that St. John's wort can ease mild (but not severe) depression, says Hyla Cass, M.D.—perhaps by inhibiting the reuptake of serotonin. Check with your doctor first, then look at a health food store for a high-quality brand such as Kira or Nature Made and take 300 milligrams three times a day. You may not feel its full effect for up to two months, and in some people, it can cause stomach upset, allergic reactions, and heightened sensitivity to the sun. Never take herbal antidepressants with any that your doctor prescribes.

culation), Dr. Cass suggests taking a B-complex supplement that supplies 20 to 100 milligrams of B_6, 500 micrograms of B_{12}, and 400 micrograms of folic acid. Take it with food.

Feel better with fish. Cold-water fish, such as salmon and tuna, are packed with omega-3 essential fatty acids, which help the brain receive serotonin. But they also contain eicosapentaenoic acid (EPA), one of the components in fish oil that has been shown to help reduce feelings of worthlessness. Since you'd have to eat a boatload of fish to get the antidepressant effects of EPA, your best bet is to eat fish several times a week and take 1 gram (1,000 milligrams) of fish-oil supplements (available at health food stores) twice a day. Just be sure your supplements contain at least half EPA and half docosahexaenoic acid (DHA). Since fish oil can thin your blood, avoid it if you take aspirin or prescription blood thinners.

Breathe hard. A study at Duke University Medical Center revealed that people with major depression who exercised aerobically for 30 minutes three times a week experienced the same relief from depression as people who took antidepressants.

There are several reasons for this effect. First, aerobic exercise forces oxygen into your cells, increasing energy production. Second, it signals the brain to release "feel-good" brain chemicals called endorphins, which boost mood. Finally, it enhances sleep and curbs weight gain, both of which can increase energy.

Hit the switch. If SAD is a problem, try what's called a dawn simulator—essentially a bedside lamp whose glow increases gradually from dim to more intense light, mimicking a natural sunrise in mid-May. All you do is program the fake dawn to start 1 to 3 hours before you awaken, and your body detects the changing light through your closed eyelids. Look for 250-lux models on the Internet and in catalogs and stores that sell personal health care products.

Get a helping hand. Preliminary studies indicate that massage may help reduce symptoms of depression, perhaps by combating a buildup of the stress hormone cortisol, says Valerie Raskin, M.D., clinical associate professor of psychiatry at the University of Chicago Pritzker School of Medicine. To enhance the effect, use some mood-boosting herbal oils, such as bergamot, geranium, jasmine, neroli, or ylang-ylang, all available at health food stores.

Tea Time

Stop and Pick the Flowers

Flowers do more than make our world a more beautiful place: Their fragrance, color, and chemical makeup can also lift our mood. Passionflower, lavender, vervain, borage, rosemary, and skullcap, with their beautiful purple and blue flowers, can be just the thing for chasing the blues away. Try making a tea with one of these herbs, or use two or three in combination. Steep 1 teaspoon of either a single dried herb or mixed herbs in 1 cup of boiling water for 10 minutes, then strain. Drink two or three cups per day.

March forward. When you feel yourself beginning to slip into darkness, don't panic—and don't even think about it. Just act. As quickly as you can, slip on your sneakers and head outside for a brisk 10-minute walk, literally counting your steps in a 1-2, 1-2 military fashion. This simple focused, almost meditative activity will not only crowd out negative thoughts, it will also encourage your brain to release endorphins to help lift your mood, says Ellen McGrath, Ph.D., executive director of the Psychology Centers in New York City and Laguna Beach, California.

Plan a girls' night out. Studies at the University of California, Los Angeles, indicate that when one woman spends time with another woman, her body releases a brain chemical called oxytocin that counters the kind of stress that can contribute to depression.

Get the point. A study from the University of Arizona found that three months of twice-weekly acupuncture treatments reduced depression in more than half of the women tested, although researchers aren't sure why. It's possible that insertion of the thread-thin needles stimulates the release of mood-lifting endorphins or corrects a chemical imbalance involved in

Healing Rays

If you exercise outdoors, you may boost the natural antidepressant effect of your workout, says Marie-Annette Brown, R.N., Ph.D., professor of nursing at the University of Washington School of Nursing in Seattle. Exposure to sunlight—even on dim, overcast days—helps boost levels of vitamin D, which then helps the body maintain higher levels of serotonin. In fact, even in a downpour, there is 30 times more light outside than in, she says.

depression. Ask your doctor to recommend a reputable practitioner in your area.

Swallow SAM-e. SAM-e (short for S-adenosylmethionine)—a compound that helps regulate the breakdown of feel-good hormones—may be an effective mood booster for people with mild to moderate depression. "You get results with SAM-e in less than a week with no major side effects," says Robert Brown, M.D., professor of psychiatry at Columbia University Medical School in New York City. Check with your doctor first, then look for quality brands such as Nature Made coated tablets (to reduce the risk of stomach upset) at health food stores. If you don't see results in a few days, gradually increase your dose, but never take more than 400 milligrams four times a day. Once your mood stabilizes, gradually reduce the dose to 400 milligrams twice a day.

Act happy, feel happy. Remember the famous restaurant scene in the movie *When Harry Met Sally*, when Meg Ryan noisily shows Billy Crystal how she can fake an orgasm? "I'll have what she's having," says a nearby patron (whose part was played by Crystal's real-life mom!). You can "fake yourself out" to lift your mood, too. Put on your favorite music, dress in your best clothes, stand up straight, and go about your day as if it were the best day of your life. If your depression is severe, however, be realistic—and get help. Putting a happy face on a serious problem is denial, and that's unhealthy.

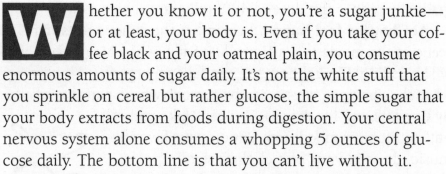

Diabetes

Beat the Sugar Blues

Whether you know it or not, you're a sugar junkie—or at least, your body is. Even if you take your coffee black and your oatmeal plain, you consume enormous amounts of sugar daily. It's not the white stuff that you sprinkle on cereal but rather glucose, the simple sugar that your body extracts from foods during digestion. Your central nervous system alone consumes a whopping 5 ounces of glucose daily. The bottom line is that you can't live without it.

But here's the rub. If you're healthy, your body extracts exactly the right amount of glucose from foods and stores the rest. For folks with diabetes, though, too much glucose stays in the blood and creates all sorts of problems.

A LIFETIME OF CONTROL

Diabetes is serious, but in most cases, it's controllable. It develops when the pancreas either doesn't produce enough insulin, your body can't use the insulin that's available, or both. In either case, too much glucose stays in the blood.

Many people can manage their diabetes with diet and exercise. Others may need oral medications or injected insulin to regulate their blood sugar levels.

The biggest problem people with diabetes face is the challenge of keeping the condition under control, says Karen Nichols, D.O., an osteopathic physician in the Chicago area. "It's always there. There are no days off. You always have to behave," she says. Looking down a long road of constant attention to diet, exercise, and blood sugar levels creates stress for many people with diabetes. "It's a challenge," Dr. Nichols adds.

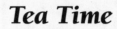

Tea Time

Be Bearish for Bearberry

Bearberry has been traditionally combined with bilberry in a tea to treat diabetes. Add 2 parts bilberry tincture to 1 part bearberry tincture and take 10 to 20 drops of the mixture in a glass of water between meals.

GET IN THE DRIVER'S SEAT

There are two types of diabetes. Type 1, sometimes called juvenile diabetes, generally begins in childhood or young adulthood and is considered an autoimmune disorder. Type 2, or adult-onset diabetes, accounts for 95 percent of cases and is becoming epidemic in the United States. From 1990 to 1998, there was a 33 percent increase in cases of type 2 diabetes—and for the first time in history, this "adult" form showed up in young people. What's more, experts estimate that there are about 5 million people with the disease who haven't yet been diagnosed.

If you're one of those trying to handle this devastating disease, you'll obviously want to work closely with your doctor. Here are some of the best ways to stabilize blood sugar levels and help keep diabetes under control, with your doctor's guidance.

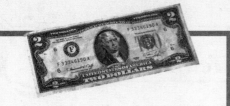

The $2 Deal

Get to Know Ginseng

A Canadian study published in the journal *Archives of Internal Medicine* showed that taking 3 grams (3,000 milligrams) of American ginseng (*Panax quinquefolius*) with meals can lower blood sugar by 20 percent! This is a breakthrough study because it was the first to test an herbal product using accepted scientific criteria, according to Andrew Weil, M.D., director of the Program in Integrative Medicine at the University of Arizona in Tucson.

The theory is that ginseng may slow digestion, decreasing the rate of carbohydrate absorption into the bloodstream. Researchers also believe American ginseng may modulate insulin secretion, but they don't yet know whether Asian ginseng (*P. ginseng*) will give the same result. If you have diabetes, talk to your doctor before using this herb.

Make some tea. Bilberry, goat's rue, fenugreek, and devil's club can be used as a tea to help reduce blood sugar. Combine equal parts of the herbs and steep 1 heaping teaspoon of the mix in 1 cup of boiling water for 15 minutes, then strain out the herbs. Drink between meals. One caution: When using any therapies that may alter blood sugar, you must monitor your blood sugar levels more frequently than normal. Check with your physician if you're taking any blood sugar–altering medications.

Shed those pounds! More than half of Americans are overweight—and every extra pound raises the risk of diabetes by 4 percent! Fight back by deciding once and for all to lose those pounds, and make exercise an everyday event. A healthy weight and two 15-minute walks a day can make the difference between being able to do what you want in old age and living as an invalid.

Stay positive. Hate testing your blood? Dr. Nichols believes the best approach is to take it one day at a time and to create your own positive reinforcement along the way. When your diabetes is out of control, she says, you need to check your blood sugar level as often as four times a day. When you stay on top of the disease, though, you can often limit the testing routine to just three times a week. So keep at it, and give yourself a pat on the back when your discipline pays off.

Go natural. There is a movement now among desert Native Americans, who have high rates of diabetes, to return to their original diet of plants such as beans, squash, cactus, and mesquite. These low-fat, low-sugar, high-fiber, high-complex-carbohydrate foods are more healthful than today's highly processed, packaged foods. Studies have shown that people on such a diet in Arizona and Australia have more stable blood sugar levels and lower cholesterol than most of us who eat a "normal" diet.

The lesson here, however, is not that you need to start munching on cactus. It's that a natural, whole-foods diet that's heavy on grains is far more likely to help blood sugar control than one of fast food and refined sugar.

Don't count on starches. A Harvard study published in the Journal of the American Medical Association noted that people who eat lots of starches to avoid fats may unwittingly set themselves up for diabetes. Study participants drank a lot of soft drinks and crowded their plates with potatoes, white bread, and white rice—all of which have almost no fiber. The

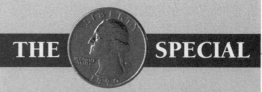

THE SPECIAL

Carry That Water Bottle!

If you have diabetes, you need to drink lots of water to prevent dehydration and replenish the fluids and nutrients you lose during exercise. Drink a glass of water before you begin your workout, then take a break every 20 to 30 minutes for more. A high-glucose sports drink can help prevent your blood sugar from dropping too low, and you can use it like water when you're active.

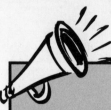

HOLLER FOR HELP

The Bad Sugar Blues

Uncontrolled diabetes damages the eyes, kidneys, nerves, gums, and blood vessels—and sets the stage for heart disease and stroke. Don't take chances: If you have early diabetes symptoms—such as excessive thirst, excessive hunger, increased urination, and weight loss—see your doctor immediately.

result? They had 2¹/₂ times the rate of diabetes found in people who ate less of these foods and more fiber, specifically from whole grain cereals. So don't let a fat phobia lead you to overload your diet with carbs. Ask a registered dietitian to explain the proportions—and portions—that will help keep your blood sugar balanced.

Dump the smokes. Nicotine raises blood sugar levels on its own, so it's definitely time to quit if you're still sucking down smoke. If it's been a while since you tried to quit, see your doctor. Today, there are all sorts of new stop-smoking aids available, and one of them can work for you.

Hit the gym. Or the walking trail or the swimming pool. Vigorous exercise helps improve your sensitivity to insulin. If you exercise regularly, you can even lower your need for injections. Exercise withdraws glucose from the blood for energy, which lowers your blood glucose levels. It also delays or even halts cardiovascular disease, the leading killer of people with diabetes. The ongoing Nurses' Health Study at the Harvard School of Public Health shows that moderate activity, such as walking, protects you as well as tougher workouts, as long as you burn around the same number of calories—so if you want to walk instead of run, just exercise longer. If you already have diabetes, walking will help control your blood sugar and manage your weight.

Scout out sweets. Always be prepared. Diabetic coma and hypoglycemia, two life-threatening complications of diabetes, can usually be avoided with regular blood testing. When levels change, you can adjust your insulin, diet, and exercise accordingly. To be safe, you should always carry a few lumps of sugar or a candy bar. This is especially important when you're exercising or are more physically active than usual, which may sometimes cause a change in the balance of sugar and insulin. Also, be sure to wear a medical alert bracelet or carry a card that identifies you as having diabetes.

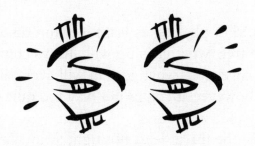

Diarrhea

Shun the Runs

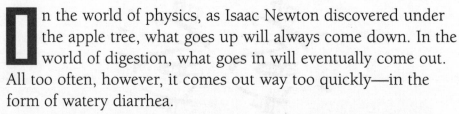

In the world of physics, as Isaac Newton discovered under the apple tree, what goes up will always come down. In the world of digestion, what goes in will eventually come out. All too often, however, it comes out way too quickly—in the form of watery diarrhea.

Don't blame the flu, at least not right away. Viral infections that settle in the intestine are a common cause of diarrhea, but so are dozens of other things, including bacteria, stress, or simply dietary indiscretions, such as eating a whole bunch of cherries in one sitting.

STEM THE TIDE

It's easy enough to "dry up" diarrhea with an over-the-counter drug that contains loperamide hydrochloride, such as Imodium, but doctors don't recommend this approach very often. For one thing, diarrhea is your body's way of giving harmful substances the boot. More important, you can almost always control it with drug-free approaches. Here's a bunch of inexpensive alternatives that experts suggest.

Spoon up some yogurt. It's brimming with healthful bacteria cultures that restore balance in the intestine and help tame the trots. If you're not a yogurt fan, take a probiotic supplement that contains lactobacillus GG (LGG). One study found that LGG could shorten the normal course of diarrhea from eight days to a more tolerable two. If you can't find LGG, any probiotic supplement that contains lactobacillus will help.

Spit out the gum. Many chewing gums are made with the artificial sweetener Sorbitol, which can cause diarrhea. If you want to chew gum, read labels to find a Sorbitol-free brand.

Dump the dairy. You'll need to give up milk and other dairy products until you're feeling better. When you have diarrhea, your intestines' ability to digest milk and other dairy products is impaired. Likewise, you'll want to avoid citrus and vegetable juices, alcohol, and caffeine, which also make things worse.

Bind with bananas. Along with rice, apples, and toast, bananas and other bland foods will help you recover from diarrhea, doctors say. Another option is eating chicken-rice soup to replenish the sodium and potassium you've lost.

Make nice with rice. The next time you prepare a batch of rice, add an extra 1½ cups of water to the pot. When the rice is cooked to the texture you want, drain off the extra water, chill it if you like, and drink it for a hydrating, binding tonic. If you need a sweet-

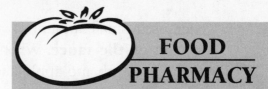

FOOD PHARMACY

Feel Better with Barley

Bland though it may be, barley can slow intestinal motion and curb diarrhea. To make it tasty, prepare pearl barley according to the package directions and add 1 cup to beef broth. The mixture will replace lost fluids and electrolytes in addition to calming your innards.

ener, use a small amount of sugar or honey.

Get on the sauce. When nothing else seems to work, let carob and applesauce come to the rescue. Mix 1 teaspoon of carob powder in ¼ cup of applesauce and eat it slowly. You may need two or three doses throughout the day.

Tame your sweet tooth. "For some people, sugar in any form—whether it's the fructose in fruit or the lactose in milk—is simply not well digested and can cause intestinal distress," says Christine Boorean, N.D., a naturopathic physician in Portland, Oregon.

Pamper with peppermint. Peppermint is a natural menthol and antispasmodic. Try a cup of calming peppermint tea to relax the muscles of your digestive tract and relieve the spasms that trigger diarrhea. Just stir 1 teaspoon of leaves (fresh or dried) into 1 cup of boiling water and simmer for 10 minutes. Strain out the leaves and enjoy. Drink as many as three cups a day after meals.

Relax your intestines. Valerian, an herbal sedative long recommended as a sleep tonic, can settle intestinal spasms and is especially helpful if you're doubled over with crampy diarrhea, says Dr. Boorean. She suggests you take one or two capsules, or 100 to 300 milligrams, a day for as long as you have symptoms. Since valerian is a sleep aid, it can cause drowsiness, so it's best to take it before bedtime, and don't take it if you're using any other kind of medication, particularly antidepressants or anti-anxiety drugs.

Soothe with slippery elm. This herb soothes the mucous membranes of the bowel with few or no side effects. Stir 1/4 teaspoon of slippery elm powder into a cup of applesauce and eat it three or four times a day. Or add 30 to 40 drops of tincture to a glass of water and drink it every 2 hours until your diarrhea stops. Both forms of the herb are available at health food stores.

Take away the burn. "If you have burning diarrhea, marshmallow tea can minimize your irritation by attracting moisture to the intestinal walls," says Dr. Boorean. Look for the tea or powder at a health food store. Make the tea according to the package directions and drink a cup several times a day until the burning subsides. To use the powder, add a teaspoon to a flavored gelatin product and snack on it throughout the day.

Go for garlic. "Garlic is one of the best ways to fight infection internally—whether your diarrhea is caused by a flu virus or bacteria that you picked up from food," says Michael DiPalma, N.D., a naturopathic physician in Newtown, Pennsylvania. Since cooking garlic neutralizes its healing properties, pick up some garlic capsules at a health food store or drugstore and take 200 to 400 milligrams three times a day until your diarrhea subsides.

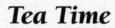

Tea Time

Dry Up with Blackberry

"The tannins in the blackberry root dry the mucous membranes in your intestine and bind up the bowel," says Michael DiPalma, N.D. Check your health food store for blackberry tea (the real McCoy, not simply tea flavored with blackberry) and follow the package directions. Drink several cups a day.

Rest easy with GSE. Made from the pulp or seeds of grapefruit, grapefruit seed extract (GSE) can knock out any bacterium, parasite, or virus that may be behind your diarrhea. "Add two drops to a glass of water and take it twice a day until you've killed whatever you picked up," suggests Skye Weintraub, N.D., a naturopathic physician in Eugene, Oregon. Never take GSE straight, or it may wipe out the beneficial bacteria along with the troublemakers, and don't use it if you're taking cholesterol-lowering medication.

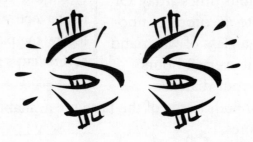

Diverticulitis

Turn Down Intestinal Pressure

Voice mail, mobile phones, and computers, along with packaged desserts and take-out Chinese food, didn't exist a century ago. And for the most part, neither did diverticulitis, a potentially serious intestinal infection. Coincidence? Probably not.

Until the 1900s, when the Industrial Revolution changed Americans' dietary habits, people ate natural foods such as fruits, whole grains, and vegetables. They had easier bowel movements and relatively low intestinal pressure. When highly processed foods became a large part of the typical diet, the intestine had to work a lot harder to move stools along—and that led to all sorts of problems.

The colon should be smooth and taut, but as it ages, the walls get progressively weaker. Pressure in the colon forces small bubbles, called diverticula, to bulge outward, like bubbles on an old tire. The bubbles themselves aren't necessarily painful, but if you have diverticulitis, they get infected and often cause intense cramping, along with constipation or diarrhea.

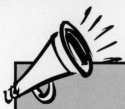

SIMPLE SOLUTIONS

If you've been diagnosed with diverticulitis, you're going to need medical help—antibiotics to quell infection, for example, or even surgery to remove the damaged areas. In most cases, however, it doesn't have to go this far. You can ease discomfort and prevent future flare-ups with inexpensive home approaches. Here are the best ones.

Stop the spasms. Chamomile tea has been used as a digestive herb throughout history. Its gentle astringent action and antispasmodic effects relax and heal the gut. Use 1 teaspoon per 1 cup of hot water and steep for 3 to 5 minutes. Drink two or three cups per day. People with ragweed allergies may be sensitive to chamomile.

Soften and soothe. You can ease inflamed intestinal tissues and soften stools with a slippery herbal concoction. Grind equal parts of marshmallow root, flaxseed, and slippery elm (often found in powder form) in a coffee grinder. Stir 1 rounded teaspoon into an 8-ounce glass of water and drink immediately. Repeat once or twice daily, following each dose with another full glass of plain water. For added benefit, mix in unfiltered apple juice for its bowel-soothing pectin content.

Eat more fiber. Soluble fiber, found in apples and other fruit, keeps stools soft for easier passage through the colon. Insoluble fiber, found in whole grains and vegetables, adds bulk, which means stools require less muscle contraction and pressure to move through your bowel. Adding more of these good-for-you foods to your diet can help prevent flare-ups (and you may find that your hips will lose some bulk, too). Since increasing fiber in your diet can cause uncomfortable bloating and gas, though, do it gradually.

Heed the call. When you feel the urge to move your bowels, head right for the throne. Putting off a bowel movement can lead to impacted stool. When that happens, you'll need more force to move things along, which increases the pressure on your colon.

Don't be scared of seeds. Until recently, many doctors suggested avoiding foods with small seeds, such as tomatoes and strawberries, and stringy foods, such as celery, because they thought particles might lodge in the diverticula and cause inflammation. This is now a controversial point, and no evidence supports it. Go ahead and enjoy these seedy, fiber-rich foods—they're good for you!

Fill up on fluids. A high-fiber diet requires lots of liquids, according to experts at the Mayo Clinic in Rochester, Minnesota. Fiber acts as a sponge in your large intestine, so if you don't drink enough, you could become constipated. Aim to drink at least eight glasses of water every day.

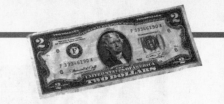

The $2 Deal

Drink Your Fiber

If you can't seem to get enough fiber from foods, your doctor may recommend a fiber supplement, such as Citrucel or Metamucil. Drinking one of these products mixed with 8 ounces of water or juice can add 4 to 6 grams of fiber to your diet daily.

Dry Eyes

Help Your Parched Peepers

When your eyes are so dry that the mere act of blinking feels like the rasp of sandpaper, and you can watch *Old Yeller* without shedding a tear, you can be pretty sure that you're heading for trouble.

Your eyes are naturally a little misty. Tears are constantly flowing across their surface, washing away grit and keeping the tender tissues lubricated. But as we age, tear production decreases (even if you cry more than ever at weepy movies). The result: Hot, dry, sore eyes that feel as parched as the Sahara.

Contact lenses are a common cause of dry eyes. Some medications, especially decongestants, antihistamines, blood pressure medications, and tranquilizers, can cause it. So can living in a dry, dusty climate.

SOOTHE AND LUBRICATE

Since dry eyes can be a sign of serious illnesses, including lupus and rheumatoid arthritis, check with your doctor just to be safe. In most cases, though, you can get relief at home without hauling out your credit card. Here's what doctors advise.

Warm them up. Heat opens clogged oil glands in the eyelids, so placing a warm compress over your eyes may induce some moisture. Just run some hot—but not too hot—water over a small towel, wring it out, and lay it over your closed eyes.

Splash and rinse. When you are in a dry, dusty climate, rinse your face and eyes often with cool, clean water. This will ease irritation and add some moisture to offset the arid atmosphere.

Brighten up. Eyebright is a favorite for any ailment of the eye, and a warm compress of eyebright and fennel seeds can be very refreshing. Make a tea by 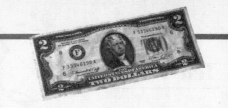 adding 1 teaspoon of eyebright and 1 teaspoon of fennel seeds to 1 cup of hot water. Add a clean cloth and steep for 10 minutes. Wring out the cloth and apply it to your eyes for 20 minutes once or twice daily.

Don some shades. If you have a fan blowing near you, wear sunglasses or regular glasses, even indoors. Breezes can evaporate moisture on the surface of your eyes. Any glasses will help, but wraparound shades offer the best protection.

Wear eye protection. Use goggles when you swim, especially in chlorinated pools. Ever notice how red people's eyes look when they've been in the pool too long? That's because

The $2 Deal

Bottled Tears

Using "artificial tears" eyedrops regularly will restore the film of moisture over your eyes, but ask your doctor which products are best and how often you should use them. Some eyedrops can blur vision, so choose those made with saline (salt) or synthetic cellulose. Some contain vasoconstrictors that help relieve bloodshot eyes, but these products can dry your eyes further and increase redness and soreness when used for more than three days, according to experts at the Mayo Clinic.

Tea Time

Berry Healthful

Bilberry has a long history of use for eye complaints. High in bioflavonoids, the herb helps strengthen eye tissues and reduce swelling. Make a tea using 1 teaspoon of dried bilberry per cup of hot water. Steep for 10 to 15 minutes, then strain; drink two or three cups a day.

chlorine can irritate the eyes and dry them out.

Humidify the air. Use a humidifier if you live in a dry climate or work in a place that's very dry. Adding moisture to the air will help combat the effects of the dryness. Be sure to keep the humidifier clean so you don't add other eye irritants, such as mold spores, to the air.

Think like a camel. Drink lots of water to keep your body well hydrated, especially if you live in

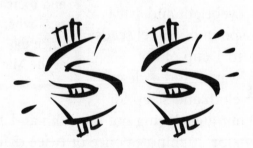

a dry place where your body moisture evaporates quickly. This will help keep your own natural tear supply flowing freely.

Dry Skin

Pump In the Moisture

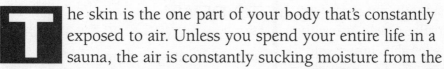

The skin is the one part of your body that's constantly exposed to air. Unless you spend your entire life in a sauna, the air is constantly sucking moisture from the skin's surface. If you happen to live in a dry climate or are exposed to drying indoor heat in winter, your skin probably feels as dry and crackly as an old paper bag.

Doctors have a fancy name for dry skin. They call it xerosis, which simply means that so much water has evaporated from the top layer of the skin (the stratum corneum) that it feels like a shriveled autumn leaf.

As we get older, the uppermost layer of our skin naturally loses some of its ability to hold water, explains Jeanette Jacknin, M.D., a

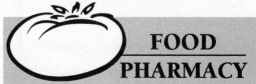

FOOD PHARMACY

Moisturize with Fish

Boost your intake of cold-water fish, such as tuna and salmon, and take 2 tablespoons of flaxseed oil (available at health food stores) daily, says Jeanette Jacknin, M.D. Both provide omega-3 essential fatty acids, which help your skin retain water to keep it plump, supple, and smooth.

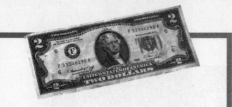

The $2 Deal

Slather on Shea

Made from the shea nut of the karite tree, shea butter is loaded with vitamins A and E and may even protect the skin from oxidative damage. Perhaps its best quality, though, is that it's a thick emollient that sinks into the skin and feels smooth, not greasy like petroleum jelly. Check at health food stores for shea butter sold alone or combined with other skin care ingredients.

dermatologist in Scottsdale, Arizona. In fact, by age 65, more than half of us have xerosis, she says.

While natural aging isn't within our control, many other factors that contribute to dry skin are dry indoor heat; prolonged sun exposure; long, leisurely baths; frequent air travel (the air on planes is always very dry); and the overuse of citrus-, alcohol-, or menthol-based skin care products.

FROM DRY TO DEWY

Almost always, you can treat dry skin without spending a fortune on fancy skin care products. The equation is simple: Add things that seal in moisture and take away things that encourage evaporation, says Leslie Baumann, M.D., associate professor of dermatology at the University of Miami School of Medicine in Tampa. Here are dermatologists' top picks.

Select the right soap. Check your health food store for oil-based bars that contain super-moisturizing olive oil or coconut oil; are not labeled as soap (which is drying); and are scented with palmarosa, rosewood, and/or sandalwood. All of these can help stimulate oil production.

Change the oil. After bathing, pat your skin to remove most of the water. Then, while it's still damp, slather on almond or sunflower oil (the same oil you use for cooking). Both are brimming with vitamin F, which provides plenty of unsaturated fatty acids that may help regulate the oil glands. If you'd rather not smell like a Caesar salad, simply add a few drops of lavender oil.

Take your time. We are often so rushed that we barely have time to apply moisturizer after a shower when our bodies are damp. Give yourself a few more minutes for a mini-massage, and rub a moisturizer all over your body. Take your time. The massage will stimulate blood flow to your skin, which helps the moisturizer be more effective.

Bathe in an oil slick. Add a fragrant bath oil to your bathwater, soak, pat yourself dry, and moisturize (but be careful not to slip in the tub). Experiment with bath oils to find the ones that feel best to you. In places where your skin is extremely dry, such as your feet, rub on some additional moisturizer, then wear socks to bed so you won't get your sheets greasy.

Take a hint from Mister Ed. Oats aren't only for eating. You can also treat yourself to a whole-body oat mask. Make a big pot of oatmeal, let it cool to a tolerably warm temperature, and slather it on from head to toe. Leave it on for 20 minutes, or until dry, and rinse. Better yet, soak it off in a warm tub. For ease of removal, lightly oil your skin before applying the oatmeal.

Honey, pass the milk. A milk-and-honey massage is one way to start your day off on the right foot! Mix equal parts of honey and milk and, starting at your feet, massage the lotion into your thirsty skin. This is best done in the shower, where you can simply rinse off when you're done.

Dry Skin

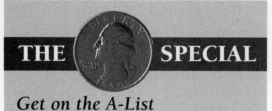
Get on the A-List

Vital for proper skin growth and repair, vitamin A is one of a family of natural and synthetic derivatives known as retinoids, which are the primary ingredients in many prescription anti-aging drugs such as tretinoin (Retin-A). You can get pretty much the same protection (at a fraction of the cost) simply by filling your plate with foods rich in beta-carotene (which converts to vitamin A in the body), such as cantaloupe, carrots, and apricots.

Fill your internal rain barrel. You need lots of water to keep all parts of your body working well, including your skin. It's really quite simple: The more water you drink, the more water is available to pump up and out to your epidermis. So don't be stingy with the water—drink a minimum of 8 to 10 glasses a day.

Enjoy an herbal steam. An herbal facial steam can deep-six dryness—especially if you use a type of oil that encourages oil production in your skin, says Kathi Keville, an herbalist in Boulder, Colorado. Simply bring 3 cups of water to a boil, then remove the pot from the stove. Add 1 drop each of rose, geranium, rosemary, fennel, and peppermint herbal oils to the water. Drape a towel over your head and tuck the ends around the pot so the steam is captured inside a "mini-sauna." Be careful not to get close enough for the steam to burn your face, and limit your steam sessions to about 5 minutes once a week.

Prime your skin with primrose. EPO, or evening primrose oil, contains the essential fatty acids linoleic acid and gamma-linolenic acid, both of which may alleviate dryness and reduce the potential for future water loss. Check your health food store for EPO and take 1,000 milligrams (about a tablespoon) of oil three times a day, says Dr. Jacknin, or get gel-caps and follow the directions on the label.

Smooth your skin with E. As an ingredient in lotions or as oil, topical vitamin E—particularly the form known as alpha tocopherol—reduces skin roughness, the length of facial lines, and wrinkle depth. When it's combined with topical vitamin C in the form of ascorbic acid (which seems to help promote the growth of collagen, the skin's underlying support), the effects may be enhanced. Check your health food store for skin care products that include both these vitamins.

Alcohol-based toners strip away much-needed oils, but rosehip oil has a high linoleic acid content, which studies show can both tone and moisturize skin. Look for rosehip oil at a health food store, douse a cotton ball, and dab the oil all over your face, neck, and upper chest.

Pass up the petroleum. For years, dermatologists have lauded petroleum jelly as the thickest emollient and therefore the best treatment for very dry skin. Now there's evidence that moisturizers with large amounts of glycerin (which has a less greasy feel) may work just as well, if not better. "Glycerin appears to increase space between cells in the stratum corneum, creating a reservoir of moisture-holding ability that makes the skin more resistant to drying," says Dr. Baumann. Look for glycerin in commercial moisturizers or simply make your own. Get some pure glycerin from a health food store and combine 1 part glycerin with 2 parts rosewater.

Brush up oil production. Starting at the soles of your feet and moving up your legs toward your heart, gently rub your body in a circular motion with a super-soft, dry-bristle brush. Then do the same with your hands and arms. "Brushing will help stimulate your sebaceous glands to produce more sebum and will remove dead skin that makes your skin look dry, dull, and old," says Dr. Jacknin.

When paste ain't safe. If your lips always seem to be dry, check out the ingredients in your toothpaste. If it contains cinnamate—a flavoring agent that can be drying—you've nailed the culprit. Simply switch to a brand that's cinnamate-free. Also avoid tartar control toothpastes, which, like long-lasting lipsticks and mouthwashes that contain alcohol, can be drying.

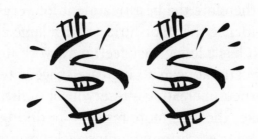

Soften with sesame. Indian women have long used sesame oil, which is rich in both vitamin E and linoleic acid, to moisten and soften dry, cracked hands and feet. Dr. Jacknin suggests pouring 1/2 cup of sesame seeds and 1/4 cup of warm water into a blender and processing for 3 minutes. Strain the lotion, apply it to your skin, and leave it on for as long as possible. Rinse first with warm water, then with cool water, and blot dry. You can also buy sesame oil at a health food store—but making it yourself will save you big bucks.

Earaches

Now "Ear" This!

A dults get ear infections sometimes, but they're a lot more common in kids. And if you really want to get, well, an earful of complaints, talk to almost any parent. You'll hear a long litany of complaints about missed school days, last-minute visits to the doctor, and the difficulty of giving eardrops to pain-racked children who won't stop screaming.

Most ear infections occur when cold germs settle in the eustachian tubes, the narrow passageways between the throat and eardrums. In kids, the tubes are nearly horizontal, which means that it's hard for mucus to drain out. As mucus accumulates, internal pressure rises, which is why ear infections are so painful.

Ear infections gradually taper off as children get older because their heads and necks get longer, causing the eustachian tubes to assume a more vertical position. The more easily the mucus drains out, the less likely it is that infections will occur.

IMPROVE THE FLOW

In the majority of cases, ear pain is caused by simple infections—often triggered by a cold, allergies, a sinus infection, or

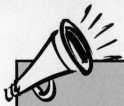

HOLLER FOR HELP

Protection from Infection

Ear infections are hardly ever serious, but that doesn't mean you should ignore them (as if you could!). If the infection isn't eliminated quickly, there could be scarring or other damage that can result in hearing loss. "Besides being painful, an infection in the ear can cause long-term damage to the ear's delicate mechanisms," says Emily A. Kane, N.D.

As long as the pain is mild, it's okay to wait a day or two before seeing a doctor. But if the pain is severe or comes on very suddenly, go to an emergency room, Dr. Kane advises.

simply moisture. You'll almost certainly need to see a doctor, but you won't have to sell the family car to afford a bunch of visits to a specialist. There's a lot you can do at home to reduce irritation and even eliminate the germs. Here's how to get started.

Heat away the pain. Gentle heat is probably the most soothing home treatment for aching ears, says John W. House, M.D., president of the House Ear Institute in Los Angeles. For adults, the easiest approach is to use a heating pad. Set it on low, cover it with a towel or pillowcase, and lie down for a while with your ear against the pad. As long as the pad doesn't get too hot, it's fine to lie there for 20 to 30 minutes, or until the pain subsides. Set a timer so you don't fall asleep.

If you don't have a heating pad, or if it's your child who's hurting, you can gently heat the ear with a hair dryer set on low. Hold the dryer at least 6 inches away from your ear, which should feel comfortably warm but not hot, Dr. House advises. If your ear starts getting too warm, it's time to stop the treatment.

To check the temperature for a child, put one hand over her ear when you turn on the dryer. Gradually move the dryer away until the airflow on your hand feels warm but not hot.

Count on analgesics. Aspirin, ibuprofen, and acetaminophen aren't just for headaches. They quickly ease ear pain and help control the fever that often accompanies infections, says Dr. House. These medications are very safe as long as you follow the directions on the label. There is one exception, however: Don't give aspirin or ibuprofen to children, because these drugs can increase the risk of Reye's syndrome, a serious neurological illness. Acetaminophen is safe for children of all ages.

Add potato punch. The next time you have an earache, reach for a simple spud. Cut the potato in half, microwave it until it's soft, and let it cool to a comfortable temperature. Then hold the cut end against your ear for 10 to 15 minutes. The heat is very soothing, and the potato may help draw excess fluid from inside the ear. "I've tried it on kids with earaches, and though I'm not sure why, it really does work!" says Emily A. Kane, N.D., a naturopathic physician in Juneau, Alaska.

Beat it with an oil blend. Rubbing oil behind your ear (where your lymph glands are located) or placing a cotton ball saturated with oil inside your ear may soothe the ache and help stimulate the lymph glands to remove infectious agents. "Many of my patients find that something called sweet oil—which is really olive oil with other oils such as lavender, tea tree, chamomile, and hops mixed in—works really well," says Michael D. Seidman, M.D., director of neurotologic surgery at Henry Ford Hospital in Detroit. Check your health food store for sweet oil, or simply make your own. Just combine the oils in equal amounts.

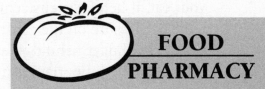

FOOD PHARMACY

Weep and Heal

A warm onion is an old-time remedy that soothes an earache—and perhaps stimulates the flow of mucus—with warm, moist heat. Simply heat an onion in the microwave (boiling works, too), then let it cool slightly, put the toasty sphere in a clean cotton sock, and rest your sore ear against it.

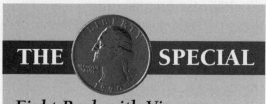
Fight Back with Vinegar

Anytime you're going to swim in a body of unchlorinated water, such as a lake, a river, or the ocean, take along a mixture of 2 drops of vinegar to 2 drops of rubbing alcohol (a drying agent), suggests William Warnock, N.D. Dry your ears well, then dribble the solution into them after each dip.

Snort some saltwater. Dissolve as much table salt as you can in a glass of warm water without the water becoming cloudy, then pour a little of the saltwater into the cup of your hand and sniff the mixture into one nostril, then the other. Repeat several times. "This nasal wash acts as a natural decongestant to shrink swollen tissues and unplug the eustachian tubes," says William Warnock, N.D., a naturopathic physician in Shelburne, Vermont.

Rub for relief. A natural way to reduce pain-causing congestion is to massage the outer part of your ear. It helps the eustachian tubes drain normally, which reduces pressure on the eardrum, says Dr. Kane. Simply put your index finger behind your ear and your middle finger right in front of the little triangular flap (the tragus) that covers the opening of your ear canal. Stroke with both fingers down toward the outer corner of your jaw, squeezing your fingers together as you pull. "This dislodges congestion and really promotes good drainage," says Dr. Kane.

Do some steam-cleaning. Eucalyptus is an herbal decongestant that may help ease the pressure in your eustachian tubes and nudge drainage of fluid that has been dammed up in the middle ear—especially if you combine it with steam, which also encourages the flow of mucus. Fill a bowl with boiling water, add several (as many as 10) drops of eucalyptus oil (available in health food stores), and drape a towel over your head and the bowl to capture the steam. Lean over the bowl (but not so close that you scald your skin) and inhale the mist for at least 5 minutes. You can also place a few drops of eucalyptus oil in your bathwater, but don't put it directly into your ears.

Try the garlic cure. It's a natural antibiotic, says Dr. Warnock. Simply mash a garlic clove with a fork and saturate it with several drops of olive oil. Let the mash absorb the oil overnight, strain out the garlic, and warm the oil so it's pleasantly tepid, not hot. Tilt your head so your sore ear faces up and plop two or three drops of the oil into your ear. Lie down—again, with your sore ear up—and let the oil settle for 2 or 3 minutes before you raise your head. Do this a few times a day, and your discomfort should disappear within a day or two.

Prevent pain with boric acid. "If you're prone to ear infections, ask your pharmacist to mix up a 3 percent boric acid, 70 percent alcohol solution," says Dr. Seidman. Squeeze a few drops into your ears every day, he says, to keep yourself infection-free. The boric acid will acidify the ear canal, discouraging any bacterial or fungal invaders from venturing down that path, while the alcohol will dry it up.

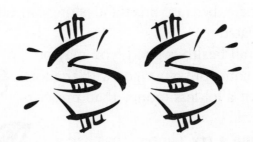

Erectile Dysfunction

Restore the Vigor

For millions of American men, the introduction of Viagra—known affectionately as vitamin V—was the biggest thing since wide-screen TV. The National Institutes of Health estimates that 10 to 20 million American men between the ages of 40 and 70 experience erectile dysfunction, but fewer than 10 percent of them do anything about it. That's unfortunate, because erectile dysfunction can usually be successfully treated.

If your overall health is good, you may be able to restore some of your vigor with the following tips—for a lot less money than prescription drugs.

Give ginseng a try. Ginseng has had a reputation for being an aphrodisiac throughout the history of folk medicine. If you'd like to try it as a tonic, make a tea by adding 1 heaping

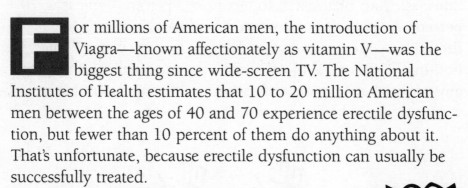

teaspoon of Asian ginseng (*Panax ginseng*) to 1 cup of hot water and steeping for 15 to 20 minutes. Drink one cup a day. If you try this, be sure to check with your doctor first, especially if you have high blood pressure. Also, be aware that the herb makes some men jittery.

Order 'em on the half-shell. Are oysters really an aphrodisiac or simply a sexual placebo? Men who slurp them off the half-shell in the hope of gaining extra sexual vigor may be successful because they believe it will work. But it's interesting to note that oysters are rich in zinc, which the prostate needs to manufacture seminal fluid, according to Marcus Loo, M.D., clinical associate professor of urology at Weill Medical College of Cornell University in New York City. You can also load up on zinc by eating other shellfish, poultry, wheat germ, vegetables, grains, and yogurt.

Check in with a therapist. If you are troubled by frequent erection problems, ask your family physician to recommend an expert in the condition, then schedule a few visits. It could make all the difference.

Bring it into the open. When a man's penis doesn't cooperate, it can be an embarrassing experience. This is, after all, a chief barometer of manhood. Don't try to resolve the problem all by yourself, though; be sure to involve your partner in the

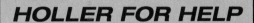

HOLLER FOR HELP

More Than a Bedroom Problem

It's important to see your doctor if you've started having erection problems. They're often caused by other—sometimes serious— health problems, including diabetes, high blood pressure, and spinal cord injuries. So get a checkup right away. Catching problems early could save your life as well as your sex life.

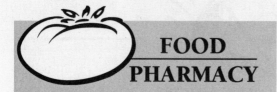

FOOD PHARMACY

Order Another Pizza

Why are Italian men reputed to be such great lovers well into their seventies and eighties? According to James F. Balch, M.D., author of *Prescription for Nutritional Healing*, studies of Italian men show they eat pizza and many other foods with lycopene-rich tomato sauce. A Harvard study published in the *Journal of the National Cancer Institute* showed that increased lycopene levels help maintain prostate health, which in turn promotes sexual performance. To get more lycopene, you should eat five servings of cooked tomato products a week, according to Dr. Balch.

process as well. She has as much at stake as you do. If she doesn't understand what's going on, she's going to be less than enthusiastic about sex—and the last thing you need is an inhibited partner.

Step on the scale. And lose weight if you don't like what you see. Erectile dysfunction increases in direct proportion to your waistline. A study presented at the annual meeting of the American Urological Association revealed that 34 percent of men ages 51 to 88 had erection problems. After adjusting for age, smoking, and hypertension, the researchers found that men with larger waistlines were more likely to experience problems than slimmer guys. In fact, men with waists of 42 inches are twice as likely to have erection difficulties as men with 32-inch waists.

Exercise your libido. Inactive men are more likely to have erection problems than those who exercise at least 30 minutes a day. "Even though erectile dysfunction affects an estimated 30 million American men, little research has been done about how modifiable lifestyle factors may contribute to the condition," says Eric Rimm, Sc.D., of the Harvard School of Public Health. There's some evidence, however, that exercise may help. The bottom line? Make exercise a priority, and you're more likely to make love.

Work on your mood. If you're depressed, you're twice as likely to have erectile dysfunction, according to a study of 1,200 men between the ages of 40 and 60 that was reported in the journal *Psychosomatic Medicine*. The study used data from the Massachusetts Male Aging Study conducted between 1986 and 1989 by a research institute with funding from the National Institute on Aging and the National Institute for Diabetes and Digestive and Kidney Disorders. If you are down in more ways than one, see your doctor about getting some help for depression.

Circulate. The high-fat foods that contribute to blocking arteries to your heart also affect those to your penis, which are a lot smaller and clog more quickly. Smoking impedes blood flow, including blood flow to the penis. Good health and good sex belong together, so cut out the fats and the butts to keep your blood circulating to all the right places.

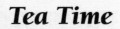

Tea Time

A Potent Brew

The herb ginkgo is used to increase circulation and may be helpful in some cases of erectile dysfunction. Combine it with two or three male tonic herbs, such as saw palmetto, horsetail, and true unicorn root. To make a tea, add 1 heaping teaspoon of herbs to 1 cup of boiling water and steep for 10 minutes. Strain and drink one or two cups daily. Tonic herbs are slow acting, and you may need to take the tea for several weeks before seeing improvement. If you are taking blood-thinning medications, don't use ginkgo without your doctor's okay.

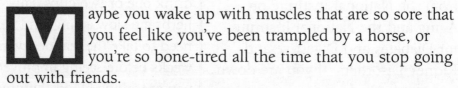

Fibromyalgia

Fight the Pain

Maybe you wake up with muscles that are so sore that you feel like you've been trampled by a horse, or you're so bone-tired all the time that you stop going out with friends.

Welcome to the lonely world of fibromyalgia. Unfortunately, nearly everyone with this mysterious condition finds it almost impossible to get others to understand what they're going through. Even some doctors don't seem to get the picture. More than a few people with fibromyalgia have gone to specialists, only to be told "It isn't a real condition"—even though a major study about it was published in the *New England Journal of Medicine*.

STILL A MYSTERY

Fibromyalgia is baffling to the experts who study it. What causes it? Your guess is almost as good as theirs. It's possible that fibromyalgia is somehow related to brain chemicals such as serotonin (linked to depression) and substance P (linked to pain).

What doctors do know is that it can be incredibly painful.

Most people with fibromyalgia experience an aching, burning sensation in their muscles. They're usually exhausted all the time, possibly because the pain makes it hard to get a good night's sleep.

Because fibromyalgia doesn't seem to cause changes in your body that can be detected by x-rays, blood tests, or other diagnostic techniques, the only way your doctor can tell if you have it is to rule out other causes for the pain. If no other problems are detected and you've had widespread aching that's lasted for at least three months—plus a minimum of 11 "tender points" that scream at the slightest pressure—there's a good chance that you have fibromyalgia.

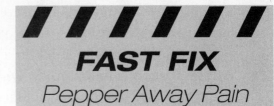

FAST FIX
Pepper Away Pain

Here's a hot tip: Over-the-counter capsaicin creams contain the same spicy ingredient that's found in red pepper. When you apply the cream to your skin, it quickly blocks a chemical (substance P) that transmits pain signals to your brain. The cream will sting a bit, so be careful to keep it away from your eyes or any areas of broken skin, and wash your hands thoroughly after using it.

WAYS TO FIND RELIEF

As of now, there is no cure, and there isn't likely to be one until doctors figure out just what causes the condition. What they have found, however, is that most people can control symptoms with a variety of self-help techniques, along with prescription medications for pain or sleep problems in some cases. Just be prepared to be patient: What works for one person with fibromyalgia won't work for everyone. You'll probably have to do some experimenting to find what's best for you. Here are a few strategies that experts recommend.

Get your muscles moving. You know how much it hurts when you pull a muscle in your leg, back, or shoulder. The problem isn't so much the initial injury as it is how the muscle responds: It tightens to prevent further damage—and tight muscles are sore muscles. In people with fibromyalgia, the muscles are essentially stuck in a short, contracted position, says Jacob Teitelbaum, M.D., a fibromyalgia researcher in Annapolis, Maryland, and author of *From Fatigued to Fantastic*. One way to ease the pain is to get the muscles to relax by doing regular stretching exercises or simply by staying active.

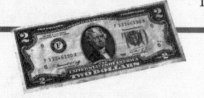

The $2 Deal

Feel A-OK with HTP

An amino acid called 5-HTP, sold in health food stores, promotes the production of a brain chemical called serotonin, which helps promote good sleep. "Take 300 milligrams at night for 12 weeks," says Jacob Teitelbaum, M.D. "It will significantly improve pain and help you sleep." The supplement may interact with antidepressants and other drugs, he adds, so check with your doctor before trying 5-HTP, especially if you're taking any medications.

The idea is to stretch the affected muscles slowly, says Dr. Teitelbaum. When you're going for a walk, for example, take long, slow strides at first. Try to feel a good stretch in all the muscles in your legs. Regular stretching will help "train" the muscles not to contract in painful ways.

Just don't stretch too much at once. "If you try to stretch through the pain, the muscle will pull back and make the problem worse," Dr. Teitelbaum warns.

Log plenty of snooze time. Sleep does more than give you much-needed rest. It also gives your body a chance to repair tiny muscle tears that occur during the day. It's essential to get at least 8 hours of sleep each night, says Dr. Teitelbaum, so set a reasonable sleep time and stick to it. Don't let late-night gatherings or classic movies on TV keep you up too late.

Wind down gradually. A lot of us get so wound up during the day that it's almost impossible to fall asleep. One thing that can help is to practice a soothing nighttime ritual a few hours before going to bed. Turn the lights down. Turn off the TV and loud music. Light your favorite scented candles and make a conscious effort to relax—by taking a long, soothing bath, for example. If you do this every night, your body will get into the habit of unwinding as you prepare for sleep.

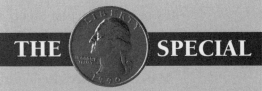

Modify your medicine. Over-the-counter sleep aids that contain the active ingredient diphenhydramine can be very helpful when you need extra sleep. The problem with these products is that they can leave you feeling hungover the next day. To get the benefits without the problems, take a much lower dose than the amount listed on the label, says Milton Hammerly, M.D., medical director of complementary and alternative medicine at Centura Health in Denver and author of a book on fibromyalgia. "Even a dose as low as 25 milligrams works for some people," he says.

Cool down or heat up. Both work for muscle pain flare-ups caused by fibromyalgia, but you'll have to experiment to decide

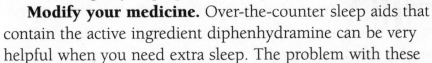

THE SPECIAL

Get Your Minerals

Two minerals in particular, calcium and magnesium, are critical because they help ease muscle pain. As a bonus, taking them at night can help you sleep. Check with your doctor to see how much will work for you. Some people report that taking 500 milligrams of calcium and 250 milligrams of magnesium an hour or two before going to bed is helpful. Magnesium may cause diarrhea in some people; if this occurs, reduce the dose.

which end of the thermometer works best for you. Apply either a heating pad set on low or a cold pack for about 20 minutes when your muscles are hurting. Take a break for a half-hour, then apply it again.

Here's the rub. Many people with fibromyalgia see their massage therapists at least as often as they see their doctors, because massage is an excellent way to reduce discomfort. Just be sure to get a light, gentle massage. Overly vigorous handwork often seems to make the pain worse, says Dr. Hammerly.

Treat it gingerly. It's thought that fibromyalgia causes painful muscle inflammation. The solution, of course, is to treat it, well, gingerly. A cup of ginger tea contains inflammation-fighting compounds called gingerols—and it tastes good, too. Just steep a few slices of fresh ginger in a cup of boiling water for about 10 minutes, strain, and sip the tea until it's gone.

Work out slowly. There's no question that regular exercise can reduce fibromyalgia flare-ups. Since exercising vigorously can make the pain worse, the trick is to warm up those muscles first, then exercise at a moderate pace. Walk slowly before jogging, for example, or swim slow laps before revving up the speed.

Don't overdo the analgesics. Ibuprofen, aspirin, and other over-the-counter standbys for pain don't seem to help very much for fibromyalgia, says Dr. Teitelbaum. "Only about 10 percent of people with fibromyalgia benefit from them."

Eat more fish. The oils found in cold-water fish help your body overcome painful inflammation. "Eat three servings of salmon, tuna, or sardines a week," says

Dr. Teitelbaum. If you're not a fish eater, and you're not taking aspirin or prescription blood thinners, you can substitute fish oil or flaxseed oil, which both contain the same beneficial oils. Follow the dosage directions on the label.

Join a group. It's common for people with fibromyalgia to feel isolated and depressed because no one really understands what they're going through. Others who have the condition do understand, so getting together with people who are fighting the same battle is a great way to cope. To find a fibromyalgia support group in your area, visit the Arthritis Foundation Web site at www.arthritis.org.

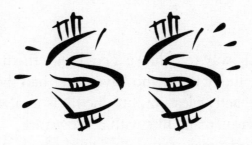

Flu

Don't Get Clobbered

The only way to confuse a cold with the flu is to be one of the lucky ones who have never had the flu. A cold isn't exactly pleasant, but the flu is in a whole different category: The virus really hits with a vengeance.

Your symptoms may start with a mild cough, a headache, or a few sniffles, but that's just the beginning. Before long, you'll know that this is no ordinary cold. The flu can knock you right off your feet with fever, chills, aches, and a racking cough, along with a sore throat and congestion.

Flu usually hits from late fall into winter, although it can occur at any time of year. The virus is easily passed from one person to another, and it tends to last for a week or more.

FIGHT THE VIRAL VILLAIN

If you act quickly, you can almost stop the flu in its tracks by getting antiviral medications from your doctor. The problem is, most people don't even know they have the flu until a few days have passed, and by then the drugs won't work.

For most people, the best remedies are also the oldest: Get

lots of rest and try to stay comfortable while your body takes care of the viral invader. Here are some super suggestions for reducing your discomfort and healing more quickly.

Welcome a fever. Nobody enjoys having a fever, but that high temperature is doing you a favor. "An increase in temperature is one of the most potent defenses your body has against viruses," says Christian Dodge, N.D., a naturopathic physician and faculty member at Bastyr University near Seattle.

In other words, lowering fever with aspirin or other drugs may actually prolong your illness. Unless you're just too uncomfortable or the fever's very high (above 102°F), it's best to leave it alone.

Sip some slippery elm. This herb forms a slick coating that can soothe a sore throat faster than you can shout "Relief!" You can buy the powdered form at a health food store and make a slightly sticky tea by adding 1 teaspoon of the powder to a cup of hot water. Or take slippery elm lozenges, also sold at health food stores. Sucking on a lozenge will keep your throat coated and comfortable for hours.

Enjoy a salt soak. The flu is almost always accompanied by

HOLLER FOR HELP

When You Need to Worry

If you're generally healthy, flu doesn't usually require a trip to the doctor. The rules change, however, for children, people over age 55, and those with underlying health problems that could complicate recovery. Anyone with heart disease, immune system problems, lung disease, or other serious health conditions should call a doctor at the first sign of symptoms. Even if you're in great shape, talk to your doctor if you don't start feeling better within about a week. It's not uncommon for viral flu to lead to a secondary bacterial infection. You may need antibiotics in order to recover.

muscle aches and pains. A quick way to get relief is to soak in a bath spiked with Epsom salts. "They contain magnesium, which is good for relieving muscle tension," says Dr. Dodge. Pour about a cup of the salts into the bathtub while the water's running.

Cool and soothe. It won't affect the underlying fever, but applying a cold compress to your skin will make you feel a lot more comfortable. Soak a washcloth in cool water, wring it out, and put it on your forehead or neck. When it warms up, soak it again and repeat the process.

Feel better with menthol. Slathering a menthol rub over your chest is a traditional remedy for flu, and it seems to help with aches and pains as well as congestion, says Dr. Dodge. "The active ingredient is eucalyptus, and it works very well." You can make your own herbal rub by adding 6 to 12 drops of oil of menthol, eucalyptus, or camphor (available at health food stores) to an ounce of olive or almond oil.

Suck down the fluids. Lots of liquids are in order when you're battling the flu. When you're not adequately hydrated, your symptoms feel worse, and your immune system won't

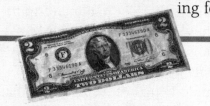

The $2 Deal

Heal with Echinacea

This flu-fighting herb contains polysaccharides, which boost the body's infection-fighting cells. Echinacea is most effective when taken as a tincture (an extract diluted in alcohol, which is available at health food stores) so it flows directly into your bloodstream rather than being digested. Take 30 drops of tincture every 2 hours for a week, then switch to 20 drops three times a day, for a total of 10 days. Don't use echinacea if you have an autoimmune disease such as lupus, rheumatoid arthritis, or multiple sclerosis, or if you are pregnant or nursing.

function as well as it should. Water is the best choice; try to drink at least eight glasses a day.

Eat light. Big, heavy meals aren't a good idea when you're sick, because your body will put more energy into digestion than into stomping the virus. Nor do you want to go hungry, because your body needs nutrients in order to recover. A good compromise is to plan your menu around soups, vegetable juices, and other easy-to-digest foods.

Hold the milk. "Avoiding dairy foods is a good idea when you're sick," Dr. Dodge says. Milk, cheese, and other dairy products tend to make mucus thicker, which increases congestion and other symptoms.

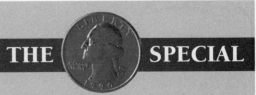

THE SPECIAL

Peel an Onion

If flu has your nose stuffed to the rafters, harness the power of the humble onion. The same vapors that make cooks weep can help clear up your congestion, so start peeling and let them work their magic. Once you're breathing easier, chop the onion and toss some into a salad for lunch: Onions contain compounds that strengthen your immune system.

Tank up on nutrients. Some of the vitamins and minerals you should be getting every day—including vitamins A, C, and E and the minerals zinc and selenium—are especially important when you're contending with the flu, because they strengthen your immune system.

You can't count on the amounts of vitamins in foods when you're sick; you need supplemental amounts. Drop by a drugstore and pick up a multivitamin/mineral supplement that provides 100 percent of the recommended daily amount of each of these important nutrients.

Have a mini-steam. Inhaling steam is a great way to open up your congested airways and soothe the irritated tissues. Just

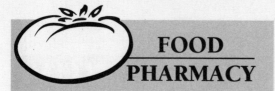

FOOD PHARMACY

Gobble Garlic

As powerful as it is pungent, garlic is great for spurring your immune system to fight off a flu virus. Since raw garlic has the highest concentration of immune-boosting components, chop up a few cloves and toss them into your favorite hot soup. By the time the soup's cool enough to eat, the garlic will have softened and added its flavor to the meal.

heat a pot of water on the stove, carefully move it to a table or counter, then lean over and breathe in the steam (but don't get close enough to burn your face). If you want, you can drape a towel around your head and shoulders to trap more steam.

To get even more relief, add a few drops of eucalyptus oil, available at health food stores, to the water. You'll benefit from the herb's germ-fighting properties.

Rest—and keep resting. It's a prime requirement for defeating flu. Even once you start feeling better, ease back into your life slowly, suggests Dr. Dodge. "Doing this can help prevent a relapse," he says.

Get the vaccine. If you're at high risk for getting the flu—you're elderly, work in a health care setting, or have chronic health problems—you should get the flu vaccine annually, says Dr. Dodge. The vaccine isn't 100 percent effective at preventing flu, but if you get the shot and practice good preventive measures—such as washing your hands frequently and supporting your immune system with a good diet—you'll dramatically improve your odds of getting through flu season unscathed.

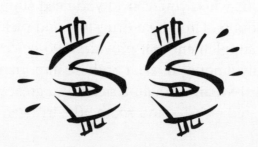

Folliculitis

Solutions to a Hairy Problem

Here's a thought that you might want to tuck into the back of your mind until Halloween: No matter how often you wash, every inch of your skin is teeming with bacteria. It sounds creepy, but it also makes sense. After all, one of the main purposes of your skin is to act as a Great Wall that keeps out the bacterial barbarians.

Like any wall, however, skin sometimes cracks or breaks down. When that happens, bacteria that normally live harmlessly on the skin's surface get underneath. If these vagabond germs find their way into a hair follicle (a tiny chamber that produces a single hair), they can quickly cause infection. When the infected follicles turn into small, yellow, fluid-filled bumps, you have a condition known as folliculitis.

BANISH THE BUMPS

Folliculitis is usually no big deal. As long as only a small area of skin is affected, you can take care of it at home, and it usually clears up in about five days. If it doesn't, your doctor will probably give you a topical steroid to control inflammation and an antibiotic to knock out the underlying infection. In most cases, though, you won't have to buy high-priced prescription drugs to control it. Once you know what's going on, folliculitis is almost always easy to treat at home. Here's how.

Scrub out infection. If you know you're prone to folliculitis, soap and water should be two of your new best friends. Frequent washing is the best way to minimize the number of infection-causing germs.

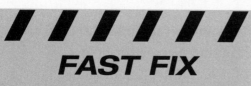

Using ordinary soap is fine, but antibacterial soap has a little extra oomph, says Valerie Callendar, M.D., clinical assistant professor of dermatology at Howard University College of Medicine in Washington, D.C. During outbreaks, wash the area once or twice a day.

Mix a mighty combo. "I have some patients mix a hydrocortisone cream with an antibiotic cream," says Dr. Callendar. Hydrocortisone controls inflammation, itching, and swelling, and antibiotics kill the germs. You can buy the creams over the counter. Squeeze equal amounts of each into the palm of your hand, mix them together with your finger, and apply them wherever the bumps are making their unwelcome appearance.

Turn down the heat. People

often think that bathing or showering in very hot water will kill aggravating bacteria. It doesn't work that way. In fact, hot water makes skin irritation even worse. You'll be a lot more comfortable if you use warm or even cool water until the outbreak is over.

Nix the cosmetics. Makeup and skin care products may irritate and aggravate skin that's trying to cope with a folliculitis outbreak. For faster healing, stop using them until your skin is back to normal.

Heal your hose. If you take the time to read the directions on the detergents used to wash hosiery, you'll see that stockings should be left in the water for only a few minutes, "but some people leave them soaking overnight," says Dr. Callendar. The excess levels of detergent act almost like folliculitis factories by changing the bacterial balance on the skin. To be safe, soak your delicate items no longer than necessary to get them clean, she advises.

Replace your razor. During a folliculitis outbreak, it's easy for a razor's edge to be contaminated with bacteria. Each time you shave, you can push hordes of bacteria under your skin. To prevent this, buy some disposable razors and use each one only once during outbreaks.

Quell the germs. The healing herbs echinacea and goldenseal spell double trouble for the bacteria that cause folliculitis, says Heidi Weinhold, N.D., a naturopathic physician in the Pittsburgh area. They kill some germs on contact, and they cre-

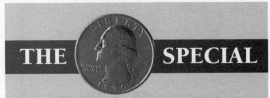

THE SPECIAL

Soak in Oats

If the itching of folliculitis is making you crazy, a colloidal oatmeal bath can put you at ease. "Oatmeal baths work very well," says Valerie Callendar, M.D. Most drugstores carry brands that are easy to use; you just add the mix to a warm bath. Or you can fill a sock with regular oatmeal, tie the top, and let it soak in the bathwater.

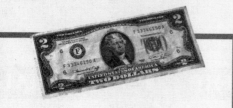

The $2 Deal

Cover Up with Clay

Natural clay packs, available at many health food stores, are useful for fighting folliculitis, says Heidi Weinhold, N.D. "They help dry out the skin and pull out toxins produced by the infection," she says.

Most clays are left on the skin until they dry, she adds. Don't substitute hobby or modeling clay, though. Natural clay packs contain special ingredients that you need for really effective relief.

ate an unfavorable environment for future populations. The easiest approach is to buy an ointment that contains both herbs at a health food store or drugstore, then apply it several times a day until the outbreak is over.

Clean the hot tub. There's nothing more relaxing and invigorating than soaking in a hot tub. Unfortunately, it's also a good way to come down with folliculitis. "Bacteria can live in the hot-tub jets," says Dr. Callendar. To keep the little critters from making the journey from the water to your skin, you need to disinfect the tub and the water frequently, following the manufacturer's directions. "It takes some work, but it's worth it," she says.

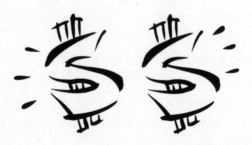

Gallstones

Strategies to Stop the Attacks

It's hard to imagine that something smaller than a grain of sand could trigger pain that rivals that of childbirth, but that's what a lot of people say about gallstones. The tiny granules cause such intense pain that they've been known to make even tough men cry.

"It's some of the worst pain you've ever dreamed of in your life," says Rowan Hamilton, Dip.Phyt., professor of botanical medicine at Bastyr University near Seattle.

ON THE MOVE

Bile, a digestive fluid that your body uses to digest fats, is stored in a small pouch called the gallbladder. Bile usually stays in liquid form, but sometimes one of the substances it contains, such as cholesterol, forms a

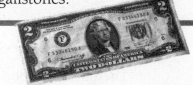

The $2 Deal

Tame It with Turmeric

The spice turmeric, commonly used in Indian cooking, is a traditional gallstone remedy. If you don't care for the taste of turmeric but still want the benefits, you can take 50 to 100 milligrams in capsule form three times a day, preferably with meals.

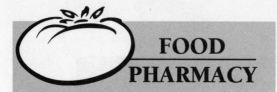

FOOD PHARMACY

Slug a Garden Cocktail

Because the liver and gallbladder are intimately involved with digestion, it makes sense that food therapies can give them a little boost. A traditional way to help the gallbladder work more efficiently is to drink vegetable-juice cocktails that include celery, parsley, beets, carrots, radishes, and lemon. Mix and match the ingredients to suit your taste and drink about two cups a day, says Rowan Hamilton, Dip.Phyt.

hard little crystal, or gallstone, that floats around in your gallbladder. Most gallstones don't cause symptoms; you can have them for your entire life without ever knowing it. Sometimes, however, a stone lodges in one of the ducts leading out of the gallbladder. When that happens, you're going to experience a world of hurt.

The crazy thing about gallbladder attacks is that they're totally unpredictable. You may be in agonizing pain for a few minutes or a few hours. You may have three attacks a day for three weeks, then never have another. There's just no way to tell.

NO MORE STONES

There's some good news and bad news about gallstones. The good news is that as long as you're not having symptoms, you don't have to worry about them. The bad news is that the main—and by far the best—treatment for symptomatic stones is to have your gallbladder removed. It's a fairly simple "band-aid" procedure, and most people are back on their feet in a day or two. But who wants surgery if it can possibly be avoided?

If you've had gallstones in the past, your doctor may give you a medication that helps dissolve any new ones in the gallbladder. Another approach involves using painless sound waves to break up the stones. Yet another option, the one doctors often recommend first, is to make some simple, inexpensive lifestyle changes that can help prevent stones from recurring. Here's what they suggest.

Trim the fat. The more fat in your diet, the more bile your liver will generate to digest it—and the greater your risk for gallstones. Studies have shown that people who get no more than 30 percent of calories from fat are less likely to get gallstones than those who eat more fat. "Look for foods that have less than 5 grams of fat per serving," suggests Leslie Bonci, R.D., a Pittsburgh dietitian and spokesperson for the American Dietetic Association.

Divide your meals. Most of us were raised on three square meals a day. If you divide the same amount of food into smaller, more frequent meals, though, you'll be less vulnerable to gallstones because the gallbladder won't secrete as much bile at once, Bonci says. "You should eat something every 3 to 4 hours," she adds. "For instance, instead of eating a sandwich, a bowl of soup, and a piece of fruit for lunch, you might have a cup of soup and half a sandwich, then eat the rest later on."

Diet smart. We've all seen those ads for diet plans that promise to change us from Titanic to Twiggy in a few weeks. But crash diets are bad news for the gallstone prone. "Rapid weight loss increases the risk of gallstones," explains

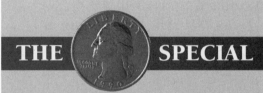

THE **SPECIAL**

Suck Up the C

One study that examined data from 13,000 people found that women with low levels of vitamin C were more likely to get gallstones, according to Joel Simon, M.D., assistant professor of nutrition at the University of California, San Francisco. That's why it's important to add foods rich in vitamin C to your diet. Citrus fruit and juices are your best sources—a whole orange, for example, offers 70 milligrams of vitamin C.

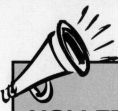

HOLLER FOR HELP

Signs of Trouble

A gallbladder attack can often be mistaken for a heart attack. Gallstone pain begins in the lower right abdomen and shoots upward to the shoulder and around the back to the right shoulder blade. If you have any unusual abdominal pain that won't go away, fever, sweating, chills, yellowish skin, yellowing of the whites of your eyes, or clay-colored stools, see your doctor immediately.

Even if you've had gallstone attacks in the past, don't assume that everything's going to be fine when you have your next one. Extreme pain may be a sign that your gallbladder is infected, which can be life-threatening without immediate treatment.

Michael F. Leitzmann, M.D., Dr.P.H., an epidemiologist in the department of nutrition at the Harvard School of Public Health. "If you're planning a weight-loss program, it's a good idea to contact a health care provider for advice on how to lose weight gradually," he says.

Count on castor oil. A quick way to help ease the pain of gallstone attacks is to relax with a castor oil pack. First, rub castor oil over the painful part of your abdomen. Cover it with a layer of plastic wrap, then put a heating pad set on low on top of the wrap. Relax for an hour or two, then remove the pack and wash off the oil. The soothing warmth won't eliminate gallstone discomfort, but it will make it a lot easier to live with until you can see your doctor.

Flush 'em out. Small gallstones can often be flushed from the gallbladder if you drink enough water, 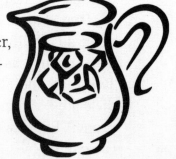 says Richard Kitaeff, N.D., a naturopathic physician and director of the New Health Medical Center in Edmonds, Washington. "I recommend drinking six to eight glasses of water a day, and more is probably better," he says.

Eat naturally. Studies suggest that processed foods, especially refined sugars, may be associated with an increased risk of gallstones. You'll be less likely to have trouble if you replace the processed foods in your diet with fresh fruits, vegetables, whole grains, and other wholesome, natural foods.

Get moving. Since research shows that the more active you are, the less likely you'll be to develop gallstones, it pays to increase the time you spend exercising to 2 to 3 hours a week. Need more motivation? Think about 20-20 (not the TV show). Walk briskly for 20 minutes a day, five to seven days a week, and you'll reduce your chances of developing gallstones by 20 percent, according to studies.

Manage your meds. If you're taking cholesterol-lowering drugs, you may be on the gallstone A-list. These drugs cause the gallbladder to excrete excess cholesterol, which in turn can raise the risk of stones. Don't stop taking the medicine, of course, but talk to your doctor. Together, you may be able to come up with a plan that will lower cholesterol without the need for medications.

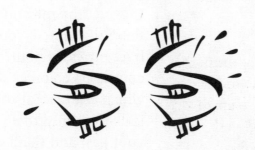

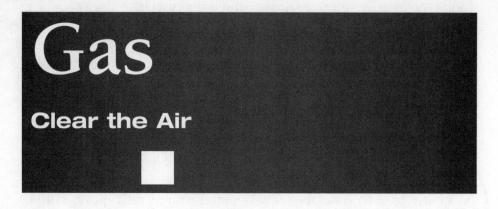

Gas

Clear the Air

Now, don't blame the dog. Intestinal gas may be embarrassing, and it's certainly unpleasant when the windows are closed, but it's a natural part of digestion—for people as well as our four-legged friends. Pointing the finger at Rover might get you off the hook, but what will you say—or do—the next time?

Flatus, as gas is known among doctors, is a result of swallowed air and the fermentation process triggered by intestinal bacteria. Food that enters your digestive tract provides nourishment for enormous colonies of bacteria, which emit clouds of smelly chemicals. Basically, their gas becomes your gas, and that's where the problem starts.

Excess gas isn't only a social problem, it's also uncomfortable

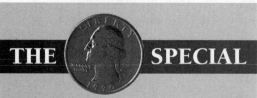

THE SPECIAL

Bet on Basil

This herb makes a sweet drink that can reduce painful and embarrassing gas. Make a tea by steeping 2 tablespoons of chopped fresh basil or 2 teaspoons of dried basil in 1 cup of freshly boiled water for about 15 minutes. Strain and sip.

because it puts painful pressure on your intestine.

FIGHT THE FLATULENCE

Of course, there are times when we all generate more gas than we would like. While you can't get rid of it altogether, there are a number of strategies for keeping it at manageable levels. Here are a few tips you may want to try.

Enjoy leisurely meals. Believe it or not, most people release about 2 pints of gas a day. "Half of that is swallowed air," explains Sean Sapunar, N.D., a naturopathic physician and clinical faculty member at the Bastyr Center for Natural Health near Seattle. There would be a lot less swallowed air—and expelled gas—in the world if everyone would eat the way their mothers told them: Take small bites, don't talk while you're eating, and eat slowly. "Hurried eating increases the amount of air you swallow," Dr. Sapunar explains.

Dump the antacids. Low stomach acid can cause gas problems because it may interfere with normal digestion, says Dr. Sapunar.

Be bitter. Bitter herbs have been used for thousands of years to improve the digestive process, but you don't have to eat pounds of arugula or dandelion to get the benefits. "I advise patients to sip a little Angostura bitters," says Dr. Sapunar. This classic after-dinner drink is available in most supermarkets.

Rely on Beano. This over-the-counter product is made from a plant enzyme that breaks down the sugars in food. Put a few drops of liquid Beano on your first bite of food or take a Beano tablet before eating. You'll enjoy your meal without that bloated feeling. There are also activated charcoal products that will absorb gas, but because they could also absorb any medications you take, you should check with your doctor before using this alternative.

Cultivate culture. The live cultures (called acidophilus) in some yogurts break down milk sugars and keep a balance of healthy bacteria in the digestive channels. Read labels to be sure the yogurt you buy contains acidophilus, and eat it often for better digestive health.

Stroll after meals. Regular exercise promotes bowel function and helps your body digest food. Flopping your butt down on the couch after dinner encourages food to ferment, creating gas.

De-gas strong foods. Add anise, fennel, or ginger to "gassy" vegetables such as brussels sprouts, broccoli, and cabbage. Along with enhancing flavor, these herbs offset the gas-producing effects of these healthy foods.

Bubbles are trouble. We all have gas to spare, so the last thing you want to do is pump more gas into your system by drinking carbonated beverages. It's fine to enjoy a soft drink or soda water now and then, but the more you drink, the

Tea Time

Intestine Protection

For centuries, people of many cultures have used natural gas-fighting, or carminative, herbs to tame the effects of poor digestion. You can take advantage of these herbal gas busters by whipping up an after-meal tummy-taming tea. Just mix equal amounts of caraway seeds, fennel seeds, and aniseed. Crush 1 teaspoon of the mixture and add it to a cup of freshly boiled water. Steep for about 20 minutes, strain out the seeds, and sip.

gassier you're going to be.

Take the gas out of beans.
On the scale of gas-producing foods, beans, along with broccoli, cauliflower, and other high-fiber foods, are almost off the chart. What you may not know is that these foods cause trouble mainly for people who don't eat them very often. Adding beans to your menu more frequently will often cut down on the excess emissions. And that's good news for everyone!

Rub away cramps. Relieve gas pains with a simple rubbing solution containing antispasmodic herbs. Add 4 to 6 drops each of lobelia and catnip tincture to 2 tablespoons of olive oil, then gently massage it into your abdomen in a clockwise pattern.

Sweeten with cinnamon. To make a gas-busting after-dinner drink, steep a stick of cinnamon in boiling water for about 10 minutes, then let the tea cool slightly. Discard the cinnamon and sip the tea.

Digest with lemon. Lemon water slips your stomach into gear and helps your digestive system work more efficiently. When you're having trouble with gas, squeeze the juice from a slice of lemon into a glass of water and drink it before and after meals.

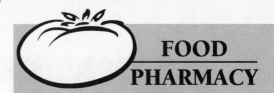

FOOD PHARMACY

Visit the Tropics

Relief from gas may be as close as the nearest pineapple. Along with papaya, it contains natural enzymes that improve digestion and help reduce excess flatulence, says Sean Sapunar, N.D. Eating as little as one serving of tropical fruit daily may be all you need to clear the air. And as long as you're not taking blood thinners, you can also take enzyme supplements (bromelain or papain), which are available in health food stores.

Gingivitis

Be a Chum to Sore Gums

It's not just a figure of speech when dentists say that gum disease can sneak up you. They mean it quite literally because the stuff that causes gingivitis—the term doctors use for gum inflammation—is invisible. It can lurk on your teeth for days, months, or even years, releasing acids that slip beneath the gums. If the process isn't stopped, the gums may shrink and pull away from the teeth. Eventually, they can get so weak that the teeth loosen and fall out.

The clingy film that causes all this trouble, called plaque, is constantly produced by bacteria that live in the mouth. Redness, bleeding, and soreness are the first signs that plaque is out of control. In other words, by the time you notice something's wrong, you already have gum disease.

PUT YOUR GUMS IN THE PINK

Here's the good news. Gingivitis is entirely reversible—and you probably won't have to write a fat check to your dentist. All you have to do is be more diligent about flossing and brushing. Severe gum disease always requires a dentist's care, but there is no reason at all to let things go that far. If you follow these tips, you'll keep your gums in the pink—and totally free of pain.

Swish with salt. Plain salt is a wonderful gum healer. Add ¼ teaspoon to ¼ cup of warm water. Stir until the salt dissolves, then use as a mouthwash two or three times daily.

Make your own paste. If you want to clear up a persistent case of gingivitis, try this inexpensive but very effective gum paste. Shake about 1 teaspoon of baking soda into a small dish and drizzle in just enough hydrogen peroxide to make a paste. Then work it gently under the gum line with your toothbrush. Leave the paste on for a few minutes, then rinse well.

Brush 'round and 'round. Don't make the mistake of using too much elbow grease when you brush. You're not trying to sandblast the sides of a building, just

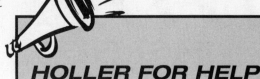

HOLLER FOR HELP
Save Your Choppers

When gingivitis isn't stopped, it progresses to a condition called periodontal disease, or periodontitis. It occurs when a long-time buildup of plaque causes chronic irritation and inflammation—and it means your gums are in really bad shape. Unless it's stopped, periodontitis weakens the gums and supporting bones so much that there's a risk of losing your teeth. Signs include gums that have pulled away from your teeth, discharge between your teeth and gums, or a change in the way your teeth come together when you bite. If you have any of these symptoms, go to a dentist immediately.

break up the thin layers of plaque that may have formed. To be sure you get it all, move the brush in little circles rather than up and down, says Emily A. Kane, N.D., a naturopathic physician in Juneau, Alaska. If you've only recently started having problems, a week or two of gentle brushing is often enough to erase the pain.

Bag the old brush. Don't forget to change your toothbrush a few times a year. Old brushes are often full of bacteria, which means you could actually be causing more problems. You can also clean your brush periodically. "From time to time, I soak my toothbrush in hydrogen peroxide overnight to kill bacteria," says Dr. Kane.

Go electric. You're supposed to brush your teeth for 2 minutes or more, but it's easy to cut the time short when you're in a hurry. Some electric toothbrushes are a great help with this because they have a built-in signal mechanism that reminds you to work on all four areas of your mouth for 30 seconds each.

Water your mouth. Water stimulates the production of saliva that you need to fight excess mouth bacteria. Be sure to drink 8 to 10 glasses of water a day.

Eat a nice slice. Oranges, along with pineapple and grapefruit, are rich in vitamin C, which is essential for gum health. Eating vitamin C–rich foods can benefit your gums, especially when they're recovering from gingivitis.

Fix it with folic acid. This B vitamin helps repair and replenish gum cells that have been damaged by gingivitis. The best way to get enough folic acid (the recommended amount is 400 micrograms a day) is to take a daily multivitamin.

Paint on some goldenseal. This herb helps protect against infection while strengthening the tissues of the gums and mouth. Use a small, unused paintbrush to apply goldenseal tincture (available at health food stores) to your gums once or twice daily. Goldenseal can be irritating, so test first by dabbing just one spot on your gums with the brush. If no irritation shows up by the next day, go ahead and paint away.

Follow this sage advice. Myrrh, sage, and calendula tone and protect tissues against infection. Two or three times a day, add 5 drops of each tincture to a small amount of warm water, swish it around in your mouth for several minutes, then spit it out.

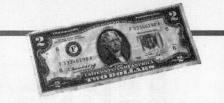

The $2 Deal

Join the Queue for Q

Talk to your doctor about taking coenzyme Q_{10} (CoQ_{10}). This supplement increases the amount of oxygen that's available to cells inside your mouth. The extra oxygen helps gum cells grow and reproduce, and it kills gum-damaging bacteria. Until your gums are better, consider taking 30 to 200 milligrams of CoQ_{10} daily.

Rinse with chamomile. A swish of chamomile tea will bring soothing relief to sore gums. Steep a tea bag in hot water for 10 to 20 minutes, then let the tea cool. Take a mouthful, swirl it around for about 30 seconds, then swallow it or spit it out. Continue the process until you've used all the tea. Don't use chamomile if you are allergic to ragweed.

Bark up the right tree. Two herbal tinctures, prickly ash bark and Jamaican dogwood, are traditional favorites for reducing gum pain. Moisten a cotton ball or swab with the tincture and apply it where it hurts two or three times a day.

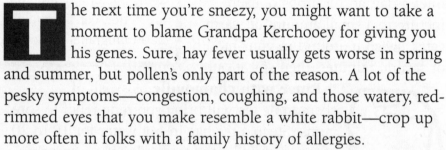

Hay Fever

Super Schnoz-Soothing Strategies

The next time you're sneezy, you might want to take a moment to blame Grandpa Kerchooey for giving you his genes. Sure, hay fever usually gets worse in spring and summer, but pollen's only part of the reason. A lot of the pesky symptoms—congestion, coughing, and those watery, red-rimmed eyes that you make resemble a white rabbit—crop up more often in folks with a family history of allergies.

Of course, every season does give us something to sneeze at. Airborne pollens pounce in the spring, grasses make us gasp in the summer, and leaf molds float merrily through the brisk fall breezes. Unfortunately, lots of other things are blowin' in the wind, such as increasing air pollution from industry and automobiles. Add the global warming that's confusing the seasonal clock, and it's Allergies 'R Us!

CHEMISTRY GONE AWRY

Hay fever is nothing more than an extreme immune reaction. Inhale a simple speck of pollen, for example, and your immune system may react as though your body were fighting off a pack of wolves. Racing to the rescue (when there's no real threat), your immune system cranks out quantities of a disease-fighting protein called immunoglobulin E (IgE). The IgE charges through your bloodstream like Paul Revere, signaling the release of chemicals such as histamine and alerting special cells in the linings of the throat, nose, and lungs to pump up their production of mucus. This is why your eyes and nose run.

DRY UP THE DRIPS

Drugstore shelves practically collapse under the weight of all the hay fever drugs out there. Medications can do only so much, though. Anti-inflammatory nasal sprays usually work, but only if you begin using them weeks before allergy season starts. Decongestants clear your sinuses and shrink swollen nasal membranes, but taking them for too long causes rebound congestion.

The other problem with over-the-counter drugs, as hay fever sufferers know all too well, is that they cost a bundle. Fortunately, as long as you don't have asthma, there are better solutions—home remedies with no side effects that also won't break your bank! Here's what doctors advise.

Dig into blackberries. They're loaded with quercetin, a natural chemical that halts the production of histamine, the substance that makes people with allergies sneeze, wheeze, and generally feel miserable. Isn't it wonderful that blackberries ripen just as hay fever season starts?

Breathe better with ginkgo. Ginkgo is a celebrity herb best

Horseradish perks up the senses and clears air passages from the nose right up into the sinuses. This powerful root is best taken raw. Just grate some into a glass of tomato juice, mix it up with your favorite salsa, or, if you're very brave, eat it right off a celery stalk.

known for improving memory, but its pretty little leaves can help with more than just one ailment. They contain ginkgolides, a medicinal component that helps fight allergies. Try a tea made of ginkgo leaves to clear up your runny nose and itchy eyes. Steep 1 teaspoon of dried leaves in a cup of boiling water, then strain out the herb. Let the tea cool, add some honey, and you're good to go. One caveat: Check with your doctor first if you're taking any kind of blood-thinning medication—even aspirin.

Relieve ragweed miseries. It's not surprising that nature provides its own remedies just when allergy season hits. Spring greens and flowers often make the best potions for allergy relief. Look in your neighborhood for nettle, eyebright, cleavers, and elderflowers. Pick them fresh and steep ¼ cup of herbs in 1 quart of water overnight. Strain out the herbs, then drink the liquid throughout the day.

Soothe your sinuses. When those headachy, runny-nose, sneezy allergies hit, try placing a dab of soothing salve on your temples. Choose a salve that contains an herbal oil, such as lavender, eucalyptus, or peppermint. The scent will soothe and relax you while the oil opens your respiratory passages and eases congestion.

Scrub with eucalyptus. Some folks swear that they can clear a stuffy nose with eucalyptus soap, just by using it for their daily shower. It may be that the scent permeates the nose with the hot steam. Pick up a bar at your favorite bath shop and give it a try.

Seal out the culprits. During

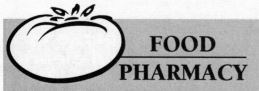

FOOD PHARMACY

A Hot Tip for Congestion

If a bowl of hot-and-sour soup or a dish of spicy chili doesn't clear your stuffy nose, probably nothing will. Spicy food is almost like a Roto-Rooter service for clearing out blocked nasal passages. The "heat" loosens mucus and gets it on the run, usually out your nose.

pollen season, keep the windows of your car and house closed, and stay in air-conditioned spaces whenever possible. Be especially cautious during early-morning hours—pollen counts are at their highest between 5:00 and 10:00 A.M. Never hang your clothes to dry outside, where they can collect pollen, and wash your hair every night to keep from contaminating your pillow-case with the stuff.

Cut the collecting. Swear off eBay and stop filling your house with tchotchkes. The dust they col-lect is just an extra trigger for your hay fever. The culprits include books, drapes, figurines, blinds, carpets, dried flowers—nearly every object in the house. Instead, go for a lean decor.

Fire up the washer. Dust mites are major allergens, and even the cleanest households are full of these microscopic crit-ters. The problem is that they love to sleep in your bed, which is full of cozy places for them to accumulate, so wash your bedding often. Have you ever seen a dust mite magnified a million times? It's a scary little crea-ture—not something you'd like to sleep with on a regu-lar basis. The mites live in bedding made with synthetic mate-rials as well as feathers, but you can wash the synthetics fre-quently to drown the little buggers. Unless you can find a down comforter that's hypoallergenic and washable, buy synthetics for your bed.

FAST FIX
Steam Your Sniffer

Soak a washcloth in the hottest water you can stand, wring it out, and lay it across your nose and sinuses for a while. If you keep the cloth as hot as you can, it seems to work on the same principle as hot soup or spicy food: It loosens and liquefies mucus.

Headaches

Dull the Pounding

You overslept. The kids shrieked and fought for the TV remote. You can't find your purse. And to top it all off, your husband dropped the coffee pot. In the middle of all this craziness, you might notice that your head is starting to throb—and you know from painful experience that within a few minutes, this minor headache could escalate into a major-league skull banger.

Tension headaches are the most common type of head pain, and they're aptly named. Whenever you're tense, muscles in your scalp, neck, and shoulders contract and tighten up. Tight muscles have to pull against something, and it's often your head that feels the squeeze.

TAKE AWAY THE TENSION

Nearly everyone gets headaches sometimes. It's worth checking with your doctor if you get them all the time or if the pain interferes with your daily activities, but you'll probably be able to manage most headaches on your own. The vast majority of headaches (about 95 percent) are "primary" headaches, which means that they aren't caused by some dangerous underlying illness.

It's fine to take aspirin, ibuprofen, acetaminophen, or other over-the-counter headache medications as long as you're not sensitive to them. Keep in mind, however, that these drugs don't eliminate the underlying problems, and they may cause side effects that are more uncomfortable than the headaches themselves. Doctors usually advise starting with gentler approaches. Here are their top picks.

Rub in some lavender. A drop or two of lavender oil massaged into the temples can help relieve a headache. If you have sensitive skin, apply a thin layer of vegetable oil or lotion before using the oil. Better yet, massage the lavender into the pad of muscle between your thumb and index finger—an acupuncture point for headaches.

Willow works wonders. Willow bark contains salicin, which metabolizes in the body like aspirin, its synthetic cousin. Chew some fresh willow twigs to ease the pain of a headache. If there's no willow tree nearby, try the more powerful tea or a tincture (30 drops of tincture every 4 to 6 hours). Obviously, people who are sensitive to aspirin should choose another remedy.

Discover the sole solution. It's hard to imagine that foot problems could cause head pain, but that's exactly what happens sometimes, especially in women. "Wearing high heels or shoes without good support can cause muscle strain that causes

You don't want a heavy-duty workout when your head is hurting, but gentle exercise, such as walking or yoga, will relieve tension headaches fast. Exercise helps eliminate muscle-tensing stress hormones from your body and stimulates the release of painkilling chemicals called endorphins.

headaches," says Chris Meletis, N.D., chief medical officer of the National College of Naturopathic Medicine in Portland, Oregon. Always buy shoes with plenty of padding, he advises. If you wear high heels, slip out of them now and then to give the muscles in your legs and feet—as well as in your scalp—a chance to relax.

Heat the upstairs. You've probably seen movies or television shows that portray headache sufferers holding comically large ice bags on their heads. Ice can certainly help in some cases, but heat is usually better for tension headaches because it causes muscles to relax instead of contract, says Terri Dallas-Prunskis, M.D., codirector of the Illinois Pain Treatment Institute in Chicago. She recommends putting a heating pad or a washcloth soaked in warm water on the areas that hurt. You can also hang out in a bath or shower for 10 to 15 minutes.

Put your fingers to work. A quick way to ease tension headaches is to press your fingers firmly where it hurts while flexing those muscles against the pressure. Doing this a few times helps tense muscles relax, says Dr. Meletis.

Suppose that your shoulder muscles are unusually tight, and you're feeling the pain in your scalp. Press your fingers into the muscles and shrug your shoulders at the same time to increase the pressure. Next, while maintaining the finger pressure, relax your shoulders for a few seconds, then

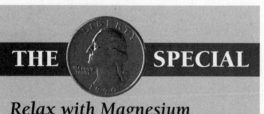

THE SPECIAL

Relax with Magnesium

This common mineral appears to promote muscle relaxation, says Chris Meletis, N.D. The next time you have a tension headache, take anywhere from 250 to 750 milligrams of magnesium and see if it helps. Start by taking the lower amount and increase the dose only if you don't get relief, he advises. Taking more than 400 to 500 milligrams of magnesium a day can cause diarrhea in some people. If this occurs, reduce the dose.

shrug them again. The combination of pressure and relaxation knocks out tension in a hurry, Dr. Meletis explains.

Try high-speed C. Vitamin C has powerful anti-inflammatory properties, which is important because inflammation plays a role in some tension headaches. You can try taking 1,000 to 2,000 milligrams of vitamin C at the first sign of a tension headache. If it's going to work, you should feel the benefits within an hour or two. If you have stomach or kidney problems, though, you shouldn't take high amounts of vitamin C. Also, to avoid diarrhea or stomach upset, take it in two or three smaller doses throughout the day.

Sit straight. If you spend a lot of time slumped in a chair or hunched over a keyboard, your head will pay the price. Poor posture is among the most common causes of tension headaches. "When you're sitting, you want your legs to be at a 90-degree angle to your hips," says Dr. Dallas-Prunskis. "Keep your shoulders back, and don't let your head hang backward or forward; keep it in line with your spine."

Kick the salt. A lot of women get tension headaches during the week to 10 days before their menstrual periods. Eating salt during this time can make things worse because it promotes fluid retention and sometimes raises blood pressure. You may find that cutting back on salt—not only when you're premenstrual but throughout the month—will prevent a lot of headaches, says Dr. Dallas-Prunskis.

Here's an acupressure technique from traditional Chinese medicine that can literally help in a pinch: Grip the skin between your thumb and index finger and give it a firm pinch. "Pressing that area often takes the pain away," says Terri Dallas-Prunskis, M.D.

Don't focus only on the saltshaker, she adds. Only a small percentage of the salt we eat is added at the table. Most is found in processed foods—canned soups, for example, or those hurry-up lunches at fast-food restaurants. If you eat plenty of natural foods, such as fruits, vegetables, and whole grains, you'll almost automatically reduce your salt intake to healthier levels.

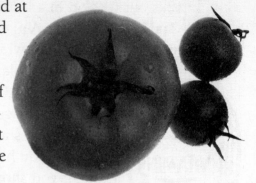

Can the coffee. Coffee is the most popular pick-me-up in America, but that pleasant morning jolt comes with a price. Your body literally gets addicted to caffeine, and you may start experiencing headaches or other withdrawal symptoms as soon as 2 hours after having a cup. Switching to decaf is one solution, but if you can't bring yourself to give up caffeine entirely, at least cut back to a cup or two a day. You'll still get the pleasant lift, but without the headaches later on.

Tea Time

A Pain-Quelling Combo

For tension headaches, try gentle pain- and stress-relieving herbs for fast relief. Combine equal parts of tinctures of ginger, Jamaican dogwood, and wood betony. Take 15 to 20 drops of the mixture every 30 minutes for relief of acute pain, up to four times in 24 hours.

Count ceiling tiles. Sleeping on your back is the best position for supporting your head and neck muscles. Sleeping on your stomach, on the other hand, means that your head is turned to the side for hours at a time. This can be a real strain on the neck—and a pain in the head. "Imagine how you'd feel if you had to stand for hours with your head turned to the right or left," says Dr. Dallas-Prunskis. "You'd end up with quite a headache."

Pop for a new pillow. Some

pillows do an excellent job of supporting your head and neck, while others are so soft that you might as well be sleeping on air. Firm pillows are usually best for preventing tension headaches, but you'll have to experiment to find the pillow that works best for you.

Flex and stretch. A good way to prevent tension headaches is with stretching exercises. Focus on your neck, because that's where tension headaches often originate. Several times a day, gently turn your head from left to right as far as you comfortably can in each direction. Then lower your chin toward your chest, hold for a moment, and tilt your head all the way back until you're looking at the ceiling. This exercise is especially helpful on those days when you've been chained to the computer or stuck in rush-hour traffic, and your muscles are tighter than usual.

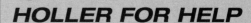

HOLLER FOR HELP

The Sledgehammer

If your headache is so intense that it feels as if you've been hit with a sledgehammer, or if a bad headache doesn't go away, check with your doctor. Strokes, high blood pressure, and adverse reactions to medications can cause this type of headache.

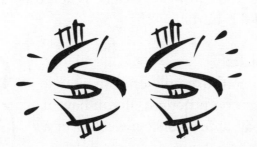

Heartburn

Extinguish the Flames

You probably already know that heartburn has nothing to do with the heart, but it's easy to understand how it got the name. When that miserable, burning feeling flares, usually at night or after meals, it can literally feel as though your heart's on fire.

The source of the burning is stomach acid that surges upward into your esophagus, the tube that carries food from your mouth to your stomach. There's a valve at the bottom of your esophagus that's supposed to prevent this upsurge, but sometimes it doesn't work very well. When this happens, you'll know it. *UGH*—it hurts!

RAPID RELIEF

If you get heartburn only once in a while, don't give it a second thought. If you have it more often—say, at least once a week over a period of months—you need to check with your doctor. For one thing, heartburn is too painful to live with every day. For another, the

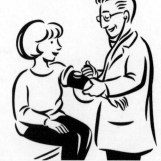

constant irritation can lead to all sorts of health problems.

In most cases, though, you can manage heartburn yourself—without spending all of your cash on over-the-counter products. Here's what you need to do.

Suck down some fluid. Water is one of the best remedies for heartburn because it dilutes the burning acid and flushes it back into the stomach, says Roy Orlando, M.D., chief of gastroenterology and hepatology at Tulane University Health Sciences Center in New Orleans. Chug it every chance you get.

Moo-ve away from milk. Milk has a reputation as a stomach soother, but it can actually make heartburn worse by increasing acid production, so avoid it like the plague.

Stand up to it. Everything that goes up has to come down. It was true for Isaac Newton's apple, and it's equally true for stomach acid that splashes upstream. To help gravity do its job, stand up at the first pangs of heartburn. You'll feel better when the acid drains back into your stomach.

Quell it with chamomile. This flavorful tea is an excellent heartburn remedy because it contains anti-inflammatory substances that soothe irritation. It also settles your stomach after heavy meals. Look for

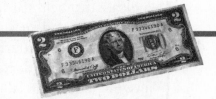

The $2 Deal

Licorice Cools the Burn

Licorice root soothes stomach fires and increases circulation to help healing at the same time. Look for chewable tablets of de-glycyrrhizinated (DGL) licorice, which do not contain glycyrrhizin, a component of licorice root that may cause spikes in blood pressure. Chew two to four tablets before meals or follow the label directions.

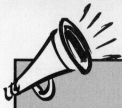

HOLLER FOR HELP

Don't Get Burned

People who have frequent heartburn are at risk for cancer of the esophagus. Chronic heartburn that's accompanied by weight loss, trouble swallowing, or visible blood when you cough or have a bowel movement can indicate that acid has already caused serious damage. If you have chronic heartburn, play it safe and see your doctor right away.

In addition, emergency room doctors see a lot of people with heartburn who think they're having heart attacks. Don't laugh, though; even doctors can't always tell the difference right away. The bottom line: Go to the emergency room immediately when you have chest pain, especially if you have a history of heart problems, if you smoke, or if you have other risk factors for heart disease.

it and other soothing herbal teas, such as slippery elm, marshmallow, and plantain, at health food stores. If you're allergic to ragweed, however, avoid chamomile.

A heavenly healer. The herb angelica has the power to cool your heartburn. You can make a tea (it tastes a bit like celery) by putting 1 teaspoon of dried herb or 3 teaspoons of crushed fresh leaves in 1 cup of boiling water. Steep for about 10 minutes, strain out the herb, and enjoy a cup after meals.

Try meadowsweet. It's a digestive herb that protects and soothes the stomach lining while reducing excess acidity. Sip a cup of meadowsweet tea between meals. To prepare it, steep 1 heaping teaspoon of dried herb (available at health food stores) in 1 cup of hot water for 15 minutes, then strain and drink.

Take a hint from hip-hop. Tight clothing presses on the

stomach and literally pushes acid uphill. So get comfortable: Loosen your belt a few notches, untuck your shirt, or undo a few buttons. Less pressure means less heartburn.

Get your jaws moving. It may not be polite at formal gatherings, but chewing on a stick of gum is a great way to stop heartburn fast. Chewing increases the flow of saliva, which acts as a natural acid neutralizer.

Tame the acid. Over-the-counter antacids will do the trick. There are dozens of brands, and they all work equally well at stopping heartburn. Liquid antacids work better than tablets because they neutralize more acid, says Jana Nalbandian, N.D., a naturopathic physician and faculty member at Bastyr University near Seattle.

Trim the squares. Eating gargantuan meals almost guarantees heartburn because all of that food in the stomach requires enormous quantities of digestive acids. You'll be much less likely to get heartburn if you eat five or six small meals a day instead of gorging yourself on two or three large ones.

Tip your bed. A lot of people get heartburn after going to bed because lying prone puts the stomach at the same level as the vulnerable esophagus. An easy solution is to raise the head of your bed a few inches by putting boards or sturdy, wide blocks under the legs.

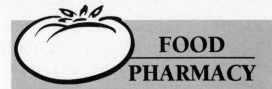

FOOD PHARMACY

Cure It with Cabbage

A head of cabbage will help you get ahead of heartburn. This vegetable is loaded with glutamine, an amino acid that appears to promote healing in the digestive tract. People who eat cabbage several times a week may be less likely to experience heartburn than those who never eat it. If cabbage isn't to your taste, you can buy powdered glutamine at a health food store.

Eat early. As you'd expect, the production of stomach acid peaks soon after meals. You're a lot more likely to get heartburn when you eat late and go to bed within an hour or two. If you can, eat earlier in the evening so that most of the food is digested by the time you hit the hay.

Catch the culprits. Caffeine, alcohol, and chocolate are notorious for causing and aggravating heartburn. You don't necessarily have to give them up, but a little moderation may bring blessed relief.

Give up the mints. Peppermint, spearmint, and other mints may freshen your breath, but they also trigger heartburn by relaxing the muscle in the esophagus that's supposed to keep acid out.

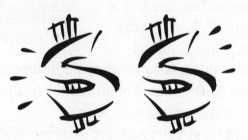

Eat lean. Fatty foods stay in the stomach for a long time and trigger the release of more acid. Drop the fat and switch to leaner meals.

Hemorrhoids

The Bottom Line

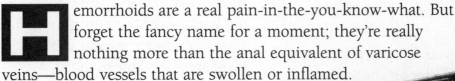

Hemorrhoids are a real pain-in-the-you-know-what. But forget the fancy name for a moment; they're really nothing more than the anal equivalent of varicose veins—blood vessels that are swollen or inflamed.

Of course, that little explanation won't make you feel one bit better when the pain is so intense that you can't sit down, or when the itching keeps getting worse—and you can't even scratch in public!

NO MORE VEIN PAIN

The main cause of hemorrhoids is straining during bowel movements. Sitting for a long time can also contribute to them, as can lack of exercise or not getting enough fiber in your diet.

For the most part, hemorrhoids

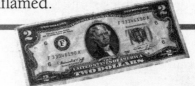

The $2 Deal

Heal from the Inside Out

Available in health food stores, mild-tasting aloe juice is a traditional remedy for digestive problems because it soothes your system right where it counts. Drink a glass a day until your hemorrhoids are gone.

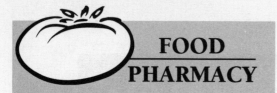

FOOD PHARMACY

The Fiber Fix

The indigestible fiber in fruit, vegetables, legumes, and whole grains soaks up water in the intestine like a sponge. A high-fiber diet makes stools softer and easier to pass, so you strain less and put less pressure on tender hemorrhoids.

Doctors advise getting 30 to 35 grams of fiber daily, but you don't have to put your produce on a scale to be sure you get the right amount. When you fill your plate, salads or vegetables should take up about a quarter of the space. Also, snack on vegetables or fresh or dried fruit during the day.

aren't serious. They almost always go away on their own, usually within a few days. But there are a few things you need to be aware of. While it's common for hemorrhoids to bleed a little, it's impossible to know for sure if blood in the toilet bowl is from a hemorrhoid or something a lot more serious, such as colon cancer. Never ignore blood in the stool—see your doctor right away.

In most cases, though, you can take away the pain of hemorrhoids—and keep them from coming back—without contributing to your doctor's retirement fund. Here are a few things to try.

Soak away pain. A soak in the bathtub is just the ticket for hemorrhoid pain, and it doesn't have to be lengthy. A 10-minute bath will relax the muscles surrounding the hemorrhoids and reduce irritation and discomfort, says Rajesh Vyas, N.D., a naturopathic physician in Morgan Hill, California.

Soothe with a spud. To reduce pain and swelling, place a potato poultice on hemorrhoids that protrude from the anal opening. Grate 1 to 2 tablespoons of raw potato, wrap it in cheesecloth, chill, and apply.

Ease the ouch with okra. Even if you're not a big fan of okra, it's one of the best foods for soothing as well as preventing hemorrhoids. For one thing, it's loaded with fiber. It also has a naturally slimy texture that augments the natural coating of mucus in the intestine, says Dr. Vyas. "It's a good excuse to eat lots of gumbo," he adds.

Say ahh with aloe. Aloe gel is one of the most soothing treatments for hemorrhoid pain. Apply a little to your finger and dab it directly on the tender spots. It may help the tissue heal more quickly, and it will lubricate the area so there's less irritation. You can buy the gel at a health food store or simply squeeze some from a freshly cut aloe leaf.

Keep a regular schedule. Having regular bowel movements is among the best ways to prevent constipation, which in turn prevents vein-damaging straining. For starters, get in the habit of having bowel movements at the same time every day. For most people, nature's call comes early, usually after breakfast or a cup of coffee. Don't ignore your body's signals. If you wait until later to go, your intestines will have to work harder than they should.

Don't force things. Since straining to have bowel movements aggravates hemorrhoids, don't try to force the issue. "Your body knows when it's time to go," says Dr. Vyas. "If you miss your regular time, let your body decide when it's ready."

His advice: If you don't get

HOLLER FOR HELP
Catch the Clots

It's not uncommon for little blood clots to form inside hemorrhoids. While they aren't serious health threats, they can be excruciatingly painful. If your hemorrhoids are making you miserable, your doctor may recommend having any clots removed. It's a simple office procedure that just takes a few minutes and eliminates the pain immediately.

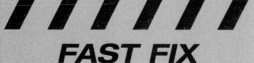
results within 10 minutes, it's time to get off the throne. There's no prize for success and no penalty for coming back later to try again.

Reduce your reading time. That's right, get those *National Geographics* and Jerry Baker catalogs out of the bathroom. They only encourage you to spend too much time on the toilet.

Tank up. Getting enough water throughout the day will go a long way toward making stools softer and easier to pass. Everyone needs different amounts of water, but a good goal is at least 5 full glasses daily; 8 to 10 may be even better.

Cool the pain. Soak a washcloth in cold water, wring it out, and hold it against the affected area until the cloth warms. Don't rub. Rinse the washcloth out, douse it in cold water again, and reapply. Repeat until the pain and itching stop.

Baby yourself. The discomfort of hemorrhoids can make a baby out of anybody, so even if you're a big bruiser, be bold and venture into the baby goods aisle for some baby wipes. They're softer than any toilet paper and help you avoid irritating an already uncomfortable area.

Get off the couch. People who exercise regularly are less likely to get hemorrhoids than those who spend most of their time lounging. Twenty minutes of exercise a day, even if it's no more than a slow walk, helps your intestines work more efficiently and with less straining.

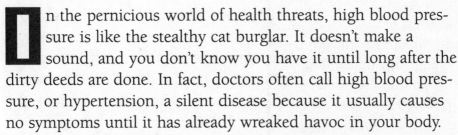

High Blood Pressure

Lower It Naturally

In the pernicious world of health threats, high blood pressure is like the stealthy cat burglar. It doesn't make a sound, and you don't know you have it until long after the dirty deeds are done. In fact, doctors often call high blood pressure, or hypertension, a silent disease because it usually causes no symptoms until it has already wreaked havoc in your body.

To understand high blood pressure, imagine a nice, new garden hose. All smooth and flexible, warm from the sun. It coils and uncoils easily, does its job. But what happens if you neglect it and leave it out year-round to suffer the weather? Yep, after a season or two, it hardens, stiffens, doesn't work very well—and may eventually spring a leak.

In a way, your arteries are like that. The "tension" in hypertension is about them. Your arteries must continually contract and relax to accommodate the powerful force of blood pumping into your heart—60 to 70 times a minute, and that's while

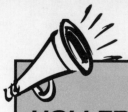

The first step toward controlling your blood pressure is to understand the numbers used to define it. Pressure is expressed as two numbers, one over the other. The upper number (systolic pressure) is a measurement of the pressure during the contraction of the heart as it pumps blood into arteries. The lower number (diastolic pressure) indicates the pressure as the heart relaxes between beats.

Blood pressure varies within a normal range during waking hours and should be around 120/80 millimeters of mercury (mm Hg). When it stays above 140/90 mm Hg for a period of time, it is considered high, can damage the surface of blood vessels, and can lead to cholesterol being deposited on artery walls. Many doctors suggest you start trying to lower your pressure well before it gets to that level.

you're resting. When the blood is moving at too high a pressure, it literally wears out the arteries. Down the line, untreated hypertension can also damage your heart, which gets bigger as it works harder to pump. Eventually, it can become more inefficient. Your kidneys and eyes take a beating, too, and a stroke can damage your brain.

A LIFETIME OF CARE

These dire consequences are unnecessary. Although it's dangerous, high blood pressure is also highly treatable. Because it sneaks up without symptoms, though, once your doctor says you have it, you have to make a commitment not to go into denial. Just do what's necessary to keep it under control.

If you have high blood pressure, you need to be under a doctor's care, and you may need a variety of prescription drugs to control it. But doctors have also learned that lifestyle factors can be just as important as drugs—and they're a whole lot cheaper. Here's what you need to do.

Stop the stress. If you are easily stressed, your body repeatedly pumps adrenaline into your bloodstream, causing a rise in blood pressure. Take an honest look at your stress level, and take control. You can commit yourself to reducing the stress in your life. Regular exercise, yoga, and meditation are good places to begin.

Heal with hawthorn. Hawthorn berries are widely used for their gentle hypotensive effects, and combining them with other anti-spasmodic herbs and relaxants can augment their effect. Combine equal parts of hawthorn, mother-wort, passionflower, and skullcap, then steep 1 heaping teaspoon of the mixture in 1 cup of hot water for 15 minutes. Strain and drink two or three cups daily.

Lower pressure with lime. Lime blossoms may be effective when your high blood pressure is associated with tension and stress. Toss 1 heaping teaspoon of blossoms into 1 cup of hot water and steep for 15 minutes, then strain. Drink one to three cups per day.

Lay off the licorice. Here's an instance where the artificial is better than the real thing. Natural licorice can raise blood pressure and wash potassium from the body, according to an Icelandic study. It's found in some herbal teas, dark beers, and candy. So, if

Both aggressive, let-it-all-hang-out folks and the quiet types who repress their anger are likely to send their blood pressure soaring, according to Nancy Snyderman, M.D. If you tend to respond to negative events by acting like either Clara Clam or Rick the Raging Bull, pick up a copy of *LifeSkills*, by Duke University psychiatrist Redford Williams, M.D. By following his simple anger-management techniques, you'll not only lower your blood pressure, you'll also change your life.

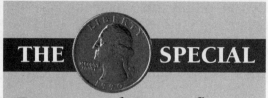

THE SPECIAL

De-stress with Passionflower

This herb is one of Mother Nature's best tranquilizers. When you need to be rescued from anxiety or stress—and the high blood pressure that can result—try a cup of passionflower tea. Simply steep 1 or 2 teaspoons of the dried herb in 1 cup of boiling water, steep for 20 minutes, strain, and drink.

your blood pressure is a little iffy, read labels and buy only licorice made with artificial flavoring.

Shake the salt. Reducing sodium intake definitely helps people with hypertension, and not just those especially sensitive to it, a Harvard Medical School study showed. That's why doctors suggest you consume less than 1,500 milligrams of sodium a day. Bear in mind that just 1 teaspoon of salt contains 2,400 milligrams.

Watch out for stowaways. Many packaged, prepared, and junk foods are loaded with sodium—some are as much as 85 percent sodium! Always read labels before you buy lunch meats, soups, canned foods, packaged meals, frozen dinners, and other prepared foods. There are healthy, low-sodium alternatives to these foods, but avoid fast foods altogether, except for an occasional salad (be prepared, and tote your own bottle of low-sodium dressing).

Pump up the produce. A diet low in salt but high in fruits, vegetables, and low-fat dairy products can lower blood pressure as much as medication can, according to research. Load up your shopping cart and stock your fridge with a variety of these products.

Fruit is especially good because its fiber apparently works even better than the fiber from vegetables and grains to lower systolic blood pressure (the top reading), studies show. Strawberries, blueberries, and peaches are especially good examples. And in some studies, strawberries lowered diastolic pressure (the bottom reading), too. So top your morning oatmeal or cold cereal with these fruits and reach for a fruit snack later in the day—every day.

Forgive and forget. Forgiveness is good not only for your soul but also for your body. A study led by Kathleen Lawler, Ph.D., a psychologist at the University of Tennessee in Knoxville, tracked blood pressure and heart rate as people talked about betrayals in their lives. When some participants reported forgiving a grievance, their readings returned to normal, while the readings of those who held a grudge remained high. Across the board, men were more likely to forgive than women.

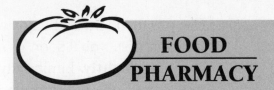

FOOD PHARMACY

Beat It with Bananas

The potassium in bananas prevents thickening of the artery walls and works in conjunction with sodium, an electrolyte, to regulate your body's fluid levels. Those fluid levels are important because an excessively high volume of fluid in your arteries can elevate your blood pressure. Bananas are particularly high in potassium, so reach for one every day to keep your potassium levels healthy. Also enjoy other good potassium sources, including apples, string beans, peas, beans, and fat-free milk.

If you find it hard to forgive, remind yourself that the word does not mean excuse, forget, or condone. It simply means that you release yourself from the anger and resentment you've been holding—literally, in your heart.

Get moving now! We're not naming names here, but many people with high blood pressure are couch potatoes. Even moderate exercise will help—as long as you do it for 30 minutes four or five times a week. Check with your doctor before you start, then pick a regular exercise program you will enjoy and stick with it. (Even if you don't like it at first, you'll soon grow to love feeling fit.)

Drink lightly. Limit daily alcohol consumption to one 12-ounce beer, one 4-ounce glass of wine, or one drink made with 1.5 ounces of hard liquor. More than that can send your blood pressure moving up the scale.

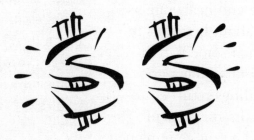

Pamper yourself with pets. Some studies have shown that having pets to care for and love lowers high blood pressure. A cat purrs, and you purr. A dog looks into your eyes, and you melt. If you don't already have a pet, visit a humane society or other shelter and choose a four-legged creature to share your life.

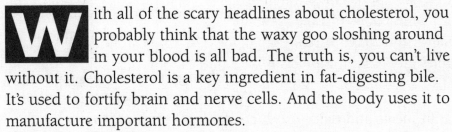

High Cholesterol

Get the Fat Out of Circulation

With all of the scary headlines about cholesterol, you probably think that the waxy goo sloshing around in your blood is all bad. The truth is, you can't live without it. Cholesterol is a key ingredient in fat-digesting bile. It's used to fortify brain and nerve cells. And the body uses it to manufacture important hormones.

Cholesterol itself isn't the problem. It's the amount. When there's an excess of the fatty stuff in your blood, it clings to artery walls like sludge in a drainpipe. And—no surprise—it's hard for the heart to pump life-giving blood when the main channels are clogged.

We talk about cholesterol as if it were a single substance, but there are actually several different forms. Low-density lipoprotein (LDL) is the nasty stuff that hangs onto artery walls. High-density lipoprotein (HDL) is the good stuff that grabs excess LDL from the blood and carts it to the liver for disposal. Thus,

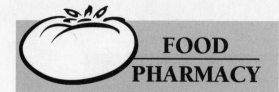

FOOD PHARMACY

Magic Margarines

Even though traditional margarines raise cholesterol more than just about anything else, some new brands, including Benecol and Take Control, actually lower it. They contain a cholesterol-like plant fat that blocks the absorption of cholesterol in the small intestine. As a result, the level of harmful LDL cholesterol drops by 7 to 10 percent. The American Heart Association says 2 tablespoons of Benecol or 3 tablespoons of Take Control daily is enough to have significant cholesterol-lowering effects.

the key to controlling cholesterol—and lowering your risk of heart disease and stroke—is to do everything you can to lower levels of harmful LDL while boosting levels of beneficial HDL.

LOOK TO YOUR DIET

The new generations of cholesterol-lowering drugs are very helpful, but some of them cause muscle pain or other side effects. They also cost a bundle. In most cases, before your doctor advises you to take drugs to lower cholesterol, he'll give you detailed advice about natural strategies. They often work—and are a lot less expensive than heart surgery! Here are the best ones to try.

Change your bread spread. We already know that the saturated fat in meats and dairy products damages arteries, so too much of those foods can sabotage a heart-healthy diet. Even worse are the hydrogenated oils and trans fats used in margarine, according to Walter Willet, M.D., chairman of the nutrition department at the Harvard School of Public Health. Research has shown that people who load up on margarine can see rises in cholesterol of 14 points—which translate to a 10 percent increase in heart attack risk. Give up margarine now, or look for trans fat–free products when you shop. (See "Magic Margarines" on this page.)

Bet on barley. Researchers at Texas A&M University tested the effect of barley bran flour, barley oil capsules, and wheat flour on men and women with high cholesterol levels. All the participants followed a low-fat diet for about a month. The result: Those who used either kind of barley significantly lowered their cholesterol levels and their blood pressures.

What's the magic ingredient in barley? It's beta-glucan, a type of fiber that study after study has shown lowers cholesterol. (By the way, it's also what gives barley its creamy texture.) Barley also boasts tocotrienol, a substance that deactivates an enzyme that tells the liver to produce artery-clogging LDL cholesterol.

Eat lean. In a study of 145 men and women with mild to moderately high cholesterol, researchers at three major medical centers compared the effects of eating lean white meat with those of eating lean red meat on the participants' cholesterol levels. For about nine months, one group ate a diet in which 80 percent of the meat was lean red meat. The other group ate lean white meat. After a four-week break, the groups switched the types of meat they were eating. During the entire study, the participants were instructed to follow a healthy eating plan recommended by the American Heart Association.

'Chokes Clobber Cholesterol

Ever since Roman times, globe artichokes have been used in traditional European medicine for liver complaints. With its liver-protective, cholesterol-reducing, and appetite-stimulating actions, the artichoke is an excellent all-around digestive herb—especially if you have trouble digesting fat and often feel bloated or nauseated after rich meals. Simply add the plant to your diet (skip the buttery dipping sauce!) or take it as a dried extract (2 grams three times a day). If you have gallbladder disease, talk to your doctor before eating artichokes, and if you're allergic to them, skip this remedy (even the extract) altogether.

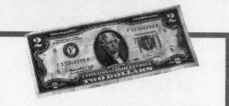

The $2 Deal

Go Nuts

The Mediterranean diet is good for the heart, but substituting a handful of walnuts (8 to 11 a day) for some of the oil in that diet could be even better. Walnuts can lower cholesterol even more than olive oil, according to a study reported in the journal *Annals of Internal Medicine*. The nuts lowered the risk of coronary heart disease by 11 percent, reports lead researcher Emilio Ros, M.D. Furthermore, researchers at the Hospital Clinic Provincial de Barcelona note that walnuts incorporated into the Mediterranean diet reduced HDL cholesterol by almost 6 percent more than the Mediterranean diet alone did.

The result: Whether the participants ate red or white meat, they lowered their levels of LDL and improved their levels of beneficial HDL. "A heart-healthy diet containing up to 6 ounces of lean red meat daily can positively impact blood cholesterol levels," says lead researcher Michael H. Davidson, M.D.

Forgo the fast food. Hydrogenated oils and trans fats are widely used in fast food (especially French fries) and most commercially prepared snacks (like cookies), according to Dr. Willet. Forget the fries on your next lunch break, and get into the habit of reading labels on cookies and other snack foods.

Mind the Mediterraneans. Scores of studies and many doctors agree that the heart-healthiest diet is the one Mediterranean populations enjoy. Consisting mostly of vegetables and fruit, beans, fish, nuts, and plenty of olive oil, Mediterranean meals have a positive effect on both cholesterol levels and blood pressure. Add generous amounts of these foods to your low-fat diet, and you'll lower both your total and LDL cholesterol levels by twice as much as people who eat ordinary low-fat meals, according to study results presented to the American Heart Association.

Eat less—but more often. It may seem surprising, but the more often you eat, the lower your cholesterol may be. In a study of men and women between the ages of 50 and 89, those who ate four or more meals a day lowered their cholesterol by 2.5 percent compared with participants who ate only once or twice a day.

The power of pectin. It binds up cholesterol, preventing its absorption in the blood. Good sources include apples, grapefruit, carrots, prunes, and cabbage.

Lower it with lemon. Living in a toxic world, as we do, can overburden the liver and compromise its ability to metabolize fats and cholesterol. Perk it up a bit by squeezing a lemon into your daily water ration. The lemon juice helps prod your digestive system, including your liver, and encourages it to go to work.

Filter out trouble. Apparently, the rumors about coffee raising cholesterol levels are not true. The cholesterol connection

The Garlic Cure

It's the real deal for lowering cholesterol, with the ability to drop levels by up to 15 percent, according to many scientific studies. To keep your arteries free and clear, try a glass of garlic tea or juice once a day. Follow it up by chewing a big sprig of fresh parsley, so you don't asphyxiate all your friends!

Another idea: Peel and chop a clove or two, let it rest on the cutting board for at least 10 minutes, then slip it into anything from soups and stews to salads and poultry dishes. Letting the clove rest allows the cholesterol-lowering compounds to form.

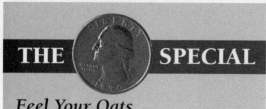

Feel Your Oats

Make it a daily habit to eat a breakfast with lots of soluble fiber, of which oatmeal's a great source. Savor a bowl every day, and you'll lower your cholesterol, according to more than 40 scientific studies. Not only is it rich in a type of fiber called beta-glucan, it also fills you up, according to Joseph Keenan, M.D., of the University of Minnesota Medical School.

actually comes from the brewing method. When coffee's unfiltered, as it is when it's made with a French press, it can add as many as 20 points to your cholesterol tally. Scientists believe that two compounds in coffee—cafestol and kahweol—are to blame. Brewing through paper or gold-plated filters is said to remove these troublemakers, so if you prefer the French press method, just strain the brewed coffee through a filter before you drink it.

Ditch the sticks. Along with all of its other terrible consequences to your health, smoking raises cholesterol levels by increasing the stickiness of blood platelets, which makes clotting in narrowed arteries more likely. It also reduces the blood's capacity to carry oxygen and damages the lining of coronary arteries, most likely by contributing to the formation of plaque. Consider this for motivation: When you quit, your risk of heart disease drops rapidly, as does your cholesterol. If you haven't tried in a while, see your doctor for help.

Know your beans. They contain soluble fiber that not only lowers cholesterol but may also make your arteries more flexible, according to a study presented at an American Heart Association meeting.

Hives

Wipe Out Welts

O kay, we all know that beauty is skin deep, but *beauty* isn't the first word that comes to mind when you're dealing with an outbreak of hives. Those nasty little bumps can make you look as though you fell into a vat of polka dots. On the other hand, you'll probably be too busy scratching to stare in the mirror anyway!

Hives are usually an allergic reaction to food or medication and should be checked by a doctor. They can also pop up after you touch a plant such as stinging nettle or are stung by an insect. Hives can erupt on any part of the body—even in the mouth—but they're usually on the skin, and, boy, are they visible! In some cases, the red wheals may be as large as 1 inch in diameter.

Most hives develop within hours of contact with a trigger substance, but sometimes they appear days later, particularly if you're reacting to a medication. One way to tell is that a drug reaction usually starts around the head and face and spreads downward.

DITCH THE ITCH

Hives usually don't stick around very long, but why put up with them longer than you have to? Here's what doctors recommend to soothe and save your skin.

Attack with antihistamines. Hives can fade within minutes or last for days or weeks. But you can fight back. Start with the first line of defense by taking an over-the-counter antihistamine such as diphenhydramine (Benadryl). In most cases, it will ease the reaction. A topical anesthetic ointment or lotion may also provide relief. If the problem persists, ask your doctor whether a prescription antihistamine might prevent additional eruptions.

Soothe with oats. To reduce the itchiness of hives, soak for 10 to 15 minutes in a bathtub full of warm water to which you've added some finely ground colloidal oatmeal. This over-the-counter bath powder stays suspended in water and won't clog your drain—but it will fix your itch.

Mend with mint. You may find some temporary relief from those hot, itchy hives by dabbing them with cool mint tea. Stir 1 teaspoon of dried or fresh leaves into 1 cup of boiling water and simmer for 10 minutes, then strain. After the tea has cooled, rub it on your skin as a healing lotion.

Screen for tartrazine. It's the technical name for a food dye known as Yellow Number 5.

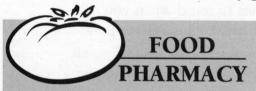

FOOD PHARMACY

Nix the Niacin

Eating foods high in niacin increases the chance of hives. The most common foods that cause this reaction are niacin-rich shellfish, nuts, and berries, but you may also be sensitive to poultry, seeds, cereals, and breads. Boycott these foods for a week to see whether niacin could be your trigger. If it is, work out a new diet with your doctor.

Reading food labels can help you avoid this common cause of hives. This not-so-mellow yellow is found in cheeses, artificial fruit drinks, and often in the coatings of vitamins or candy.

Search for the source. When hives first hit, try to remember everything you've recently eaten. If you can identify the trigger early, you can avoid a more serious recurrence. Drawing a blank? Keep a daily food diary until you're sure whether or not something in your diet is triggering the hives.

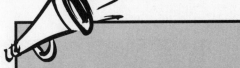

HOLLER FOR HELP

When Hives Get Heavy

If, in addition to hives, you have any swelling in your throat or difficulty breathing, speaking, or swallowing, call for emergency help immediately. You could be showing signs of anaphylaxis—a severe allergic reaction that can be fatal.

Ax the aspirin. This common analgesic is a frequent cause of hives. If you're allergic to aspirin, also try eliminating foods that contain salicylate, the active ingredient in aspirin. These include apricots, berries, grapes, raisins and other dried fruit, and tea.

Don't be a sourpuss. Foods that are processed with vinegar, such as pickles, may cause hives in some people. Give up the sour stuff for a while and see if it helps.

Chill the chick. Chickweed salve soothes itching, burning hives in no time. For extra relief, keep the salve in the fridge and dab it on cold. Another way to use chickweed is to make a strong infusion of the herb by steeping a handful of fresh chickweed in 2 cups of hot water for 15 minutes. Strain the liquid into a spray bottle, chill, and spritz it on your hives to relieve the itch.

Hot Flashes

Dial Down the Heat

Imagine leaning over a blistering stove, cooking a holiday meal for 17 of your favorite relatives. Your face turns fire-engine red, your skin sizzles with millions of hot pinpricks, and your blouse is soaked with sweat.

Now, imagine that the same thing happens when you're in the office or standing in line at the supermarket. It doesn't happen just once or twice, but day after day for months or even years.

Welcome to the hot-as-heck world of hot flashes, one of the main signs that your body is moving into menopause. Hot flashes are a by-product of fluctuating estrogen and progesterone levels, which interfere with the nerves controlling your body temperature. To compensate for loss of estrogen, your pituitary gland begins to overproduce luteinizing

THE SPECIAL

Field Some Alfalfa

Alfalfa contains plant sterols, making it an ideal choice for hot flashes. To make a tea, steep 1 teaspoon in 1 cup of hot water, then strain. Drink one cup daily.

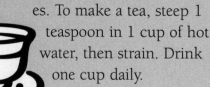

hormone (LH). The more abruptly your estrogen decreases, and the more LH is produced, the more severe your hot flashes.

STAY COOL

Hot flashes typically last about five years and stop altogether two to four years after your periods end, as your body adjusts to its new hormone levels. In the meantime, however, you don't have to walk around with a smudged face or resort to potentially dangerous—and expensive—hormone replacement therapies, which have recently been found to increase the risk of breast cancer, heart attacks, and even Alzheimer's disease. With dietary changes, exercise, and a few simple, nondrug remedies, you can not only cut the number and severity of your hot flashes, you can do so without jeopardizing your overall health.

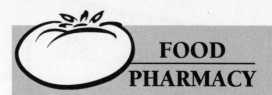

FOOD PHARMACY

Put Plants on Your Plate

Here's another reason to aim your shopping cart straight for the produce aisle: Women who eat a lot of fruits and vegetables tend to experience fewer blasts from their internal furnace because these foods contain natural phytoestrogens, according to Cornell University researchers. Foods that are especially high in phytoestrogens include apples, alfalfa sprouts, split peas, spinach, and especially soy products.

To start, avoid vessel-dilating foods such as caffeine, alcohol, and hot or spicy dishes; take a multivitamin with 400 IU of vitamin E (which has been found to cut hot flashes); and use these additional tricks for turning down the heat.

Fill up on phytos. Women in Asia get far fewer hot flashes than Western women, possibly because they eat a plant-based diet brimming with phytoestrogens, which bind to estrogen receptors in the body and reduce overall estrogen levels. To mimic their phyto-dense diet, load up on soybeans, which con-

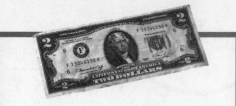

The $2 Deal

Get Ease with E

Vitamin E often helps reduce the severity and frequency of hot flashes and other menopausal discomforts. Some doctors advise starting with 400 IU twice a day. If you already take a multivitamin, be sure to note how much vitamin E it contains and figure that into your total intake. Although no one knows exactly how vitamin E reduces hot flashes, it produces remarkable results for many women with moderate symptoms. If you're taking other medications, check with your doctor before you use this much vitamin E.

tain isoflavones, the most potent phytos. In fact, studies show that eating 50 milligrams of soy a day—the rough equivalent of 1½ cups of soy milk—could slash the frequency of your hot flashes in half. Chickpeas, lentils, and flaxseed oil (try 1 tablespoon a day) also pack plenty of phytoestrogens. Women who have been diagnosed with breast or ovarian cancer should consult a doctor before consuming phytoestrogens.

Try black cohosh. In one study, most women who took this herb daily for three months had lower LH levels and 70 percent fewer hot flashes. For best results, use RemiFemin, a widely tested commercial black cohosh supplement available in most health food stores, advises Maida Taylor, M.D., associate clinical professor of obstetrics, gynecology, and reproductive sciences at the University of California, San Francisco. Take 20 to 40 milligrams a day.

Come over to red clover. According to two small studies, this isoflavone-rich herb reduces the number and severity of hot flashes by nearly half. The studies involved Promensil, a commercial preparation available in health food stores, but you can also take the herb as a tincture (60 to 100 drops three times a day). Consult your doctor before taking red clover if you have a history of breast cancer.

Turn to motherwort. The Latin name for this herb means "lion's ear," which is fitting since motherwort is a ferocious mood tamer and a powerful phytoestrogenic herb favored by women's healers to quell hot flashes and night sweats. Add 25 drops of tincture (which you can find at health food stores) to a cup of water and drink it four times a day. Don't use motherwort if you have heavy periods.

Sip some sage. At the first hint of a flash or night sweats, drink some sage tea, suggests Carol Leonard, a certified nurse-midwife and chair of the New Hampshire Council of Midwifery in Hopkinton. To make the tea, steep 1 tablespoon of dried sage (available at health food stores) in a cup of hot water for 10 minutes, then strain. Sage is what's called a hormonal stimulant and is often used to minimize menopausal discomforts such as hot flashes and dizziness. Don't use sage if there's any chance you could be pregnant.

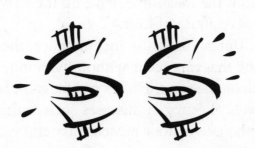

Walk on the wild side. Studies show that daily exercise—such as walking, swimming, or biking—decreases the amount of circulating LH and increases levels of feel-good brain chemicals called endorphins, which nosedive during hot flashes.

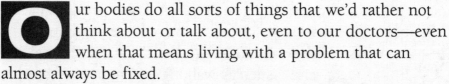

Incontinence

Banish the Bladder Blues

Our bodies do all sorts of things that we'd rather not think about or talk about, even to our doctors—even when that means living with a problem that can almost always be fixed.

Urinary incontinence is a case in point. More than 10 million Americans, most of them women, have it. Yet one study showed that it typically took 10 years—an entire decade!—before women brought the problem to the attention of their doctors. Many of them, in the meantime, gave up their favorite activities because they were afraid of losing control.

All sorts of things can cause incontinence, the accidental leakage of urine that can occur without warning, especially when laughing or sneezing. Excess weight can contribute to it. So can low levels of estrogen, diseases such as diabetes, or weakening of the pelvic floor muscle after childbirth, explains Lila Wallis, M.D., former president of the American Medical Women's Association and a specialist in women's health based in New York City.

CONTROL THE FLOW

Since incontinence can be a sign of serious underlying problems, it's essential to see a doctor right away. In the great majority of cases, though, you won't be faced with ever-escalating medical bills. Most women can get their bladders under control with some simple lifestyle approaches. Here's what your doctor will probably advise.

Chart the trouble. Keep a daily record of when and how often you leak urine, how often you urinate voluntarily, how often you feel like urinating, and what seems to cause the leaking. Share these notes with your doctor if you can't determine the cause of the trouble on your own.

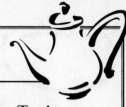

Tea Time

A Bladder-Toning Tonic

Skullcap relieves nervous tension, so it may help to restore adequate sphincter tone in the muscle that controls the bladder opening. To make a tea, steep 1 teaspoon of herb in 1 cup of hot water for 10 minutes, then strain. Drink one to three cups daily.

Suspect your medicines. Sometimes medications cause incontinence. Diuretics and blood pressure drugs can weaken the urethra and allow urine leakage. Antihistamines and decongestants may cause you to retain urine, creating a situation in which "overflow" incontinence may occur. Some antidepressants and narcotics can also cause this reaction. Keep a record of medications you take and see if you notice any connection, then consult your doctor about your suspicions.

Be good to your bowels. Severe constipation can cause you to retain urine by compressing the bladder outlet. A healthy, high-fiber diet can prevent things from compacting down below.

Give a squeeze. If your doctor believes your leaky bladder is due to a weak pelvic floor muscle, you may be able to correct

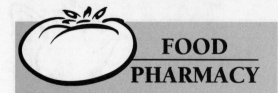

FOOD PHARMACY

Bad Bladder Foods

Could your bladder problems be related to something you eat or drink? Incontinence can sometimes be managed with changes in diet, so pay attention to the foods and beverages you consume. Try boycotting foods that irritate the bladder, such as caffeinated and carbonated drinks, alcohol, citrus fruits and juices, spicy foods, and artificial sweeteners, to see if this eliminates the problem.

the problem with simple exercises known as Kegels. Here's how to do them: While you're on the toilet, stop and start the flow of urine. This action will help you locate the pelvic floor muscle. Once you've learned exactly where it is, you can squeeze it shut and open it anywhere, not just on the toilet. Repeat your Kegels several times a day, perhaps while you're sitting at your desk or watching television.

Exercise internally. Insert a small weight, such as a clean marble, into your vagina and squeeze the muscles around it. Hold for a count of four, then relax. Repeat 10 times several times a day. For an alternative exercise, ask your doctor about using vaginal weights, which are shaped like tampons. These can be worn for 20 to 30 minutes at a time.

Don't bounce. Running and high-impact aerobics can cause leakage, which is hard to control during bouncing. If this is a frequent problem for you, try swimming or bicycling instead. These activities require less impact and create fewer leaks.

Teach your bladder new tricks. Try to wait a bit longer before you urinate, even when you feel some urgency. You can briefly stop the feeling by contracting the pelvic floor muscle. Each time you do this, you increase the time between urinations, which trains your bladder to wait.

Practice biofeedback. This simple, painless technique, usually performed in a hospital or office setting, can help you retrain your bladder. A sensor is placed in your vagina or rectum, and another is put on your stomach. The sensors read the signals given when you contract or relax your pelvic floor muscle, and you can view them on a video screen. By watching the monitor, you learn what your muscles are doing and thus can begin to control them. In a study at the University of Alabama, medication alone reduced women's episodes of incontinence by 68.5 percent, but women who used biofeedback and exercise without drugs reduced their episodes by 81 percent. If you'd like to give it a try, ask your doctor to refer you to a biofeedback specialist.

> **Always drink plenty of fluids to keep your entire urinary tract in good working order. People often believe that if they drink less, the urge to urinate will be lessened, but this isn't the case. Dehydration irritates your bladder and makes the condition worse.**

Improve with a jolt. In electrical stimulation therapy, a tiny amount of painless electric current is sent to the pelvic floor muscle and your bladder to help the muscles contract so they can get stronger. This is especially helpful if you have a very weak pelvic floor muscle. Ask your doctor if this type of therapy would help you.

Go hot and cold. Sitz baths increase circulation to the pelvic organs and may help tone and strengthen tissues. Simply prepare a comfortably hot bath and immerse yourself up to your belly button. After soaking for 5 minutes, get out of the tub, apply a cold, wet towel like a diaper, and leave it on for 5 minutes. You may repeat the sequence two or three times in a session.

The water in the bath should be warm enough so that you don't become chilled during the cold phase, but the greater the temperature contrast, the greater the toning effects. Modify the temperatures to your comfort level.

Ask about collagen. When all else fails, implants of collagen, a natural protein, can be injected near the bladder neck to bulk up the urethral tissue, narrowing the urethral opening so that the muscle has a smaller space to open and close. Several injections create a seal that prevents leaks. Talk with your doctor about this procedure. It may require more than one treatment and need to be repeated in a few years.

Don't depend on Depends. Many women seem willing to accept the advice of an aging film actress who used to hawk adult disposable diapers on television. Such absorbent products are a stopgap—a temporary measure, not a life sentence. If you do opt to use them, however, be sure to change them frequently. You can also use special deodorant products to reduce any tell-tale odors until you can change the pad.

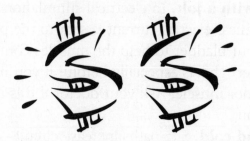

Ingrown Hairs

A Hair-Curling Tale

It's hard to believe that something the size of a hair could cause so much, well, hair-raising pain. But an ingrown hair, which curls downward instead of growing out straight, is like a sharp needle that digs deeper and deeper into the skin—not all at once, but over days or weeks. You don't feel it at first, but once bacteria take advantage of the tiny wound, you get an inkling of what pain is all about. At the very least, you develop a tender little bump.

Obviously, you'll need to see a doctor if the infection spreads and causes fever, dizziness, or other symptoms. In most cases, though, you can take care of an ingrown hair—and prevent a recurrence—without paying for your dermatologist's new fur coat. Here are a few things to try.

Wipe out the germs. It's not necessary to pull an ingrown hair out of your skin; your body will eventually expel it. But you should gently clean the affected area twice a day with soap and water, and definitely keep an eye out for infection. Warning signs include increasing redness, swelling, pain, or pus. If an infection doesn't clear up on its own in a day or two, see your doctor.

Hit it with heat and cold. To ease painful or infected ingrown hairs, alternate hot and cold compresses. Soak a washcloth in hot water, wring it out, and drape it on the sore area. Keep it there for 3 minutes, then replace it with a cold cloth for 30 seconds. Repeat the cycle two more times, ending with the cold compress.

This technique, called contrast hydrotherapy, improves skin circulation and speeds healing, says Darrell Misak, N.D., a naturopathic physician in Mount Lebanon, Pennsylvania.

Cream it with calendula. A quick way to take the sting out of irritated skin is to apply a cream that contains the herb calendula, says Heidi Weinhold, N.D., a naturopathic physician in the Pittsburgh area. Ready-made creams are available in health food stores, or you can make your own version. Just add 6 to 12 drops of calendula oil to an ounce of almond or olive oil. Rub it on the irritated area once a day until the problem is gone.

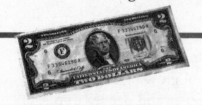

Dr. Weinhold particularly recommends using calendula in the form of a succus, which is the juice of the herb in an alcohol base. It's available at most health food stores. Apply it to the sore spots once or twice a day, using a cotton swab or a clean cloth.

Stay wet. "I recommend that

The $2 Deal

Acidify Your Skin

If you frequently get ingrown hairs or irritated bumps, you may want to use a soothing skin cleanser that contains alpha hydroxy acids or benzoperoxide to keep them at bay, says Valerie Callendar, M.D., clinical assistant professor of dermatology at Howard University College of Medicine in Washington, D.C. "They tend to be very effective."

people shave in the shower," says Dr. Misak. That keeps your skin clean and the pores open. It also reduces the chances that your skin will be irritated and allows for a closer shave, which can keep hairs from growing inward.

Wash before and after. It's important to wash with soap and water before as well as after shaving. Thorough cleansing reduces the risk that bacteria will survive long enough to colonize tiny shaving nicks or ingrown hair follicles.

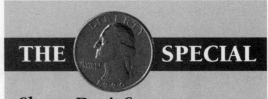

THE SPECIAL

Shave, Don't Save

You're less likely to get ingrown hairs if you shave once with a disposable razor, then throw it out. Reusing a razor makes it easier for yesterday's bacteria to get into today's shaving cut or ingrown hair follicle.

Forget the antibiotics. A lot of people insist on using antibiotic soaps and creams, but they shouldn't. These products tend to irritate your skin, including areas where hairs may be growing inward.

Turn off the juice. Electric shavers may allow you to shave without using lather or water, but they're more likely than razors to irritate your skin, Dr. Misak says. "If you're having problems, go back to blades," he suggests.

Try the sexy gen-x look. For some men with extremely curly facial hair, not shaving may be the only solution to persistent ingrown hairs. Give it a try and see how well the bearded look suits you—or at least go a few days between shaves to give your skin a much-needed break.

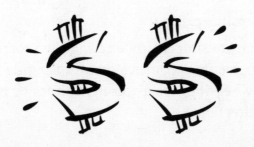

Ingrown Toenails

Solutions to "Nature's Spikes"

Mother Nature isn't all sweetness and light. She has her own form of torture—one that can reduce you to tears if you don't take care of it quickly.

The "nail" in toenail isn't just a figure of speech. Humans don't have the daggerlike claws that cats do, but if you've ever had an ingrown toenail, you know that your nails are still plenty sharp. An ingrown nail starts out like any other nail, but sometimes its sharp edge curves into the side of your toe instead of growing out straight. The more the nail grows, the deeper it digs into your skin.

PREVENT THE PAIN

Some people are simply prone to ingrown toenails—and the infection that sometimes comes along for the ride. Others get ingrown nails when they wear too-tight shoes or trim their nails in the wrong direction.

You'll have to see your doctor once a toenail starts penetrating the skin. But before that happens, here are a few tips to try.

Start with a salt soak. "An Epsom salts bath will help draw out pain and infection," says Pamela Taylor, N.D., a naturopathic physician in Moline, Illinois. Fill a basin with warm water, add a cup of Epsom salts, and soak your foot for 20 to 30 minutes.

Pack it in clay. A clay pack, available at health food stores, will help keep swelling and infection under control. "I'd use French green clay," says Dr. Taylor. "Or ask a pharmacist for pharmaceutical-grade kaolin clay."

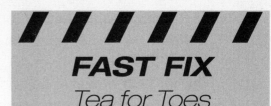

FAST FIX
Tea for Toes

Here's a tea treatment that's taken by foot, not by mouth. Put a quart of water in a saucepan, then add 1 cup of dried calendula flowers, 1 tablespoon of dried thyme, and 1/2 cup of dried lavender flowers (all available at health food stores). Simmer the mixture for 5 minutes, then let it cool to room temperature. Put it in a basin and soak your foot for about 5 minutes. "It will reduce infection and painful swelling," says Pamela Taylor, N.D.

Apply the clay to the affected toe and leave it on until it dries, usually 30 minutes to an hour. Then rinse away the clay and dry your foot thoroughly. Repeat the treatment once or twice a day.

Rub out infection. An herbal foot massage can soothe the pain of an ingrown nail and protect the area from a potentially serious infection. Start with a trip to the health food store for infused calendula oil and oregano, thyme, and lavender oils. Then combine 1 ounce of the calendula oil with 10 drops each of the others and apply the mixture all over your foot. The hands-on attention will make the area feel a lot better, and the oils will help reduce swelling and pressure around the sore nail.

Change your socks. To reduce the risk of infection, put on clean socks two or three times a day. For additional protection, add a few drops of lavender, oregano, or thyme oil (available at health food stores) to a basin of water and soak your socks in the solution overnight. The germ-killing action of the oils will help ensure that your socks don't allow infection-causing bacteria to thrive.

Let the sun shine in. Germs are never happier than when they're in a dark, tight space. To keep them under control, expose the toe with the ingrown nail to the air as often as possible. "Going barefoot is always the best," says Dr. Taylor. At the very least, take off your shoes and socks when you're lounging around the house.

Don some sandals. They're a wonderful option for airing out an ingrown toenail. Footwear made of natural materials, such as leather and cork, will probably be the most comfortable and least aggravating to your toe.

Cut it straight. If you know that one of your nails is prone to becoming ingrown, check it every week so you can cut it before it gets too long. "Trim straight across the top of the nail," says Dr. Taylor. Don't try to round the edges so the nail follows the shape of your toe; this just makes it more likely to curve into the flesh.

HOLLER FOR HELP

Fight Infection

You should never ignore an ingrown toenail for very long. Apart from the fact that it can be excruciatingly painful, there's a very high risk that the area around it will get dangerously infected.

If one of your toenails has started to penetrate the skin, get to a doctor right away—and make the appointment even sooner if you see redness, swelling, or other signs of infection. At the very least, you'll need to have the dangerous part of the nail removed, and you may need antibiotics to knock out infection-causing germs.

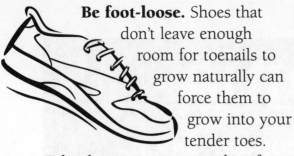

Be foot-loose. Shoes that don't leave enough room for toenails to grow naturally can force them to grow into your tender toes. Take the time to try on a lot of shoes until you find the ones that fit well and feel good.

Don't dig. It's fine to snip away a toenail that has just started to grow in the wrong direction, but you don't want to mess with a nail that's already embedded in the skin. Trying to trim it at that point is likely to damage the tissue and increase the risk of infection. To play it safe, see your doctor.

Train your nails. Here's a safe, painless way to encourage an ingrown nail to head in the right direction before it can cause real trouble. Take a small piece of cotton and roll it into a tight cylinder. Slip the cylinder under the nail right where it's touching (or almost touching) the skin. The cotton will relieve the pressure and may make the nail grow out rather than in.

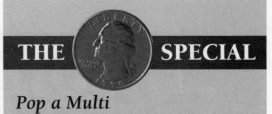

THE   SPECIAL

Pop a Multi

A daily multivitamin will help ensure that your body has the right nutrition for proper nail growth. Healthy nails are less likely to become ingrown or infected.

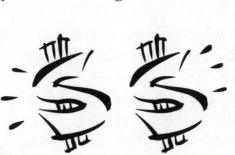

Insomnia

Shortcuts to Sounder Sleep

Whoever came up with the idea of counting sheep obviously never had insomnia. If anything, your brain is too active when the lights go out, and the last thing you need is some kind of woolly math problem.

We all have sleepless nights now and then. Doctors estimate that about a third of Americans spend at least a few nights watching the clock hands s-l-o-w-l-y revolve. In most cases, there's no mystery about what causes it. Stress is a big factor. So are lack of exercise, depression, and miscellaneous aches and pains.

Most people with insomnia don't need pricey prescription or over-the-counter drugs. These simple tips from top sleep experts will do the trick.

Wear yourself out. Physical activity during the day will help you sleep better at night. Exercise reduces stress and induces sleep by depleting chemicals that stimulate the body, such as adrenaline. Exercise also helps you fall asleep faster and sleep longer, according to Abby

King, Ph.D., of Stanford University School of Medicine in California, who has researched the relationship between exercise and sleep. Her study showed that exercise, even a brisk walk before dinner, made a big difference.

Take a hint from kitty. Catnip may turn your lazy feline into a rowdy cat, but it has the opposite effect on us humans. A little catnip tea after dinner may be just the ticket for winding down after a long day. Steep 1 teaspoon of herb in 1 cup of hot water for 10 minutes, then strain and enjoy. Note: Stash your catnip out of the reach of all cats!

Sleep by your brain clock. Sleep is malleable, like a muscle, and within limits, it can be trained and refined, according to Claudio Stampi, M.D., director of the Chronobiology Research Institute in Newton, Massachusetts. Repeat the same sleep pattern every day to set your brain clock to a good schedule. Your body will adapt to the regularity and get ready for sleep, with glands and hormones functioning and by-products breaking down. If you stay as regular as you can and don't skimp on sleep, you will feel great in the morning.

Soak up sunshine. If you fall asleep at 8:00 P.M. and wake up at 4:00 A.M. instead of 6:00 A.M., your sleep cycle is off. Spend more time outdoors during the day. That way, daylight can help your internal clock counteract its tendency to put you to sleep earlier in the evening and wake you up earlier in the morning.

Ax the aches. The reason older people sometimes

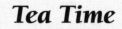

Tea Time

Calming Chamomile

Chamomile is a fragrant herbal tea with proven sleep-inducing qualities. As long as you're not allergic to ragweed, brew a cup before bed and slowly sip it. It will help your whole body, including your brain, relax and wind down.

sleep less is that they have more medical conditions, such as arthritis, that keep them awake. Don't be a stiff-upper-lipper when it comes to pain. Talk to your doctor—and do something about it.

Adjust to your sleep type. A morning person goes to sleep relatively early in the evening, wakes up early, and is most effective at doing complex tasks in the morning rather than in the evening. A night person goes to bed later, gets up later, is slower to reach full horsepower, and does better at complex tasks in the evening. If insomnia is a major part of your life, the odds are good that you're fighting your natural sleep type. Just decide which type you are and try to readjust your daily priorities so that complex tasks are scheduled for the proper time. Sleep will soon follow.

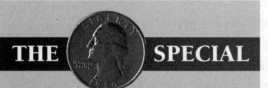

THE SPECIAL

Snooze with Valerian

Valerian, an herb also known as heliotrope, is a mild sedative that smells like stinky socks and is reputed to help you sleep. Research shows that valerian root depresses the central nervous system and relaxes smooth muscle tissue. It can be used as a tea or taken in pill or tincture form. Valerian isn't recommended if you have asthma or use sleeping pills, alcohol, antidepressants, or anti-anxiety medication.

Pull the shades. Your body needs darkness to trigger its sleep cycle. If you have a big street light shining in the window, or you have to sleep during the day because you're on night shift, close the blinds or pull opaque drapes across your windows so the light won't get through.

Follow the same routine. The best way to get to sleep more quickly is to establish and follow bedtime routines, according to Dr. Stampi. These rituals have a big influence on your ability to get to sleep and wake up according to a regular pattern. Try reading a book, breathing deeply, or sipping a cup of herbal tea. They all can work, in the same way that shaving, washing your face, and having a cup of coffee help you accelerate in the morning.

Cut the caffeine. If you find no other reason for your sleeplessness, consider your coffee habit. Keep the high-test for the morning and switch to decaf in the afternoon or evening. See if it makes a difference.

Snooze in comfort. Be as comfortable as possible for the third of your life you spend in bed. A good mattress and pillow help you enjoy your stay. Use a feather bed under your sheet for a floating-on-a-cloud feeling, and treat yourself to high-quality, smooth sheets and covers that will caress you rather than make you itch or sneeze.

Welcome some whoopee. If you can't sleep, you might as well have sex. Seriously, if sexual activity makes you sleepy, be glad. After getting worked up sexually, your body goes quite naturally into a state of total relaxation. If your significant other is sound asleep, make some romantic moves. Turn on the sexual vibrations, and you'll turn off any others that may be keeping you awake.

Relax with soothing thoughts. Use guided imagery, a form of self-hypnosis, to help yourself sleep. Listen to a meditation tape or use a progressive muscle relaxation exer-

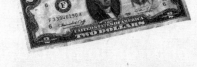

The $2 Deal

Travel to Dreamland

Native American healers invented a sleep-enhancing "dream spirits" pillow to ease one into dreamland. To make your own, put equal amounts of dried leaves of catnip, rabbit tobacco, mint, and sage into a small calico or plain cotton pillowcase and sew it shut. If you like, you can add some rosemary leaves, lavender, or mugwort. This aromatic, sedative pillow is said to make dreams more memorable, and its effects are even more noticeable in hot, humid weather.

Drugs that interfere with sleep include beta-blockers for high blood pressure, thyroid medications, bronchodilators and corticosteroids for asthma, sinus and nasal decongestants, and antidepressants. If you're taking any of these, ask your pharmacist whether a change in medication may help ease your insomnia.

cise to get deeply relaxed, then picture yourself comfortably asleep. While you're at it, imagine that you're in a more comfortable bed, in a luxury hotel, on a mountaintop, or in a gently rocking sailboat. Visualize every possible detail of the scene to increase the suggestion's power. Do this nightly for several weeks, and you'll soon be able to fall asleep more easily.

Stop trying so hard. Striving to sleep only makes the problem worse, so if you haven't fallen asleep after a little while, get up

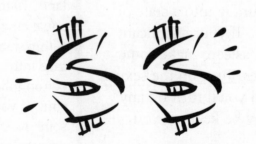

and distract yourself. Sit in another room to read or do some paperwork.

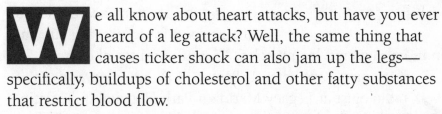

Intermittent Claudication

Get Back into Circulation

We all know about heart attacks, but have you ever heard of a leg attack? Well, the same thing that causes ticker shock can also jam up the legs—specifically, buildups of cholesterol and other fatty substances that restrict blood flow.

If a blood vessel in your leg is narrowed by fatty sludge, the muscle that depends on that vessel won't get enough blood or oxygen. This may not be a problem when you're just sitting around, because the muscle isn't demanding very much blood. When you're active, though, it calls for more fuel than it's able to get.

The result: a painful cramp that forces you to stop moving and rest the muscle. The condition is called intermittent claudication because it comes and goes. It also usually follows a distinct pattern. The pain comes on when you walk or are otherwise active, and it goes away when you relax. Another telltale

FAST FIX
Stop and Feel Better

Attacks of intermittent claudication can be intensely painful because your leg muscles are literally starved for blood and oxygen. For almost instant relief, stop whatever it is you're doing. The pain will probably go away in a minute or two, but don't use it as an excuse to call it quits altogether. Once the pain is gone, start exercising again. "There's no harm in continuing once the pain goes away," says Peter T. Beatty, M.D.

sign is the regularity of the attacks. You may feel pain whenever you're 100 feet into your daily walk, for example, or 20 minutes into your weekly bike ride.

WALK AWAY FROM PAIN

Keep in mind that anything that affects circulation in your legs could also be causing problems in your heart or other parts of your body. But that doesn't mean you have to risk bankruptcy to find relief. Along with a doctor's care, the following tips can make a real difference.

Get your legs pumping. Exercise is good for your heart, and it's just as good for improving circulation in beleaguered leg muscles. "Get 20 minutes of exercise every day," says Peter T. Beatty, M.D., an interventional radiologist at Legacy Meridian Park Hospital in Tualatin, Oregon. "It's the most important thing you can do."

The type of exercise is up to you; swimming, cycling, and walking are all great choices. "The goal is to get your heart rate up and to break a sweat," he says. If you haven't been exercising regularly, talk to your doctor before starting a new regimen. Then do it!

Chomp a clove. Garlic is both a clot buster and a cholesterol reducer. Its heating properties also make it a great circulatory tonic because it gets the blood moving to

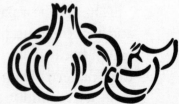

where it needs to be. Eat one raw clove per day to help alleviate claudication.

Nap with an herbal wrap. Herbalists use yarrow and peppermint to improve circulation, and after a visit to a health food store for the herbs, so can you. Steep 2 tablespoons of each herb in 2 cups of hot water for about 15 minutes. Strain out the herbs and put the teapot in the refrigerator to chill. Meanwhile, gather enough gauze, cheesecloth, or muslin to wrap your lower legs. Soak the cloths in the chilled liquid, wrap them around your legs, and rest with your legs elevated for about 20 minutes. If you do this once a day for several weeks, you'll notice quite a reduction in discomfort.

Get a leg up with hawthorn. Hawthorn, lime blossoms, and ginger are recognized for their ability to reduce the stickiness of blood platelets and enhance circulation. As long as you're not taking any other medications, use them together, or choose just one. To do the former, mix equal parts of the dried herbs, add 1 heaping teaspoon of the mix to 1 cup of hot water, steep for 15 to 20 minutes, and strain. You can drink two or three cups of this tea per day.

Eat heart smart. The same type of diet that's recommended for preventing heart disease will also go a long way toward protecting your legs.

The basics are simple enough: Quit eating fatty foods, eat

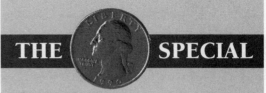

THE **SPECIAL**

Mineral Magic

Anyone with intermittent claudication should have the mineral magnesium in the medicine cabinet, says Kimberly Beauchamp, N.D. "It relaxes smooth muscles in artery walls, and it's helpful in lowering blood pressure." Check with your doctor first, then consider taking 300 to 600 milligrams daily, she advises.

five servings of fruit and vegetables a day, use olive oil in place of butter, and load up on legumes and whole grains. Eating a healthier diet will keep all of your blood vessels, including those in your legs, a whole lot healthier.

Dine on fin cuisine. Salmon, tuna, and other cold-water fish are loaded with omega-3 fatty acids. These healthful fats help prevent blood clots and may lower cholesterol. Have at least two or three servings of fish a week.

Drink green. If you have intermittent claudication, make your tea the green kind. It's a great source of bioflavonoids, natural chemical compounds that make blood vessels stronger and less vulnerable to blockages and pain. You can buy green tea bags in most stores where tea is sold; just steep a tea bag in a cup of hot water for 10 minutes, then enjoy. Try to have a cup or two every day.

Add some E. Vitamin E is a vasodilator, meaning that it opens narrowed blood vessels and allows more blood to flow through, says Kimberly Beauchamp, N.D., a naturopathic physician in Wakefield, Rhode Island. "It can allow people to walk farther without pain," she says. The recommended dose is 400 to 800 IU daily, but check with your doctor before taking E.

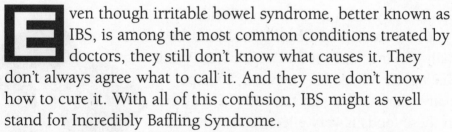

Irritable Bowel Syndrome

Get Your Gut Back on Track

Even though irritable bowel syndrome, better known as IBS, is among the most common conditions treated by doctors, they still don't know what causes it. They don't always agree what to call it. And they sure don't know how to cure it. With all of this confusion, IBS might as well stand for Incredibly Baffling Syndrome.

For some reason, people with IBS have intestines that are, well...irritable. They seem to have abnormal electrical activity that causes frequent, uncomfortable muscle contractions, or spasms. Everyone with IBS has a slightly different pattern of problems. Some people have mainly cramps, some have episodes of diarrhea and/or constipation, and others are afflicted with gas and bloating. The symptoms may occur daily for years, or they may disappear for a while, then come roaring back with no warning.

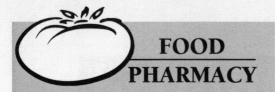

FOOD PHARMACY

Spoon Up Some Culture

Not all germs are bad germs. In fact, we couldn't get along without certain types of bacteria that live in the intestine and aid digestion. Live-culture yogurt contains beneficial *Lactobacillus acidophilus* organisms, which appear to reduce IBS symptoms. Check labels when you shop to be sure the yogurt you buy contains live cultures, and plan on having at least a few servings a week.

CALM THE CHAOS

If your symptoms are so severe that they interfere with your day-to-day life, you should see a doctor right away. If it turns out that you have IBS, lifestyle changes may be just as important as medical care. Here's what doctors advise.

Sweet isn't neat. If you have IBS, sweets are a one-way ticket to disasterville. Sugary foods appear to interfere with the normal muscle contractions that propel food through the intestine. "Cutting back on sugar is an important change for people with IBS," says Michael A. Visconti, N.D., a naturopathic physician in Orlando, Florida.

Get your fill of fiber. You should have five daily servings of fruit and vegetables. While that's good advice for everyone, it's especially important if you have IBS. The fiber in these foods is very effective at reducing symptoms.

"Five servings a day is a good start," says Dr. Visconti, but more is even better. The more fiber you eat, the less painful—and frequent—your symptoms are likely to be.

Slip and slide. When mixed with water, slippery elm powder makes a drink that will soothe your irritated gut from end to end. This is a good remedy to take first thing in the morning and last thing at night to help your tissues heal 24 hours a day.

Pour 1 cup of warm water over 1 teaspoon of powder, stir briskly, and drink immediately.

Say no to joe. Either eliminate or strictly limit the amount of caffeine you consume. Whether it comes in coffee or your favorite soda, caffeine is a bowel stimulant.

Bubbles mean trouble. Reach for noncarbonated drinks, such as fruit juice or water. The fizz in carbonated drinks can cause problems for people with IBS.

Feast less, graze more. Many people with IBS find that it helps to split their day's calories among five or six small meals rather than following the traditional breakfast-lunch-dinner schedule. Eating less food at one time puts less strain on the large intestine.

Fish for relief. Some foods can help quell the intestinal inflammation that contributes to IBS symptoms. For example, salmon and other cold-water fish, as well as ground flaxseed, contain omega-3 fatty acids, which help your body suppress inflammation.

Put on your workout shoes. You may not be up to it when your symptoms are in high gear, but 15 to 20 minutes of exercise every day is an important IBS-stopping strategy. Physical activity helps in two ways: It reduces levels of emotional stress, and it helps your bowel work more regularly. "People who exercise have a significant reduction in

FAST FIX
The Castor Cure

A castor oil pack provides rapid relief from abdominal pain and cramps. To make one, moisten a washcloth with the oil, drape it over your abdomen, and cover it with plastic wrap. Put a heating pad set on low on top of the plastic and leave it on for 20 minutes. The combination of oil and plastic traps the heat and helps reduce spasms and cramping.

Tea Time

Pound It with Peppermint

Peppermint oil, taken in capsules between meals, is a powerful anti-spasmodic and pain reliever. If capsules aren't available, try using peppermint leaves to make tea. Steep 1 heaping teaspoon of leaves in 1 cup of hot water, covered, for 10 to 15 minutes, then strain. Drink three cups daily between meals.

symptoms," says Dr. Visconti.

Take a deep breath. Studies show that meditation (which involves controlled breathing) can lower levels of stress hormones in your body and reduce anxiety and pain. But deep breathing can be soothing on its own, says Emeran Mayer, M.D., a gastroenterologist and IBS specialist at the University of California, Los Angeles. At least half of his patients who adjusted their diets and practiced deep breathing cut the severity of their symptoms. Instead of breathing shallowly from your chest, inhale deeply until you feel your abdomen expand, then slowly exhale. Repeat three more times. This is effective because when your diaphragm moves, it lowers your body's stress response.

Rub your tummy. Chronic conditions like IBS can create a vicious cycle when flare-ups are greeted with increased stress, tension, and anger toward a body that isn't behaving the way it's supposed to. A good exercise for breaking this pattern and focusing on healing your gut is to give yourself a 10- to 15-minute abdominal massage every day. To make a massage oil, mix ¼ teaspoon of lobelia oil or catnip tincture per 1 tablespoon of vegetable oil (any kind will do). Then begin at your belly button and massage in small, gentle, clockwise circles until you've covered your entire abdomen. Visualize your intestines relaxing and returning to their normal, healthy state.

Kidney Stones

Take a Stand against Sand

If you were experiencing kidney stone pain right now, you wouldn't be reading this book. You'd be on the floor, curled up in agony. Even though most kidney stones aren't much bigger than a grain of sand, every now and then one gets stuck in the narrow tubes, called ureters, that connect your kidneys and bladder. Or they irritate the urethra, the tube that carries urine out of the body. In either case, the pain can be excruciating.

According to the National Institutes of Health, about 1 in 10 of us will get kidney stones at some point in our lives. Chemicals and minerals that are normally present in urine sometimes solidify and form hard little crystals, or stones. Most are so tiny that they pass harmlessly through your

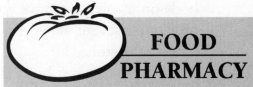

FOOD PHARMACY

Peel a Banana

Besides being just plain yummy, bananas help build a shield against kidney stones. They're packed with potassium, the mineral that can help prevent stones from forming, especially if you tend to get a lot of salt in your diet.

body without making you aware of their existence. Larger stones that get stuck, on the other hand, usually cause pain in the lower back or groin. Some people also experience nausea, blood in the urine, or an increased urge to urinate.

ROLL 'EM OUT

A kidney stone obviously isn't something to handle on your own; you need to see a doctor immediately. You'll probably need x-rays or other tests to determine exactly where the stone is. Once your doctor knows its location and size, there are a number of treatment options. He may recommend "watchful waiting"—giving the stone a little time to exit your body on its own—or give you medication to dissolve it. If the problem is severe, however, you'll probably need surgery to remove the stone.

Fortunately, your body is usually pretty good at getting rid of kidney stones. If you get them frequently, though, you need to find ways to minimize the pain—and more important, to keep them from coming back. Don't keep throwing money at specialists if you don't have to. Instead, try these tips and see if they help.

Drink up. Staying well hydrated should be a top priority for those who are stone-prone. Keeping enough water flowing through your system reduces the concentration of stone-forming minerals. Water can also help dissolve small stones that have already formed.

Heat up—or cool down. During a kidney stone attack, one of the best things you can do is apply an ice pack or a heating pad to your abdomen, lower back, or wherever you're feeling the pain. Either will take the edge off until you can get professional help.

Squeeze an orange. Anyone who's concerned about kidney stones will want to start the day with an orange or a tall glass of juice, then continue to eat oranges or quaff OJ throughout the day. The citrus fruit raises your body's level of citrates, natural chemicals that keep new stones from forming and existing stones from getting worse. Discuss this with your doctor first, though, since not all types of stones are affected by citrates.

Calm them with corn. Herbalists have traditionally recommended the herb cornsilk for kidney stones, and there's good evidence that it works. Cornsilk is a demulcent, which means that it coats and soothes irritated tissues in the body, including tissues in the urinary tract. Drink one or two cups of cornsilk tea daily when you're coping with kidney stones, advises Amy Turnbull, N.D., a naturopathic physician at the

HOLLER FOR HELP

Symptoms to Heed

Don't assume that everything's going to be fine if you've been diagnosed with kidney stones. While pain is normal, you shouldn't have fever, nausea, or vomiting, nor should the pain get significantly worse. If you experience any of these symptoms, call your doctor immediately. There's a good chance that the stone has caused an infection, and you may need antibiotics right away to keep it from getting worse.

Bastyr Center for Natural Health near Seattle. To make it, steep 1 teaspoon of herb in a cup of hot water for about 10 minutes, then strain and sip.

Take the produce express. You'll do yourself a big favor by adding more fiber to your diet. "People who have high-fiber diets are less likely to get stones," says Dr. Turnbull. You can get loads by filling up on fresh fruit and vegetables as well as legumes, whole grains, and high-fiber cereals. You want to get at least 20 grams of fiber a day, but 30 to 35 grams is even better.

Cork the bottle. Avoid alcohol when you're coping with a kidney stone. Its dehydrating effects will interfere with your body's ability to dissolve and flush the stone. The same goes for caffeine. Either will make you feel a lot more uncomfortable when your system is trying to eliminate one or more stones. "Caffeine increases activity in the nervous system, which can aggravate the pain," Dr. Turnbull adds.

Get a break with magnesium. The mineral magnesium relaxes muscles throughout your body, which can reduce pain during kidney stone attacks, says Dr. Turnbull. "Take 600 milligrams a day," she advises. This amount may cause diarrhea in some people, so if this occurs, reduce the dose.

Bring out the B$_6$. It hasn't been proven, but there's some evidence that people who don't get enough vitamin B$_6$ in their diets are more likely to get kidney stones, says Dr. Turnbull. If you've had stones in the past, an easy preventive strategy is to take a daily multivitamin that contains 100 percent of the Daily Value of B$_6$. Avoid individual B$_6$ supplements, however.

Get calcium the natural way. Some types of kidney stones are composed mainly of calcium. In the past, people who got these kinds of stones were advised to cut back on the mineral. Doctors now believe that the calcium you get from foods actually helps prevent kidney stones, although the calcium in supplements may make you more prone to them.

When you talk to your doctor, find out if your stones are the calcium variety. If they are, ask whether he recommends increasing or cutting back on calcium in your diet.

Ease them out. The herb cramp bark (viburnum) is a muscle relaxant that makes it easier for stones to move through your body. It's available at health food stores in many forms, including capsules, tinctures, and teas. Each product contains different amounts of the active ingredient, so follow the label directions to be sure you're taking the proper amount.

Take a tonic. Check the shelves at the health food store for gravelroot, stoneroot, and pellitory-of-the-wall. These herbs have long been used by herbalists as kidney tonics for people who are prone to developing stones. Make a tea by adding 1 tablespoon of each herb to 1 quart of hot water and steeping for 20 minutes. Drink it throughout the day for up to one week. Again, check the label directions before using any of these herbs. If you plan to use them for more than a few days, consult a naturopathic physician, who can advise you about their benefits and risks.

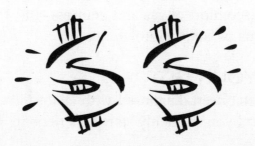

Lactose Intolerance

Drive the Devil Out of Dairy

Don't be fooled by those silly milk mustaches on sexy celebrities and models who are featured in the dairy industry's advertising campaigns. Chances are, they can't digest milk any better than you can.

Most people begin to lose their ability to digest milk and milk products at about age two, although they may not have symptoms until much later. It turns out that once our ancestors were weaned, they never got milk again, so the necessary enzyme to digest it—lactase—got programmed out of existence. And without lactase, milk can't be digested without the discomfort of gas and cramps—the main symptoms of lactose intolerance.

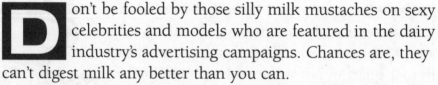

SOOTHE YOUR GUT

If you haven't been diagnosed with lactose intolerance, and you suddenly start experiencing digestive discomfort, check with your doctor; the symptoms are nearly identical to those caused by many other conditions, including irritable bowel syndrome and colitis. But if you know from experience that dairy puts you in these dumps, try these tips.

Heal with marshmallow. Marshmallow tea soothes inflamed tissues and helps heal the lining of the gut. Make a cold infusion by soaking 2 tablespoons of marshmallow root in 1 quart of cold water overnight. Strain and drink it throughout the day.

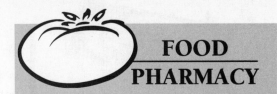

FOOD PHARMACY

Cocoa Comfort

If you have trouble digesting milk, stirring in a few teaspoons of cocoa may help, according to a study at the University of Rhode Island. Why? The cocoa may stimulate an enzyme that breaks down the lactose in milk that may be responsible for your bloating and gas.

Ferment and feel better. Traditional nomadic peoples, who continued to use dairy products as a food source beyond infancy, cultured their milk products to make them more easily digestible. If you are lactose intolerant, you may be able to handle fermented dairy products (such as yogurt and kefir) and perhaps even goat's- or sheep's-milk cheeses. If your lactose intolerance is severe, however, it's best to omit milk from your diet completely.

Look for hidden lactose. Many foods contain milk solids as filler. If you're especially sensitive to lactose, these can cause you discomfort if you ingest enough, so read food labels carefully and search out lactose-free products instead.

Have cookies with your milk. Studies have found that eating other foods with a dairy product increases the likelihood that the lactose can sneak into your body without bothering your gut.

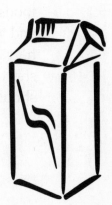

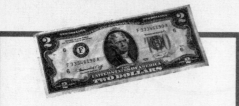

The $2 Deal

An Excellent Enzyme

Lactaid, along with several other over-the-counter products, does the work of natural lactase. Just drop a caplet in a glass of milk, then guzzle the moo juice. Follow the package directions to take it before eating cheese, sour cream, and other high-lactose foods. Your bones will benefit from the calcium, and you can enjoy your favorite Ben & Jerry's without uncomfortable after-effects.

Shop for substitutes. Look around until you find as many lactose-free products as you can—or products that are supplemented with extra lactase. There is now a brand of yogurt with added lactase, for instance. You can also buy lactose-free cheese that melts just like real American cheese. Pop it under the broiler, and you'll have a melted cheese sandwich, a tuna-cheese melt, or a baked potato topped with cheese.

Get some great recipes. Check out the Internet for sites such as www.lactaid.com, where you'll find many recipes and menu ideas to help you enjoy dairy-free living.

Replace the calcium. Because milk is such a rich source of calcium and vitamin D—major dietary bone builders—you need to find those nutrients elsewhere if you're avoiding dairy foods. Eat plenty of dark green, leafy vegetables and almonds, and add fatty fish like salmon and herring to your diet, too. If you're still coming up short on these bone basics, ask your doctor if you should take calcium supplements.

Laryngitis

Give Your Pipes Some Peace

Maybe you were a little too enthusiastic on the soccer sidelines, yelling your lungs out at your daughter's great plays. Or maybe you had a little too much fun at the pub, shouting across the table and doing your always-popular rendition of "New York, New York." But when you woke up, you felt like you had tacks in the back of your throat, and instead of "Good morning," you said something like, "Grroo...murgh."

Blame laryngitis, an inflammation of the vocal cords. It sometimes results from an infection, but usually it's simply a consequence of using your voice too much. Check with your doctor if it doesn't go away within a few days to a week. In the meantime, try these tips to start sounding like yourself again.

Give your voice a break. The most effective treatment is silence. Don't use your voice at all—not even for whispering. Trying to express yourself in squeaks and croaks just aggravates your inflamed vocal cords, actually causing them to bang together and slow your recovery.

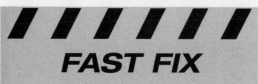
A red sage tea gargle can ease the mucous membranes of your larynx and boost your immune system. Pour 1 cup of warm water over 1 teaspoon of red sage and steep for 10 minutes. Strain, then gargle.

Suck in some steam. If you have an extreme case of laryngitis, try resting in a warm room with high humidity for a day or two. Use a humidifier if necessary, and let your worn-out throat soak up some moisture while you sleep.

Alleviate with elm. Slippery elm is used by professional singers and speakers to recover their voices and keep their laryngeal tissues in tiptop shape. To make a tea, steep 1 heaping teaspoon of dried herb in 1 cup of hot water for 15 minutes. Strain, add honey and lemon if you like, and drink three or four cups per day.

Take your thyme. An herbal steam can help soothe respiratory passages and alleviate laryngitis pain. Put 3 or 4 drops of thyme oil in a bowl of steaming hot water. Bend over the bowl—but not close enough to burn your face—and tent your head and the bowl with a towel. Breathe in deeply.

Calm a cough. The more you cough, the more you irritate your sensitive larynx. If your cough is dry and unproductive, use an over-the-counter cough suppressant such as dextromethorphan to keep your larynx from further harm. Follow the package directions.

It's a wrap! Place a warm, wet, cloth compress on your neck for 2 to 3 minutes, then replace it with a cold one. Wrap a wool scarf around your neck to keep the cold compress in place for 30 minutes.

Aim for the middle. Drink lots of water or tea, but

keep it tepid—not too hot or too cold, either of which could further inflame your vocal cords.

Keep it bland. When your throat is under siege by laryngitis, be wary of what you put down it. Avoid very spicy foods, hot soups and beverages, and any other edible irritants.

Back away from the butts. The most serious cause of laryngitis is long-term smoking. If you haven't been convinced by now that smoking is a major health risk, let the damage to your delicate vocal cords motivate you. Look into all the aids to help you quit—from prescription medications and nicotine gum to group therapy. Ask your doctor to help you find the right method for you.

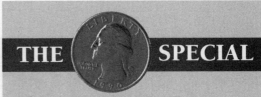

THE SPECIAL

The Carrot Cure

A carrot neck wrap may ease inflammation and help you recover your voice more quickly. Grate a carrot onto a length of cheesecloth, fold the cloth in half lengthwise, and moisten it with warm water. Wrap it around your neck, then wrap your neck with a warm towel. Leave it on for 20 to 30 minutes. For extra heat, sprinkle some red pepper on the grated carrot.

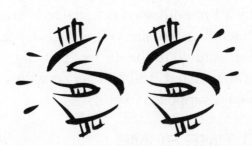

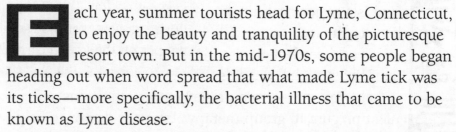

Lyme Disease

Quick Tips to Lick the Ticks

Each year, summer tourists head for Lyme, Connecticut, to enjoy the beauty and tranquility of the picturesque resort town. But in the mid-1970s, some people began heading out when word spread that what made Lyme tick was its ticks—more specifically, the bacterial illness that came to be known as Lyme disease.

Actually, Lyme disease has been around for a long time, and despite all the media hoopla, it's usually not that serious. If you're bitten by a Lyme-infected tick, bacteria enter your bloodstream. You may notice telltale symptoms, such as a red bull's-eye on your skin, and go to the doctor. You take antibiotics for a week or two. You're cured, and you get on with your life. At least, that's how it's supposed to go.

A TICKING TIME BOMB

Many people who are infected with Lyme disease have localized symptoms at first, such as pain and swelling at the site of the bite. As the infection spreads, they may experience more widespread symptoms, such as pain in their muscles and joints, fever, fatigue, and stiffness.

Here's the tricky part, though. These lingering symptoms may occur soon after the bite, or they may take years to develop. You may or may not experience localized pain. And without prompt treatment, Lyme disease can cause arthritis-like aches and pains, along with muscle stiffness. Some people develop neurological problems, such as confusion and forgetfulness.

TAKE CHARGE

You'll want to check with your doctor if you even suspect you have Lyme disease. Once you've been diagnosed, the treatment almost always includes antibiotics, but sometimes that's not enough by itself. You'll also need to take steps to make yourself more comfortable while the drugs do their work—and to make sure you never get the disease again. Here's what you should do.

Give yourself a hand. One of the best home remedies for the aches and pains of Lyme disease is to thoroughly rub the affected areas. Better yet, have someone else do the massage for you.

"Massaging painful muscle groups can help," says Sam Donta, M.D., an infectious disease specialist and professor of medicine at Boston University School of Medicine. Just be gentle, he adds. Your muscles and joints will be pretty sore, and an aggressive massage will hurt too much to enjoy.

Stay active. The pain and fatigue of Lyme disease can make

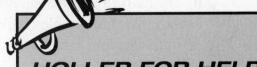

HOLLER FOR HELP

Time Counts

If you've been in tick territory, and you have some combination of Lyme symptoms—fatigue, fever, joint pain, and so on— don't take chances, says Sam Donta, M.D. Go to a doctor and request a Lyme test. The quicker you're diagnosed and treated, the less likely you'll be to have long-term problems.

it very hard to stay active; even walking across a room can seem like an insurmountable challenge. Don't give up. You have to do as much as your condition allows, says Dr. Donta. The more active you are, the more quickly you'll regain your energy. You'll even experience less pain.

Push the envelope. Once you have some momentum going with your exercise, gradually increase the challenge. "Increase the activity week after week," Dr. Donta says. You don't have to push yourself to exhaustion, though; just walk a little farther or stay on your feet a little longer. It will keep your muscles strong and make it easier to recover.

Add recovery time. You want your body to use as much of its energy as possible to fight the bacteria coursing through your blood. Do whatever you have to do to reduce the physical and emotional stress in your life.

This could mean taking a relaxing bath every day. It could mean taking naps, working fewer hours, or going to bed earlier at night. Your body has a big job ahead of it, and you want to make it easier for your natural resources to work in your favor.

Try heat—or cold. Lyme is notorious for causing symptoms that wax and wane. You may feel fine one day and totally awful the next. When you're feeling achy or tired, you may want to experiment with cold or heat treatments. Neither is best; different people respond in different ways.

For example, apply a cold pack or ice cubes wrapped in a small towel to an achy joint or muscle. Hold it in place for about 20 minutes, then repeat the treatment throughout the day. If that doesn't seem to help, try a heating pad set on low instead. Once you figure out which approach works for you, use it for soothing relief whenever symptoms are threatening to lay you low.

Don't bother with supplements. You may hear from friends or slick-looking advertisements that supplemental amounts of nutrients, especially B vitamins, are good for Lyme disease. Forget it, Dr. Donta says. For one thing, the bacterium that causes Lyme disease doesn't produce its own B vitamins; supplemental amounts could be just what it needs to keep going.

In fact, some scientists speculate that extra amounts of any nutrient could make Lyme disease worse, or at least increase recovery time. Until you're better, it's a good idea to stay away from supplements altogether.

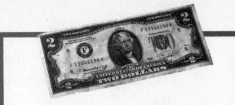

The $2 Deal

Give Thanks to St. John's

If Lyme disease is making your muscles ache, give yourself a rubdown with St. John's wort, a traditional treatment for both nerve pain and muscle soreness. Buy some St. John's wort oil at a health food store and add 6 to 12 drops to an ounce of olive or almond oil, then rub it on.

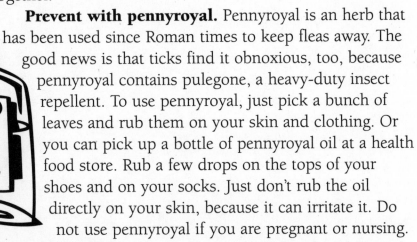

Prevent with pennyroyal. Pennyroyal is an herb that has been used since Roman times to keep fleas away. The good news is that ticks find it obnoxious, too, because pennyroyal contains pulegone, a heavy-duty insect repellent. To use pennyroyal, just pick a bunch of leaves and rub them on your skin and clothing. Or you can pick up a bottle of pennyroyal oil at a health food store. Rub a few drops on the tops of your shoes and on your socks. Just don't rub the oil directly on your skin, because it can irritate it. Do not use pennyroyal if you are pregnant or nursing.

Repel the suckers. Before you go into tick-infested areas, spray your clothes with an insect repellent that contains DEET. Read the label to be sure the bug spray you select targets ticks.

Take the middle of the road. When you're hiking in the woods, stay in the center of the trail. That way, you'll avoid brushing against trees and shrubs and be less likely to attract ticks.

Pull it fast. The quicker you remove a feeding tick, the less likely you'll be to get infected. Grasp it firmly with fine-pointed tweezers and pull straight up—not at an angle—or the head may break off and stay embedded, warns Joseph Piesman, D.Sc., chief of the Centers for Disease Control and Prevention's Lyme disease section. The tick will still be alive, so seal it in a vial or wrap it in tape before disposing of it.

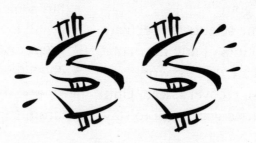

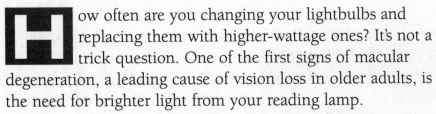

Macular Degeneration

Strategies to Save Your Sight

How often are you changing your lightbulbs and replacing them with higher-wattage ones? It's not a trick question. One of the first signs of macular degeneration, a leading cause of vision loss in older adults, is the need for brighter light from your reading lamp.

Macular degeneration tends to be mild at first. You may notice a bit of blurring when you try to read fine print, for example. With the passage of time, though, you gradually lose central vision due to degeneration of the macula, a tiny bull's-eye point at the center of the retina. By age 65, about 15 percent of us will have some macular degeneration; by age 75, the prevalence more than doubles, to nearly 33 percent.

VISION PRESERVERS

While macular degeneration is a serious condition that needs a doctor's attention, there are many ways to prevent it—without having to whip out your credit card. Here's what the experts recommend.

Avoid Ol' Sol. Wear proper sunglasses and a brimmed hat, and avoid the sun during the peak hours of 10:00 A.M. to 2:00 P.M. Also, make sure your sunglasses provide 100 percent protection from ultraviolet light. Buy glasses with the darkest possible lens color. Brown and tan offer the best balance of comfort and protection, with gray and green second best.

Pass the peppers. Bell peppers, especially the red type, pack a powerful punch of lutein and zeaxanthin. These two key plant compounds may play a role in preventing age-related macular degeneration.

Toss a salad. All fruits and vegetables contain antioxidants, chemicals that counteract the oxidative wear and tear that's always going on in your body and are especially important for preventing macular degeneration, says Alex Eaton, M.D., an ophthalmologist and retina specialist in Fort Myers, Florida. Because the macula in the eye contains a protective pigment made up of antioxidants, you need to replenish it with antioxidants found in food and supplements to offset the breakdown.

Go for the green. All produce is good, but kale, spinach, and chard are tops for protecting your

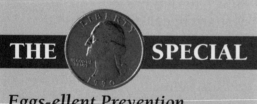

THE SPECIAL

Eggs-ellent Prevention

Lutein and zeaxanthin, the two carotenoids that are critical for preventing age-related macular degeneration, are found in eggs as well as produce, and studies show that your body absorbs them more easily from eggs than from other foods. Scramble to the kitchen and cook yourself some eggs today.

eyes. Why? They're loaded with the pigment lutein, which, in the eyes, helps filter out the light implicated in macular degeneration. A study by the National Eye Institute found that foods rich in lutein and zeaxanthin were associated with reduced risk of macular degeneration.

Go slow on fast food. Avoid those bacon cheeseburgers and other high-fat foods. Just as fat can block the arteries of your heart, it can also clog those that go to your eyes, reducing the flow of blood and nutrients to your retinas. In fact, studies reveal that many of the same factors that lead to atherosclerosis also contribute to the development of macular degeneration.

Kick the smokes. Smoking increases your risk of developing macular degeneration by two to six times, warns Dr. Eaton. It does so by depriving your retina of oxygen and constricting your blood vessels, making it more difficult for nutrients to be carried through those vessels to your eyes. Get help today to overcome this addiction.

Get ginkgo. This herb increases microcirculation in the eyes and enhances the activity of antioxidants. Make an infusion of ginkgo and bilberry (another eye-friendly herb) by steeping 1 heaping teaspoon of each in hot water for 15 minutes. Strain and drink two or three cups daily. If you are taking blood-thinning medications,

HOLLER FOR HELP

Don't Wait—Get Tested

Any abrupt change in vision should be checked by an ophthalmologist. Symptoms of macular degeneration can also be detected during routine ophthalmological checkups, so don't wait until things are all blurry before making an appointment. Get checked at least once a year. If you have several relatives with macular degeneration, ask for retinal examinations starting at age 40.

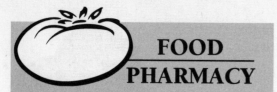

FOOD PHARMACY

Shop for Orange

Your mother was right: Carrots really are good for your eyes, and so are other orange and yellow vegetables and fruits. They are all rich sources of beta-carotene, the plant-based building block for vitamin A, so add some carrots, squash, and pumpkin to your menu, along with plenty of greens.

though, don't use ginkgo without your doctor's okay.

Fish for chowder. An Australian study found that omega-3 fatty acids may help reduce the risk of macular degeneration. Study participants who ate fresh or frozen fish one to three times a month had about half the risk of macular degeneration compared with those who ate fish less often. To make a basic chowder, first cube two white potatoes, slice two large carrots, dice one onion, and cut at least 1 pound of fish into bite-size pieces. Place the ingredients in a large saucepan and add seafood seasoning (Old Bay is good) to taste. Add enough water to cover, plus an inch more. Bring the water to a boil, then simmer until the veggies are cooked and the fish is opaque.

Soothe the strain. Warm compresses made with an infusion of chamomile or eyebright may help relieve eye strain from macular degeneration. Steep 1 teaspoon of either herb in 1 cup of hot water, covered, for 10 to 15 minutes. Strain, then saturate a clean cloth or gauze pad with the cooled solution. Cover your eyes and rest for 20 minutes.

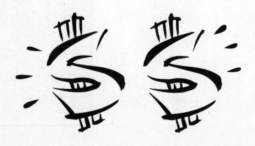

Memory Problems

Keep Your Mind Sharp

Most of us fear losing our mental abilities more than anything else that could conceivably happen with age. Okay, we could give up marathon running, walk with a cane or two, or even sport a hearing aid—but lose our brain power? Yikes!

The good news is, we can be forgetful for many reasons other than incipient Alzheimer's disease. Forgetfulness at midlife is more often a result of being busy, stressed, or short on sleep. Estrogen loss in menopause may have some small effect, as can too much caffeine or a drop in blood sugar levels. Clinical depression is a frequent cause of forgetfulness. And then there are some things that we may just not want to remember.

MANAGE YOUR MIND POWER

Just as we clean out our filing cabinets, we do the same with our mind's "memory files." Some things just become less important over time. Here's how to keep those memory files from disappearing too soon.

Eat "smart" berries. Researchers at Tufts University uncovered the first hint that blueberries may help reverse short-term memory loss. First, they divided older rats into four groups, then gave one group their usual diet and the others supplements of blueberry, strawberry, or spinach extract. By far, the blueberry group outperformed all the others on memory tests.

Now scientists are working to isolate the memory-boosting compounds in blueberries and test them on humans. In the meantime, eat blueberries so you'll remember to eat blueberries!

Have a bunch with lunch. Studies suggest that grapes contain chemical compounds that may help ward off memory loss and improve motor skills.

Sweeten your memory banks. Memory loss is most often attributed to low blood sugar and fatigue. Be sure to eat nutritious, well-balanced meals—especially a good breakfast of protein and complex carbohydrates, such as whole grain cereals and breads. You may find that your spells of forgetfulness come less often.

Fill your plate with pasta. An Italian study of diet and cognitive decline reported in the journal *Neurology* found that cognitive impairment was less common among elderly people who ate a Mediterranean diet, which includes lots of olive oil— a monounsaturated fat. As their "healthy fat" intake increased, their risk of memory problems declined.

When you cook, swap saturated, brain-fogging fats such as butter and marbled meats for healthy monounsaturated fats such as olive and canola oils. Use them not only on pasta but also in salad dressings and hearty soups.

Get your folate fix. If you don't get enough folate (the natural form of folic acid), your brain could atrophy, according to a recent study. Folate, as well as vitamins B_6 and B_{12}, may keep your gray matter going by keeping homocysteine levels in check. (Elevated homocysteine, a byproduct of methionine metabolism, is associated with Alzheimer's disease.) Pad your diet with folate-rich orange juice, broccoli and other cruciferous veggies, avocados, and legumes. Meat, poultry, whole grains, and green leafy vegetables provide vitamin B_6, and vitamin B_{12} is found mostly in meat.

Bet on beans. Along with egg yolks and cabbage, they're rich in lecithin, which produces chemicals that act as messengers for our thoughts and memories. We also need minerals such as magnesium, potassium, and boron, which are important for mental alertness. Millet, dark leafy greens (such as collards, kale, and broccoli), and figs are full of these minerals.

Get extra E. As reported in the journal *Neurology*, doctors at New York City's Weill-Cornell Women's Health Center concluded that supplements of vitamin E and C had a significant protective effect against vascular dementia (loss of cogni-

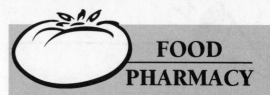

FOOD PHARMACY

Forget Less with Good Fats

Brain cells are 60 percent fat, which is needed to transmit the impulses that carry thought. In a healthy brain, omega-3 fatty acids predominate; in fact, low levels of omega-3's have been linked to depression and the risk of Alzheimer's disease. How do you get these healthy fatty acids? They're plentiful in oily fish (such as tuna and salmon), walnuts, and flaxseed. To benefit your whole body, add a handful of nuts, a serving of fish, or 2 tablespoons of freshly ground flaxseed to your diet every day.

HOLLER FOR HELP

Mind the Warning Signs

It's normal to occasionally forget names or phone numbers, but it shouldn't happen all at once—and it shouldn't interfere with your ability to live a normal life. If you're suddenly having memory lapses or experiencing mental confusion, see your doctor right away. Many physical problems, including low blood pressure, artery disease, and nutritional deficiencies, can make your mind slip.

tive function due to atherosclerosis). The study subjects performed better on tests, too. And in another study, vitamin E slowed the mental decline of patients with Alzheimer's disease.

Stop the stress. Chronic stress makes your adrenal glands pump out cortisol, a hormone that can lead to difficulty retrieving long-term memories, according to a study reported in the journal *Nature Neuroscience*. Cortisol overload is associated with memory problems, fuzzy thinking, and difficulty in concentrating and making decisions. Do all you can to control the stress in your life—and consider some counseling if you just can't seem to relax.

Get your feet moving. If you're serious about getting your exercise, you're more likely to be mentally sharp, too, since physical activity boosts the production of brain chemicals. A study of sedentary people who began taking brisk walks showed that they improved in both mental agility and concentration. So add a brisk daily walk to your routine. When your brain is well supplied with oxygen, it will remember more—and the rest of you will feel better, too.

Challenge your mind. According to the Weill-Cornell Women's Health Center, studies of healthy people suggest that ongoing mental stimulation—such as work, continuing education, extensive reading, mentally challenging games, and crossword puzzles—can keep your mind sharp. Scores of laboratory studies link mental activity and the production of protective neuro-trophins. Even Alzheimer's disease is less common among the well educated (although many smart people do get it). The explanation? Mentally active folks may have increased brain reserves, more neu-rons, and a more complex, cell-to-cell commu-nication system to draw on if some brain cells sustain damage. So take out the chess board (or learn if you've never played), write in a journal, or design that great gadget you've been thinking about.

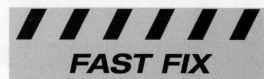

FAST FIX
Get Your Mind Minerals

Keep losing your keys? Forget where you wrote that important telephone number? Studies have shown that deficiencies of iron and zinc can interfere with concentra-tion. Boost your brain power by eating a serving of beans a few times a week—they're loaded with both minerals.

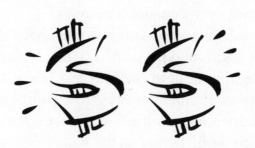

Menstrual Pain

Smooth Out Your Cycle

Women used to refer to monthly periods as "the curse." It sounds almost ridiculous today, but it's easy to understand why a term usually used in relation to mummies and witchcraft came to summarize the clockwork fluctuations of a woman's hormones.

More than half of menstruating women have menstruation-related cramps and low-back pain. The discomfort may begin before any bleeding, peak in the next few hours, then usually stop in a day or two. The intensity of the pain, known as dysmenorrhea, varies among women and can even vary for the same woman from one period to the next.

Cramps are caused by uterine contractions, and many of the accompanying symptoms, such as fatigue, headaches, and bloating, are thought to be due to an imbalance of the hormones estrogen and progesterone. Usually, progesterone is the dominant hormone following ovulation. An excess of estrogen or a deficiency of progesterone can trigger discomfort.

KILL THE CRAMPS

If you have severe menstrual cramps or changes in your normal flow, you need to see a doctor. Most women, however, don't need cutting-edge medical technology to feel better. There are plenty of strategies for handling the pain, and many of them have been working for women for centuries. Here are a few of the best.

Trust OTCs. Aspirin and other nonsteroidal anti-inflammatory drugs are inexpensive and very effective for treating cramps. They block the production of prostaglandins, body chemicals that cause uterine contractions, says Mary Ellen Mortensen, M.D., executive director for medical affairs at McNeil Consumer Healthcare in Ontario.

Take the standard dose of two caplets every 4 to 6 hours, but no more than 8 in 24 hours, says Dr. Mortensen.

Put fish on the menu. Anti-inflammatory compounds are also abundant in seafood. Have a daily serving of oil-rich fish, such as sardines, salmon, or cod, to help reduce your symptoms.

Avoid processed foods. The more fresh fruits, vegetables, and whole grains you eat, the less room there will be in your diet for packaged and processed foods. That means you'll cut out a lot of sodium, which will reduce the dis-

FAST FIX
Move Your Belly

If you've ever had an urge to explore the culture of the Middle East, here's your excuse: The movements taught in belly dancing are great for stretching your pelvis and keeping cramps at bay. "Belly dancing can be very helpful," says Jana Nalbandian, N.D. "Any exercise that gets you moving and rocking your pelvis will help."

comfort of water retention and bloating. It also means that you'll eat fewer animal-based saturated fats, which have been linked to pain and inflammation. Plus, you'll get plenty of complex carbohydrates, which will keep your blood sugar levels steady and your mood on an even keel. Consider your supermarket's produce department to be your personal garden of eatin'.

Crank up the calcium. This mineral was voted by women as one of the top treatments for premenstrual syndrome because it can soothe cramps, low-back pain, bloating, food cravings, and mood swings all at once, says Mary Hardy, M.D., medical director of the Cedars-Sinai Integrative Medicine Medical Group in New York City. Try taking 1,000 milligrams a day.

Magnesium helps, too, but you might want to go easy on it (stick with 200 milligrams once or twice a day) because too much can give you diarrhea.

Bump up the Bs. "The big vitamin for premenstrual problems is vitamin B_6," says Jana Nalbandian, N.D., a naturopathic physician and faculty member at Bastyr University near Seattle. It seems to have a positive effect on levels of serotonin, a feel-good chemical in the brain. Make sure it's in your one-a-day multi.

Alternate heat and cold. You

HOLLER FOR HELP

Catch Bad Cramps

Certain types of cramps may signal a serious medical problem, such as endometriosis or fibroid tumors, that has nothing to do with menstruation. See your doctor if cramps don't disappear after your period ends; if the pain is on only one side rather than the entire abdomen; or if you don't get relief from aspirin, ibuprofen, or related drugs.

can unkink menstrual cramps with compresses made by soaking washcloths in hot and cold water. First, place a hot compress on your abdomen for about 3 minutes. Replace it with a cold compress left in place for 30 seconds. Repeat the cycle two more times, always ending with cold. This simple technique is a very effective way to increase blood flow, which in turn reduces cramps.

Ease with oil. A castor oil pack is a traditional way to ease the pain of menstrual cramps. First, spread castor oil on the skin of your abdomen and cover it with a layer of plastic wrap. Then heat the area with a warm, moist towel or a heating pad set on low. The gentle heat penetrates deeply into your abdomen and relaxes muscles as well as cramps. One caveat: Don't use this remedy if you have heavy bleeding.

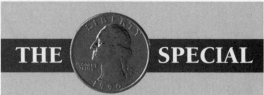

THE ![coin] SPECIAL

Munch Pumpkin Seeds

They're loaded with essential fatty acids (EFAs) that lower levels of body chemicals responsible for muscle aches and menstrual cramps. You can get the same oils by eating ground flaxseed or cold-water fish, such as salmon and tuna. Plan on having at least one of these foods daily when your symptoms are flaring up. Or, unless you're taking aspirin or prescription blood thinners, you can take EFA capsules or liquids, available in health food stores.

Experiment with exercise. Studies show that exercise eases premenstrual and menstrual symptoms, but a high-impact workout may be uncomfortable if you're cramping. Take it easy for a few days and stick to low-impact forms of exercise, such as yoga, swimming, or tai chi.

Stretch like a cat. "Yoga's great for menstrual problems because it's relaxing, and it increases circulation," says Dr. Nalbandian. One yoga pose in particular, called the Cat, is especially helpful because it targets the abdominal area. Get on your hands and knees on the floor.

Tea Time

Rave for Raspberry

Red raspberry is a uterine tonic that may help relieve cramping and pelvic congestion. To make a tea, steep 1 heaping teaspoon of raspberry leaves in 1 cup of hot water for 10 minutes, then strain. Drink one or two cups daily. Tonic herbs such as raspberry are best taken every day for several weeks.

Moving slowly and gently, tilt your pelvis and tailbone toward the floor while arching your back toward the ceiling. Hold the stretch for a few moments, then go the opposite way: Tilt your pelvis upward and let your spine curve toward the floor.

Try the Child's Pose. This is another yoga move that's good for menstrual discomfort. Kneel on the floor, then sit back on your heels. Lean forward, gently lowering your chest until it's resting on your thighs. Extend your arms in front of you until your palms touch the floor. Hold the pose for as long as you're comfortable, then slowly return to the kneeling position. It's very relaxing—and good for you, too!

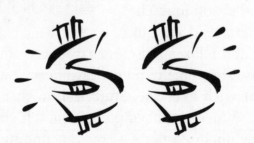

Migraines

Head Off Head Pain

It's true that migraines are a type of headache, but they really don't belong in the same category as garden-variety tension headaches. It's almost impossible to exaggerate how awful migraines can make you feel.

About 26 million Americans get migraines, and women are more prone than men to these miserable skull busters. They occur when blood vessels in your scalp dilate, or expand, and press against nearby nerves. Intense, throbbing pain is just one part of the picture. Many people are so nauseated during migraine attacks that they can't leave the bathroom. They may experience "auras"—sparkling flashes of light or zigzag lines in their field of vision. They may also have weakness or tingling in the face or other parts of the body. It's common for migraines to persist for hours—and sometimes even days.

ALLAY THE AGONY

It's generally fine to take ibuprofen at the first sign of a migraine. Over-the-counter treatments are surprisingly

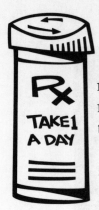

effective as long as you take them before the migraine really gets under way. Even if you have only "simple" migraines, you should talk to your doctor at some point. There are a number of prescription drugs that can stop migraines within minutes, and there are other treatments that can help keep them from recurring.

Most people with migraines, however, don't have to spend a fortune on medical care. There are plenty of effective home-care approaches that can reduce your need for high-powered medications. Here are some you may want to try.

Beware the rebound. A paradoxical thing about migraines is that the same treatments that make you feel better can also make things worse. If you take a lot of aspirin or other medication to control migraines, the pain may come back, or rebound, even more severely as soon as the medication wears off. The natural response is to take more medication, and the cycle continues.

Obviously, you shouldn't stop taking a prescription drug without checking with your doctor first, but don't automatically reach for the aspirin or ibuprofen the next time you feel a migraine coming on. You may aggravate your migraines in the long run.

Take a break. Lie down immediately in a cool, dark place when you feel a migraine coming on. Moving around will only intensify the pain.

Try the caffeine-and-aspirin combo. The combination of 130 milligrams of caffeine (that's about 1½ cups of coffee) and two aspirins relieves a headache 40 per-

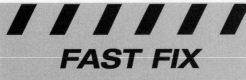

FAST FIX
Ice Is Nice

One of the quickest ways to reduce throbbing migraine pain is to put a cold pack against the part of your head that hurts. Keep it in place for about 10 minutes. Cold shrinks blood vessels and helps reduce the pounding.

cent better than the pain reliever alone, according to the National Headache Foundation. In addition to starting your motor in the mornings, caffeine helps your body absorb medications. You'll feel the full effects within 30 minutes, and they'll last from 3 to 5 hours. Some headache remedies already contain caffeine, so be sure to check the ingredients—you may need to take fewer pain relievers if you take them with coffee.

Starve your migraine. Many people with migraines find their attacks are connected to what they eat and start 1 to 24 hours after a meal. Trigger foods include alcoholic beverages, particularly red wines and beer; aged cheeses; smoked fish; sour cream; yogurt; and, alas, chocolate, even though some people crave it just before an attack. Food additives and preservatives such as monosodium glutamate (MSG) and sodium nitrate (often found in lunch meats) are known triggers, as are sweeteners containing aspartame.

To figure out if food's fueling your headaches, keep a simple diary. Write down what you eat and when, as well as when your headaches occur. You'll spot the connections. And eating regularly, three times a day, may also help fend off migraines.

Strike out against stress. A stressful situation can trigger a migraine immediately afterward—

HOLLER FOR HELP

Pain Signals

If migraine pain doesn't retreat fairly quickly, you'll want to see your doctor. This is especially true if you've had a recent head injury, if the pain occurs on both sides of your head, or if it's accompanied by difficulty speaking or mental confusion. Migraines can be a symptom of serious underlying problems, such as a brain tumor or blood vessel damage.

it's called a "letdown" migraine. If you are living a migraine lifestyle, you need to take stress reduction seriously. One way to do that is to take up regular aerobic exercise, such as walking, swimming, or bicycling. Besides taming stress, it helps maintain healthy circulation, which can also head off migraines. Whatever activity you choose, do it for 20 to 30 minutes every day, and you'll be healthier all over. Be sure to check with your doctor before you start any exercise program.

Pamper your feet. Reflexology is a type of massage therapy in which pressure is applied to places on the feet that are believed to influence other parts of the body. Find a reflexology practitioner and give the treatment a try—it may just be the answer to your desperate migraine prayers. In a Danish study, regular reflexology treatments helped 81 percent of the participants find relief from their migraines. One-fifth were even able to go off their pain medication.

Eliminate the triggers. Most migraines are triggered by external factors. Everyone's different, so you'll have to be a bit of a detective to identify the things that tend to bring them on. "Many people

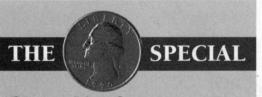

THE **SPECIAL**

Ginger: It's a Snap

Here's a time-tested kitchen cure for coping with migraines: Spice up your diet with ginger. This pungent root appears to help keep blood vessels from dilating and pressing against sensitive nerves, says Terri Dallas-Prunskis, M.D., codirector of the Illinois Pain Treatment Institute in Chicago. Even small amounts of ginger seem to be effective, she adds. You can start by adding fresh or powdered ginger to stews, rice dishes, soups, and even fresh green salads.

have more than one trigger," adds Seymour Diamond, M.D., director of the Diamond Headache Clinic in Chicago. Besides foods, common triggers include bright lights, changes in altitude, and even certain odors. Pay close attention to your environment when you feel a migraine beginning, suggests Dr. Diamond. Over time, you'll start to identify patterns, activities, or specific things that seem to bring them on.

Live by the clock. Try to go to bed and get up at the same times every day. You may even want to eat and exercise at regular times. "Keeping a regular schedule is best for most people with migraines," says David C. Haas, M.D., a headache specialist in the department of neurology at SUNY Upstate Medical University in Syracuse. "Being overtired can trigger migraines," he adds, "and so can being hungry because you skipped a meal."

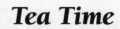

Tea Time

Nature's Aspirin

The herb willow bark contains salicin, which metabolizes in the body like aspirin, its synthetic cousin. To help calm a migraine, pick up some dried bark at a health food store, then follow the package directions to brew up some soothing tea. Don't use this herb if you're sensitive to aspirin, and don't combine it with aspirin or alcohol.

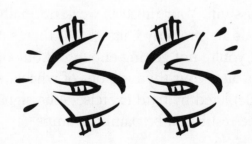

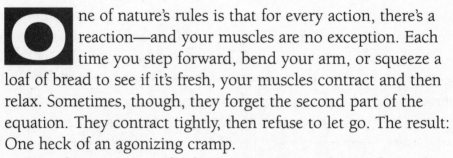

Muscle Cramps

Loosen the Vise

One of nature's rules is that for every action, there's a reaction—and your muscles are no exception. Each time you step forward, bend your arm, or squeeze a loaf of bread to see if it's fresh, your muscles contract and then relax. Sometimes, though, they forget the second part of the equation. They contract tightly, then refuse to let go. The result: One heck of an agonizing cramp.

Muscles contract and relax in response to electrical signals generated by electrolytes—minerals such as magnesium, calcium, and potassium. Your muscles work normally when levels of these minerals are properly balanced. If there's an imbalance—because you're not getting enough of one or more electrolytes in your diet, your thyroid's out of whack, or the minerals have been depleted by hard exercise—the signals essentially get crossed. The result can be painful cramps.

FIX IT QUICK

Muscle cramps rarely last more than a few seconds, but they're not something you want to put up with. For one thing, they're excruciatingly painful. More important, cramps that happen at the wrong time—when you're at the deep end of the pool, for example—can be dangerous. The next time you're clamped by a cramp, try one of these tips to get out of its grip.

Help the muscle move. A painful muscle cramp will eventually relax on its own, but the sooner you encourage it to do so, the sooner you'll get relief. Since the cramped muscle can't move itself, you'll need to use a free hand to straighten the affected leg, arm, or foot. Gently pull the muscle in the opposite direction from the cramp. Doing this a few times will usually relax the muscle and ease the pain.

Rub out the pain. Some firm fingerwork will almost always ease a cramped muscle, says Ellen Potthoff, N.D., D.C., a naturopathic physician and chiropractor in Martinez, California. "During a cramp, muscle fibers stay contracted and forget how to relax," she explains. Massaging the cramped area will break up the contraction and loosen the muscle again.

Put minerals in the bank. Your muscles need healthful amounts of calcium, potassium, and magnesium to function properly. If your stores of these electrolytes have been depleted by exercise or a poor diet, your muscles will become much more prone to cramping. To prevent this, your best bet is to take a daily multivitamin/mineral supplement that contains these and other important minerals.

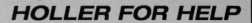

HOLLER FOR HELP
The Cholesterol Connection

If you're taking cholesterol-lowering medication, report any muscle aches, pains, or cramps to your doctor immediately. They can indicate a rare, life-threatening condition in which muscle—including heart muscle—is being destroyed as a side effect of your medication.

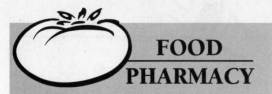

FOOD PHARMACY

Eat Green

The greener your midnight snack, the less likely you are to be rudely awakened by middle-of-the-night cramps. Leafy green vegetables, such as spinach, okra, and turnip and beet greens, are chock-full of cramp-stopping electrolytes—especially magnesium, potassium, and calcium. A daily salad or stir-fry that includes these ingredients should keep cramps at bay.

Soothe with sour. Hot vinegar is great for relaxing cramped muscles. Mix equal parts of water and vinegar in a saucepan, heat until comfortably hot, and soak a small towel in the solution. Wring it out and hold it against the painful area for 5 minutes, then replace it with a towel that's been soaked in cold water. Repeat the cycle three times, keeping the hot towel in place for 5 minutes and the cold towel in place for 1 minute, and always end with the cold treatment. By the time you're done, the cramp should be gone, or at least feel a lot better.

Gulp a sports drink. Drinks such as Gatorade contain the minerals that your muscles need to function properly. If your cramps are caused by a lack of nutrients, a swig of a sports beverage before and during exercise could prevent them from occurring (or recurring).

Stretch it out. Stretching your muscles before you exercise is essential if you want to prevent cramping. It's especially important if you haven't been active for a while.

Water your muscles. Muscles that aren't properly hydrated are more prone to cramping. "People should drink at least six to eight glasses of water a day, and more if they're going to be sweating heavily," says Dr. Potthoff. Don't wait until you're thirsty to drink, though; by the time you start to feel parched, you may already be dehydrated.

Change position often. Some cramps happen because a muscle group becomes fatigued after being in the same position for a long time. If you can schedule your day so that you can alternate long tasks with shorter ones, your muscles will appreciate the chance to switch gears. Get up from your desk a few times an hour. Rake leaves as a break from working on

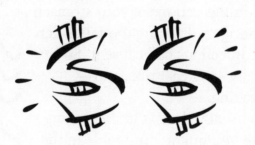

your knees in the garden. The more frequently you change position, the less likely you are to have cramps.

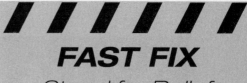

Nausea

Soothing Stomach Settlers

Good food, good drink, good friends—who doesn't love to celebrate? But all that rich food and those tasty libations can make you wish you'd spent the night at home alone, watching TV.

All sorts of things can make your stomach go topsy-turvy. Eating or drinking too much can trigger nausea. Infections can cause it. So can stress, bad smells, long car trips, and— *URP!*—going sailing.

Queasiness usually doesn't last very long, but it can make you mighty miserable in the meantime. Here are some ways to help your stomach settle down.

Snap up some ginger. Ginger is widely used as a remedy for upset stomach and nausea. You don't even have to chew the root; simply make a tea by boiling a quarter-size piece of ginger in a cup of water for 5 minutes, then strain, says Gary Null, Ph.D., an alternative healer and host of the "Natural Living" radio show in New York City.

A dilly of a cure. A home-made infusion of dill seeds can help calm an upset stomach and ease nausea. Steep 1 teaspoon of seeds in 1 cup of hot water, covered, for 15 minutes, then strain.

Beat it with broth. Here's a healing remedy that originated with Florida herbalist Martha Sarasula, M.D., Ph.D. Mix together two 12-ounce cans of vegetable broth or bouillon (or 2 cups of water with three packets of instant vegetable bouillon), two quarter-size pieces of ginger, two cloves of minced garlic, and ¼ cup of soy or tamari sauce. Bring it all to a boil, turn down the heat, and let it simmer for 30 minutes. Sip it slowly by the spoonful.

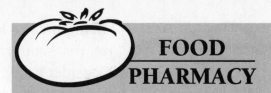

Soothe with the sweet. For nausea caused by stress and anxiety, have a cup of meadowsweet tea. Steep 1 heaping teaspoon of the herb in 1 cup of hot water, covered, for 10 minutes, then strain. Sip it slowly to settle your stomach.

Scratch and sniff. If you're feeling queasy, head for the fridge. Grab an uncut lemon and scratch into the peel. Then sniff the clean, fresh citrus scent. That's what they do in India to handle nausea!

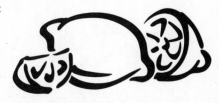

Relax with peppermint. The volatile oils in peppermint can help counteract nausea. Simply uncap a vial of peppermint oil and inhale for a few seconds. If you're feeling up to a bath, add 4 to 6 drops to your tub and slide in. Just remember to breathe deeply while you're soaking.

Bring on the bland. When your appetite finally returns, scout around the kitchen for bland food. Consider eating easy-to-digest applesauce, a little plain rice, dry toast, or even a mild cooked vegetable.

Calm with the balm. Bee balm leaves contain a compound called thymol, which helps ease nausea, vomiting, and even embarrassing flatulence. Simply combine 1 teaspoon of dried bee balm leaves with 1 teaspoon of black or green tea leaves. Put 1 teaspoon of the mixture into 1 cup of boiling water, steep for 5 to 10 minutes, and strain. Sweeten the tea with 1 teaspoon of honey, then sip.

Focus on fluids. For the first 12 hours after a bout of nausea, drink only clear liquids such as ginger ale, plain water, or soothing teas. Vomiting causes your body to lose a lot of liquid, and it's important to replace it.

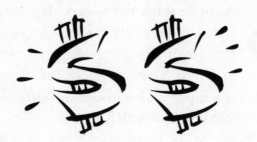

Neck Pain

Take the Creaks Out

It's not a coincidence that we use the expression "a pain in the neck" for things that really bug us. Apart from the fact that neck pain hurts, it also has a way of sticking around. Almost everything we do—driving, working on a computer, and even rolling over in bed—affects the neck to some extent. When the pain flares up, it seems impossible to find a position that doesn't make it worse.

Most neck pain occurs when your muscles are overworked. This often happens when you've been holding your head in the same position for too long—while riding in a car, for example, or working on an overdue report. Neck pain can also be caused by sharp, sudden movements, such as your head lurching forward when you slam on the brakes. In either case, the pain

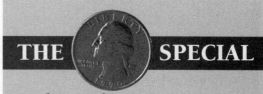

THE SPECIAL

Soak in Salts

Epsom salts baths can help ease spasms and relieve neck pain. Add 2 cups of the salts to a hot bath, sink down so your shoulders and neck are in the water, and feel the relief. Afterward, place an ice pack on your neck.

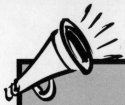

HOLLER FOR HELP

Protect the Nerves

Neck pain is almost always caused by normal muscle strain, and it's pretty easy to help the muscles relax and loosen up a bit. The obvious exception is if you've had an accident of some kind—you've been in a car crash, for example, or taken a hard fall. Neck pain that flares up after a traumatic injury must be treated by a doctor, especially if you have symptoms such as weakness or tingling in one or both arms. These are signs of possible nerve damage, and you'll need professional help to make sure things don't get worse.

means that the muscles are strained or inflamed. Sometimes, they lock up in agonizing spasms—and when that happens, you'll know it!

FIX IT FAST

Neck pain that follows an injury should always be checked out by a doctor. Most often, though, it's nothing more than sore muscles, and you don't need a fancy MRI to know what's going on—or high-tech treatments to fix it. Here's what the experts recommend.

Stretch out. A bit of a stretch can coax tense neck muscles into relaxing, says Dennis Dowling, D.O., chairman of the department of osteopathic and manipulative medicine at the New York College of Osteopathic Medicine in Old Westbury. "The stretching should be gentle enough that you can feel the muscles stretching but not increase the pain," he says.

1. Start by slowly bending your neck forward and lowering your chin toward your chest.

2. Push gently on the back of your head with your hand to increase the stretch a bit.

3. Gently bend your neck backward while pushing lightly on your forehead.

4. Gently bring your head back to its normal position, then turn it slowly to the right, then to the left.

5. Bend your neck sideways, lowering your right ear toward your right shoulder, then your left ear toward your left shoulder.

Do this series of stretches a few times a day until your neck is better, Dr. Dowling advises. Just be sure that you always move your head in a straight line, he adds. You don't want to twist your neck, which could make the pain worse.

Hit it with cold. Applying a cold pack or ice cubes wrapped in a washcloth or small towel is a great way to numb neck pain. At the same time, it will reduce any inflammation, which makes the soreness worse. Apply the cold pack for about 20 minutes every few hours until your neck feels better. Another good method is to hold a bag of frozen peas or corn against your neck. In some ways, this is actually the best approach because the bag will conform to the shape of your neck.

Take out the ouch with arnica. Arnica gel is an excellent first-aid ointment for muscle or joint pain. Apply it frequently. Arnica is for external use only; don't use it on broken skin.

Check your pillow. Does your neck hurt first thing in the morning? You may have a problem pillow that's not providing adequate support. Most people do better when they use a firm pillow that keeps the head and neck in proper alignment while they sleep. But you'll have to experiment: A pillow that provides good support for someone else

FAST FIX
Work It Out

A lot of neck pain actually originates in the shoulders and upper back, says Dennis Dowling, D.O. One of the best ways to relieve it is to give your shoulders a relaxing workout. Here's a move you can do in a hurry: Put your right arm across your chest and grip your right elbow with your left hand. Slowly pull your elbow toward the left side of your body. Hold the stretch for a moment, relax, and repeat with your other arm.

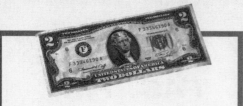

The $2 Deal

Tiger in a Tube

Tiger Balm is the one remedy from ancient Chinese medicine that everyone seems to know about. When rubbed into the skin, this potent salve creates heat to warm tight muscles and a tingling sensation to divert your attention from the pain.

may not necessarily be right for you.

Snooze on your side. People who sleep on their backs sometimes get neck pain because this position doesn't always provide enough neck support. You'll probably do better (and feel better) if you sleep on your side.

Take a look at your workspace. If you spend a lot of time sitting at a desk, be sure you can reach everything you need without having to contort your neck and shoulders. Keep your computer monitor positioned so you can read it without bending your neck. If you're on the phone a lot, use a headset rather than holding the receiver in the crook of your shoulder.

Take 5. "We have a tendency to work on things until they're done, no matter how long it takes, so we're doomed to hurt our-selves," says Dr. Dowling. As a general rule, you don't want to hold your neck in the same position for more than about 20 minutes at a time. When you're working, make it a point to take several breaks—by getting up and walking around, for example, or at least by turning your head and neck a few times each hour. (Set an egg timer so you don't forget.) On long car trips, pull over occasionally to stretch and enjoy the sights. You'll be glad you did.

De-creak with calendula. When things get to be a pain in the neck, reach for a jar of calendula cream, available in health food stores and some drugstores. Just rub 1/2 teaspoon into the skin where it aches, then lie flat with a rolled-up towel under your neck. You'll be up and at 'em in 15 minutes.

Osteoporosis

Beef Up Your Bones

For years, most of us have tried to reduce the fat in our diets in order to lose weight and lower cholesterol. In our efforts to save our hearts, however, we may have done long-lasting damage to our bones.

The dairy industry used to have us all convinced that milk is the ideal food. In some ways it is, but in trying to reduce fat, a lot of us simply gave it up. The problem is, milk is among the best sources of calcium, the bone-building mineral that you need to keep your skeleton strong. It's hardly surprising that osteoporosis, a serious condition in which bones get progressively weaker with age, is so common in this country. Most women, who are at highest risk for osteoporosis, get only about 450 milligrams of calcium

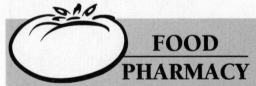

FOOD PHARMACY

Peel Some Protection

The Framingham Heart Study found that women whose diets are rich in potassium have denser bones in their spines and hips than women with potassium-poor diets. Bananas and oranges are terrific sources of this mineral.

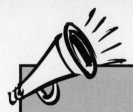

HOLLER FOR HELP

The Test That's Best

Many women don't get bone density tests until something happens—such as a broken hip—and then it's too late to reverse the damage. You should have this easy test—you simply stick your foot in a boot and read a magazine for a few minutes while a machine measures your bones—for the first time around age 35 and then each year thereafter to monitor for any changes in bone density.

If you have risk factors, such as small stature, lack of exercise, or years of smoking, ask your doctor to give you this test sooner rather than later.

daily, nowhere near the 1,000 to 1,500 milligrams that doctors recommend.

GOOD TO THE BONE

Although we can't see, hear, or feel it coming, osteoporosis can happen to anyone. While men generally have larger, stronger bones and don't experience a drop in bone mass the way women do after menopause, they're still at risk as their testosterone levels gradually decline. The good news? Osteoporosis is completely preventable. Here's how to help keep body and bone together.

Drink the moo juice. As long as you buy low-fat or fat-free dairy products, you'll get all the calcium you need without putting weight where you don't want it. One glass of milk, for example, has about 300 milligrams of calcium, while a cup of yogurt has between 275 and 325 milligrams. As a bonus, milk is generally fortified with vitamin D, which you need to help your body absorb calcium.

Bite some bones. No, not like a puppy, but like this: Eat a can of sardines or salmon with bones once or twice a week for a calcium boost. Just 3 ounces of canned salmon with bones has about 200 milligrams of calcium.

Pile on the tofu. Add ½ cup of tofu made with calcium sulfate to salads and stir-fries to get 250 milligrams of calcium. As a bonus, tofu is rich in two major types of isoflavones, compounds that act as a weak estrogen and may inhibit bone breakdown.

Go easy on the hooch. Alcoholism is a major cause of osteoporosis in men. Alcohol poisons the bone-forming cells called osteoblasts, says Sydney Lou Bonnick, M.D., director of the Institute for Women's Health at Texas Woman's University in Denton. If you do drink, do so in moderation, and not every day. One drink a day for women and two for men is considered moderate.

Shut down the soda tap. Many soft drinks are loaded with phosphorus, a mineral that interferes with calcium absorption. It's fine to have a cola now and then, but water is always a healthier choice.

Load up on D. Your body needs vitamin D—which you can get from food, a supplement, or regular exposure to sunlight—to absorb calcium. Take 400 IU of vitamin D each day if you are over age 50. If you are over age 70, you need 600 IU daily. The best food sources of D are salmon and tuna and some types of mushrooms.

Get some sun. If you spend sufficient time outdoors, you may not need a vitamin supplement. After age 50, however, our bodies have more difficulty manufacturing vitamin D from sunlight and absorbing it from food. If you do want to

THE SPECIAL

Strengthen with C

Vitamin C is an antioxidant that combats the aging process and appears to play a role in collagen production—the first step in bone formation. Eat plenty of fresh fruits and veggies to be sure you get enough. For extra protection, take a multivitamin that provides 100 percent of the recommended daily amount.

soak it up from the sun, expose your face and arms for 15 minutes before you put on any sunscreen. In northern climates, the sun's low angle from November to March prevents it from providing much benefit, so drink vitamin D–enriched milk during the winter months.

Get extra magnesium. This mineral helps promote bone health. The best sources are potatoes, seeds, nuts, legumes, whole grains, and dark green vegetables. Ask your doctor about supplements if you don't think you're getting enough in your diet.

Have some bone soup. You've heard of stone soup? Well, bone soup is better! Pick up some beef bones at the meat counter or use any other kind you prefer, such as chicken, pork, or ham. Put them in a soup pot with water, vegetables, potatoes, your favorite herbs and spices—and the magic ingredient, vinegar. It will dissolve a significant amount of calcium from the bones. Just 1 pint of soup can give you as much as 1,000 milligrams of calcium.

Shake dem bones. When your bones are challenged, they rise to the occasion. Just 60 seconds of running during a brisk walk is enough to shift your bones into a strengthening mode. Since you need to perform at least 30 minutes of weight-bearing exercise three times a week, and the American Academy of Orthopedic Surgeons says running ranks the highest for bone building, hit the

---

Tea Time

A Cuppa Bone Health

Nettle, horsetail, oatstraw, alfalfa, dandelion, chicory, kelp, and bladderwrack can all be made into bone-boosting teas. Combine equal parts of two or more dried herbs, steep 1 heaping tablespoon in 1 quart of hot water for 10 minutes, and strain. Dandelion is rich in potassium and should not be taken with potassium tablets.

pavement to walk and run your way to better bones.

Get out in the garden. According to a report in the *Journal of the American Geriatric Society*, moderate physical activity such as gardening reduces the risk of hip fracture by 20 to 60 percent. In fact, one study showed that women who did some form of leisure activity for more than 3 hours a week had about half as much chance of fracturing a hip as those who were sedentary.

Stamp your feet. No, don't have a tantrum—but do take up step dancing or get out the castanets and try some flamenco. With every step you take, the striking of your heel on a hard surface creates stress on your skeleton. In response, it strengthens and renews itself, says Judith Andariese, R.N., director of the osteoporosis center at the Hospital for Special Surgery in New York City. Going down stairs is also ideal, as is ballroom dancing—especially if you do it for 2 hours several times a week.

Build 'em with weights. Regular strength training does more than just keep you fit: The pull of your muscles as you work out stimulates your bones to increase their density. In fact, in a landmark study, 20 sedentary post-menopausal women attended two weekly supervised weight-lifting sessions of about 45 minutes each. In just one year, they gained an average of 1 percent in bone density, while the control group, who didn't lift weights, lost

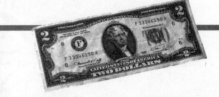

The $2 Deal

Oil Away Pain

As osteoporosis progresses, the bones in your spine can begin pinching the nerves that run between them. St. John's wort oil is specifically indicated for nerve pain. Massage a small amount into any painful areas two or three times daily. You can find the oil at health food stores.

about 2 percent in bone density. What's more, members of the weight-lifting group were soon in-line skating, playing tennis, gardening, shoveling snow, and walking—doing things they hadn't done in years! If you don't have dumbbells, you can hoist a couple of heavy cans of food. Just be sure both cans are the same weight.

Hold up a wall. Wall pushups are an easy way to strengthen the bones in your upper body. Put your hands flat on a wall, level with and about as far apart as your shoulders, and take a step away from the wall. Lean into the wall, then push your body away from it. Repeat several times at least three times a week.

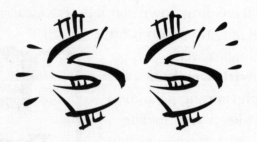

Pizza Mouth

Take a Slice Out of Pain

We eat hot foods all the time without getting burned, so what is it about pizza that almost guarantees the occasional singed mouth? Eagerness obviously has something to do with it. Take one sniff of that delicious rising steam, and it's hard to resist diving right in before it cools. Then there's the molten cheese: It's not only hot right out of the oven, but it stays hot for a long time. Yow! Instant burn.

A burned mouth is no laughing matter. It takes only a second for hot foods to sear the delicate tissues in your mouth. The area will usually heal within a few days, but it can be hard to eat in the meantime. To reduce pain and help the burn heal more quickly, here are some tips to try.

Stick to cool cuisine. The last thing your mouth needs after a close encounter with scorching pizza is even more heat. Remember, you've already burned off a protective layer of skin. Eating anything hot at that point will be doubly painful. "Stick to cool foods for a day or two when you've got a bad burn," says John Hibbs, N.D., a naturopathic physician and professor at Bastyr University near Seattle. Cool soups are good choices, as

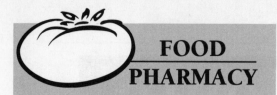

FOOD PHARMACY

B for Burns

The next time you burn your mouth with hot pizza, make the second course a fresh green salad. Spinach, arugula, broccoli, and other leafy greens are loaded with folate (the natural form of folic acid), a B vitamin that helps damaged cells grow and reproduce to repair painful damage. While you're recovering, it's also a good idea to take a supplement that contains 400 micrograms of folic acid.

are salads and sandwiches.

Chill out. As with any burn, applying ice to the area will strip away residual heat, numb the pain, and constrict, or narrow, tiny blood vessels, which will inhibit inflammation or bleeding under the surface. The best way to use ice is simply to suck on an ice cube for a while. You can also swish ice water around in your mouth for about 20 seconds several times a day.

Try a slippery swish. Slippery elm is one of the best herbal remedies for pizza mouth. "It's soothing, it reduces irritation and inflammation, and it shortens the healing time for burns," says Dr. Hibbs. Buy the powdered form at a health food store and mix it with water. Several times a day, swish the solution around in your mouth, then swallow it or spit it out.

Heal with St. John's. To help a pizza burn heal more quickly, put a tiny amount of St. John's wort oil, available at health food stores, on your finger and dab it on the sore area once or twice a day, suggests Dr. Hibbs.

Eliminate the acids. Forget oranges, pineapple, tomatoes, and other acidic foods when you're recovering from pizza mouth. Apart from causing pain, they'll increase the time it takes the injury to heal.

Stay on this side of the border. The chemical compounds

that put the heat in salsa, chili, and other spicy foods will really irritate the burn.

Avoid the crunchies. There's a good reason that people with pizza mouth often find themselves eating a lot of cottage cheese and similar foods. Anything with hard edges, such as pretzels or carrot pieces, can jab against the roof of your mouth and make the pain worse.

Protect the area. You can't stick a bandage on your tongue or the roof of your mouth, 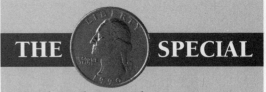 but you can cover the area with an over-the-counter adhesive gel such as Orabase. It will form a shield against irritation from acids and other pain-causing substances, says Joseph L. Konzelman Jr., D.D.S., professor at the medical college of the Georgia School of Dentistry in Augusta.

Don't bother with saltwater. A traditional remedy for mouth burns is to gargle with saltwater, but take this advice with a grain of salt, says Dr. Konzelman. Saltwater can actually increase discomfort and slow healing time. "Rubbing salt on any wound is not a good thing," he says. So don't do it!

THE SPECIAL

Heal with Bicarbonate

Rinsing with a baking soda solution will reduce acidity in your mouth. That's important because mouth acids cause additional pain, and their levels rise quickly after burns or other injuries. "Add a level teaspoon of baking soda to an 8-ounce glass of water," advises Joseph L. Konzelman Jr., D.D.S. Swish the solution around in your mouth a couple of times a day until the discomfort is gone.

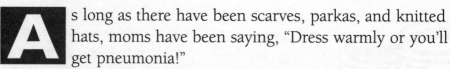

Pneumonia

Best Bets for Better Breathing

As long as there have been scarves, parkas, and knitted hats, moms have been saying, "Dress warmly or you'll get pneumonia!"

No offense to Mom, but cold weather actually has very little to do with it. Pneumonia is the general term for any infection of the lungs. Like other infections, it can be caused by bacteria, a virus, or even a fungus or parasite. As you might guess, your lungs are protected by some pretty sophisticated defense mechanisms. When those defenses are weaker than they should be—because of smoking, for example, or the natural decline in immunity that occurs as we get older—germs are more likely to proliferate.

BAD LUCK FOR THE LUNGS

The symptoms of pneumonia are pretty much the same as those of a bad cold or the flu. You may have a fever, chest pain, coughing, chills, and fatigue. In addition, you'll find it increasingly difficult to breathe as the illness progresses. Your lungs simply can't function well when they're compromised by infection-related inflammation and fluid buildup.

Even though many people with pneumonia naturally recover on their own, the fact remains that your lungs are pretty crucial pieces of equipment, and severe pneumonia is life-threatening. It doesn't pay to take chances: You must see a doctor if you even suspect you have pneumonia.

Antibiotics and other medications can knock out most serious cases of pneumonia pretty quickly, but severe pneumonia requires ongoing care, either at home or in the hospital, to ensure that your lungs make a full recovery.

SAVE YOUR BREATH

By now you're probably thinking that pneumonia sounds pretty scary—and expensive. It doesn't have to be either. In most cases, you can get back on your feet without emptying your wallet.

Here are a few ways to help you bounce back.

Stay close to water. You should never be more than an arm's length away from a glass of water while you're recovering, says Norman H. Edelman, M.D., scientific consultant for the American Lung Association and

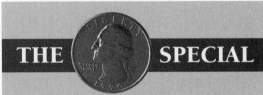

THE SPECIAL

Salt to the Rescue

Your nose and throat will probably feel intensely irritated when you're battling pneumonia. Sniffing saltwater is a quick way to ease the discomfort because it draws fluid from the tissues and encourages the inflammation to clear up, says Christian Dodge, N.D.

You can buy ready-made saline solution at drugstores, or you can make your own by mixing a few teaspoons of salt in a few ounces of warm water. Cup some of the solution in your hand, sniff it into your nostrils, then swallow it or blow it out.

HOLLER FOR HELP

Listen to Your Lungs

Pneumonia kills more than 40,000 Americans each year, so it's important to get medical help if you develop a fever, difficulty breathing, or chest pain, or if you begin coughing up blood. If you have any one of these symptoms, go to an emergency room right away.

dean of Stony Brook School of Medicine in New York. "We suggest that people drink plenty of fluids, at least eight glasses a day," he says.

Drinking lots of water dilutes all the mucus your lungs produce when you have pneumonia. You'll breathe easier, and your lungs will recover more quickly.

Take plenty of downtime. Your immune system needs every ounce of energy it can muster to defeat pneumonia, so it's important to get as much rest as you can. Pneumonia will clear up much more quickly when you take it easy, says Dr. Edelman.

Eat some eggs. They come in single-serving packages (no leftovers!), and they're stuffed with easy-to-digest protein that your body needs to recover. They also build immunity and can help prevent flu as well as pneumonia.

Sip a congestion-free tea. All liquids are helpful when you have pneumonia, but warm echinacea tea is in a class by itself. It reduces chest congestion and soothes your throat and lungs while also boosting the ability of your immune system to fight the infection. Steep a teaspoon of dried herb in a cup of hot water for about 10 minutes, then strain. Plan on drinking two or three cups of echinacea tea a day until the infection is gone and you're feeling better. Don't use echinacea if you have an autoimmune disease such as lupus, rheumatoid arthritis, or multiple sclerosis, or if you're pregnant or nursing.

Pack in the mustard. Chest pain is probably the most uncomfortable symptom of pneumonia. A quick way to ease the ache is to use a mustard pack, says Christian Dodge, N.D., a naturopathic physician and faculty member at Bastyr University near Seattle. "It will increase circulation and ease the pain."

First, mix 1 part mustard powder with 10 parts flour and enough tepid water to make a paste, then spread a thin layer on a cloth. Rub some olive oil on your chest, place a layer of cloth over it, and apply the plaster, mustard side out. Leave the plaster on for 10 minutes or less. To prevent blisters, remove it when your skin begins to redden.

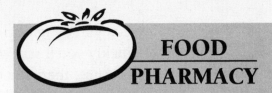

FOOD PHARMACY

Slurp That Soup

For one thing, soup increases the amount of lung-cleansing fluids in your body. In addition, it provides an abundance of healing nutrients, and it's easy to eat when you're sick and your appetite is low.

Soup has even more benefits. The warmth helps loosen mucus in your chest, and the high protein content of chicken or other meat-based soup helps your body recover. There's also some evidence that chicken soup increases the activity of immune cells that help mop up infections.

Fight back with garlic. If you like your food on the pungent side, you're in luck: Garlic is one of the best herbs for strengthening immunity and fighting infections, says Dr. Dodge. He advises eating two raw garlic cloves a day until the infection is completely gone. "If that's too intense, you can lightly bake the garlic," he adds.

Encourage coughs. The chest-racking cough that accompanies pneumonia can be agonizing, but you don't necessarily want to block it with a cough suppressant. Coughing is your body's way of expelling the gunk that's clogging your lungs. The

Pneumonia

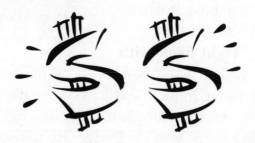

more mucus you cough up, the better you'll feel, and the more quickly you'll recover, says Dr. Dodge.

Of course, there are times when a cough is so severe that it interferes with sleep or causes intense pain; people have even broken ribs during attacks. If your cough is really bad, go ahead and use an over-the-counter cough suppressant, following the label directions.

Heal with humidity. A dry environment causes mucus to dry and thicken, impeding your recovery. Keep the air moist with a humidifier or bedside vaporizer, but be sure to get some fresh air at the same time. "If you have a window in the bedroom or wherever you're spending most of your time, keep it cracked open," Dr. Dodge suggests.

Dodge the dairy. Milk, cheese, and other dairy foods are loaded with beneficial calcium and protein, but they also tend to thicken mucus—the last thing you need when you're recovering from pneumonia. Once the infection is gone, you can go back to the dairy aisle and stock up again.

Rashes

The Best Skin-Saving Solutions

Are you one of those lucky people who have never had a rash? Nope, didn't think so. There are probably hundreds of potential causes of rashes, and no one's immune to all of them.

Insect stings can obviously cause a rash. So can poison ivy. Eczema. Reactions to jewelry. Diet. Stress. The list goes on and on. Obviously, the best treatment will depend on what's causing the rash in the first place.

Some rashes are just reddened skin. Others burn or sting. Still others are maddeningly itchy. It all depends on what's behind the rash and how your skin reacts to it.

TAKE RASH ACTION

If you keep getting rashes and you don't know why, you obviously need to see a doctor. Once you determine what's making you break out, you can take steps to avoid it. If that's not possible, your doctor may advise you to take antihistamines or use topical steroids to control the symptoms. In the

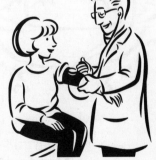

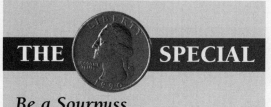
meantime, here are a few ways to defend yourself—and save a few dollars in medical bills at the same time.

Get your pencil ready. A recurring rash has so many possible causes that it may take careful observation—and a lot of notes—to get to the root of it. "Almost every chronic condition or disease has some kind of rash associated with it," says Darrell Misak, N.D., a naturopathic physician in Mount Lebanon, Pennsylvania. Ask and answer as many questions about the rash as you can. Has it been there a long time, or did it just appear? Is it a reaction to something that touched your skin? Were there any recent changes in your diet, clothing, or environment that preceded it? "The answers to these kinds of questions determine the best way to respond," says Dr. Misak.

Say ahh with oats. An almost instant way to ease a dry, itchy rash is to treat it to an oatmeal bath. You can buy a colloidal oatmeal kit at most drugstores. Add the finely ground oatmeal to warm (not hot) water, then settle in for a soothing soak. You can also fill an old sock with plain dry oatmeal, then fasten the open end to the faucet with a rubber band. Fill the tub with warm water, letting the water run through the sock. (You can fasten the oatmeal bundle and let it float in the bathtub when you're done filling it.) Oatmeal makes water soft and soothing—perfect for a painful rash.

Mend with an herbal blend. If your rash is wet and oozing, here's some help: Wash your skin, then help dry up the rash and prevent secondary infections by dusting it with an herbal powder. Mix equal parts of slippery elm powder and goldenseal powder and gently dust the mixture on the rash for soothing relief and quick healing.

Fix it with flax. People with skin conditions such as eczema are often lacking essential fatty acids. Ideally, you should get these kinds of fats (found in nuts, seeds, and cold-water fish) from your diet, but you can get quick relief by applying them directly to your skin as well. Rub a small amount of flaxseed oil into rashy areas before going to bed and after bathing, and sweet relief will soon be on its way.

Lose the heavy metal. Earrings with nickel wires and posts commonly cause rashes in people with metal allergies. You'll know if you're one of them: A metal allergy will make you itch within 20 minutes, and a rash will usually appear within a day or two. To avoid both, make sure only stainless steel needles are used for ear piercing, and buy earrings with stainless steel posts. Although stainless steel does contain some nickel, it is bound so tightly to the steel that it is safe, says the American Academy of Dermatology. In addition to your jewelry, check buttons, fasteners, and zippers. If they touch your skin, they can cause a rash.

Stay balanced. Very hot or very cold temperatures can aggravate a skin rash. You won't find the perfect environment anywhere, except maybe in the next biosphere, but if you can,

FAST FIX
Calm It with Cream

Hydrocortisone cream is an anti-inflammatory steroid cream that is safe for self-care, says the American Academy of Dermatology. It blocks the allergic skin reactions that trigger some rashes, and it can speed healing of inflamed or cracked skin, regardless of the cause. You can find it at drugstores.

HOLLER FOR HELP

Know Your ABCDs

You should always check with your doctor when you discover a new, unexplained blemish on your skin. It's probably a rash (or maybe a mole), but it could also be skin cancer. It doesn't pay to take chances.

Your suspicion level should be even higher if the "rash" displays any of the following characteristics, known as the ABCDs.

- **Asymmetry.** In other words, the two halves aren't the same size.
- **Border irregularity.** The blemish has a jagged, notched, or irregular edge.
- **Color variegation.** It's not a solid color.
- **Diameter.** It's more than 6 millimeters in diameter.

"Cancer is the biggest concern when these things happen, so don't wait," says Darrell Misak, N.D. "Get it checked."

avoid exposing your skin to extreme heat and cold. Also avoid sudden changes in temperature or humidity, which can trigger a rash.

Use safe cosmetics. Even if you've used the same brands of makeup for years without any problems, you can get a rash if the company changes the chemical ingredients. Choose products with no fillers, dyes, or added colors and those labeled "hypoallergenic."

Keep a diet diary. "Food sensitivity is a big issue with rashes," says Dr. Misak. A recurring or chronic rash could be triggered by something in your diet—dairy foods, wheat, corn, or citrus fruits, for example. Keeping a record of everything you eat over the course of several weeks and noting when the rash occurs and subsides may flush out the cause—or at least narrow the pool of suspects. "Remember, a rash can appear 24 to 72 hours after you eat the problem food," Dr. Misak adds.

Heal with hydrotherapy. This is just a fancy way of saying that you may want to use warm or cool compresses to get relief. If you have a rash that feels warm to the touch, for example, you may want to soak a small towel in cool water and drape it over the area to relieve the discomfort. If your rash feels dry and itchy, a warm compress may be more effective.

Get some R&R. Sometimes a rash appears because your body's overloaded with stress or irritating waste products. One of the best things you can do is take some time to relax and get the stress out of your life. Start by taking an hour a day to just play. Go to the zoo, head for the pool, or dig in the dirt. That may be enough to make the rash disappear

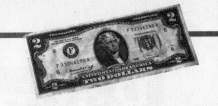

The $2 Deal

Make Time for Marigolds

Marigold blossoms are skin-friendly botanicals that are great for stopping a rash in its tracks. The next time a rash rears its ugly head, dab on some marigold oil with a cotton swab or clean cloth. Keep applying the oil, available at health food stores, until the rash is gone.

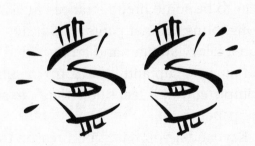

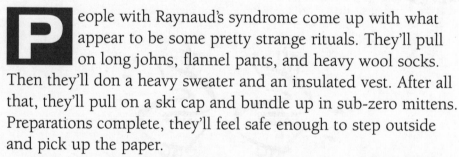

Raynaud's Syndrome

Stop the Cold Attacks

People with Raynaud's syndrome come up with what appear to be some pretty strange rituals. They'll pull on long johns, flannel pants, and heavy wool socks. Then they'll don a heavy sweater and an insulated vest. After all that, they'll pull on a ski cap and bundle up in sub-zero mittens. Preparations complete, they'll feel safe enough to step outside and pick up the paper.

If you have Raynaud's, you have good reason to fear the cold. This mysterious condition makes blood vessels in the hands, feet, or legs clamp down if they get even slightly chilled. This may cause color changes in the skin—often from white to red to blue—as well as numbness or tingling.

THERMOSTAT OUT OF WHACK

The most important parts of your body—namely, your brain, heart, lungs, liver, and other organs—are located in your head and chest, and your body is pretty efficient at protecting them. Part of this protection means keeping your core body temperature at the optimal 98.6°F.

Suppose that you step outside into a howling blizzard. Your body will detect the frigid temperatures, then take steps to ensure that your brain and trunk stay at the proper temperature. It does this in part by narrowing blood vessels in your hands, arms, feet, and legs. The restriction of blood flow to these areas ensures that more heat stays in your deeper tissues and organs.

In people with Raynaud's, however, this normal response is exaggerated, and so much circulation is rerouted to the trunk that very little blood reaches the hands or feet. This is what causes the numbness, color changes, and other symptoms.

RESTORE THE FLOW

Normal blood flow usually resumes within a few seconds or minutes, although some people may experience the effects for hours. When circulation resumes, there may be a tingling sensation or perhaps throbbing pain. Attacks

FAST FIX
Wiggle and Warm

The quickest way to stop a Raynaud's attack is to warm up your hands and feet. Doctors recommend a five-step plan—and each of the steps starts with the letter W, which makes them easy to remember.

- Wiggling your toes or fingers will restore normal circulation.
- Windmills, in which you rotate your arms in large circles, will also boost circulation.
- Warm water is a great way to unchill your hands and feet instantly. Fill the sink or a basin with water, but don't make it too hot, because that can actually prolong an attack. Soak your hands or feet for about 5 minutes, or until they're feeling better.
- Warm pits (meaning your armpits) are a handy source of heat. When your hands suddenly turn cold or numb, tuck them into your armpits and keep them there until circulation returns.
- Warmers, such as heated gloves or socks, will often stop a Raynaud's attack before it gets under way.

can be triggered by a cold day in February or even reaching into the freezer for ice cubes.

You need to see a doctor if you notice symptoms of Raynaud's. Most cases are mild, and there's a lot you can do to maintain normal circulation, says Magdalena Dziadzio, M.D., a faculty member in the department of internal medicine at the University of Ancona, Italy. Here's what doctors advise.

Keep your hands and feet warm. Avoiding extreme cold is the best way to prevent attacks. One useful strategy is to wear battery-heated gloves and socks, available in sporting goods stores, whenever you're going to be spending time outside in cold weather. "A belt-worn rechargeable battery pack can keep them powered for up to 3 hours," says Dr. Dziadzio. Those chemical hand warmers used by hunters, campers, and other outdoor enthusiasts are also good gadgets for people with Raynaud's. When you squeeze them, they release chemicals that produce instant, hand-warming heat.

Can the caffeine. The caffeine in coffee, tea, and some soft drinks causes blood vessels to constrict, which reduces crucial blood flow. You don't necessarily have to give up your favorite beverages, but you'll certainly want to limit yourself to one or two servings daily.

Protect your soles. Don't neg-

HOLLER FOR HELP

Look for the Cause

Even though Raynaud's is rarely serious, you have to see a doctor if you even suspect you have it. For one thing, the disease is sometimes triggered by other conditions, such as scleroderma, lupus, or other forms of arthritis. Even if your doctor can't identify a cause—and in most cases, there isn't a known cause—you'll get plenty of good advice for preventing and stopping attacks.

lect your feet when shopping for anti-cold clothing. "Shoes with padded soles will keep your feet warm and relieve pressure on your toes," says Dr. Dziadzio. "Pressure can also trigger the symptoms."

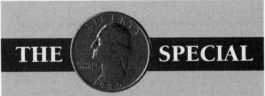

Dress for convenience. Avoid coats, gloves, boots, and other kinds of outdoor clothing that have lots of snaps, zippers, or other fasteners. You'll find it almost impossible to get them off when your hands are cold. Try on outerwear in the store and be sure you can slip it over your head, or off your hands or feet, without having to fumble with hard-to-grip fasteners.

Plan for the Arctic. To prevent Raynaud's flare-ups, you have to keep your whole body warm, not just your hands and feet. Shop for clothes made of space-age fabrics in shops catering to winter sports enthusiasts. Wear whatever you need to stay nice and toasty, from thermal underwear and tights to long coats, scarves, and earmuffs. The advantage of dressing in layers is that you'll find it easier to adjust your levels of insulation—and comfort—as the temperature changes.

Lube your circulation. Fish oil, available in capsules at health food stores, appears to encourage vasodilation, the ability of blood vessels to expand and carry more blood, says Dr. Dziadzio. People with Raynaud's sometimes notice an improvement in their symptoms when they take the capsules

THE SPECIAL

Get Your Nutrient Fix

Vitamins C and E help reduce the harmful effects of free radicals, harmful oxygen molecules in the blood that may play a role in triggering Raynaud's, says Magdalena Dziadzio, M.D. She recommends taking 100 to 400 IU of vitamin E and, if you don't have stomach or kidney problems, 500 to 1,000 milligrams of vitamin C daily.

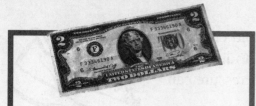

The $2 Deal

Pop for Mitts

Keep a pair of warm mittens or insulated oven mitts hanging in a handy spot in your kitchen. You can use them to take cold items out of the refrigerator or freezer. Some people even use them when they handle frozen foods at the supermarket.

daily, following the directions on the label.

Drink with comfort. Cold beverage containers are a Raynaud's attack waiting to happen. To protect your hands, slip a cold soda into an insulating foam container, or sip it through a straw. That way, you can enjoy your drink without touching the cold can or bottle.

Beware of bad vibes. Sometimes vibration can trigger an attack of Raynaud's. Causes of vibration may include using power tools, vigorous typing, or even working in the yard with a shovel or rake. Try to insulate yourself from vibration as much as possible by taking frequent breaks, for example, or using tools with thick foam handles.

Put out the smokes. You shouldn't be smoking anyway, but here's one more reason to quit: Cigarettes impair circulation and can make Raynaud's much worse. "Stopping cigarette smoking can produce immediate benefits," says Dr. Dziadzio.

Discuss medicines with your doctor. A number of medications, including a class of drugs called beta-blockers, sometimes aggravate Raynaud's symptoms. Make a list of all your medications and review it with your doctor. In some cases, just changing drugs will bring dramatic improvement in your symptoms.

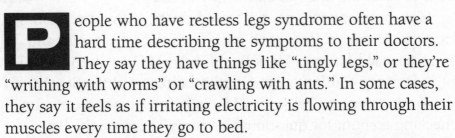

Restless Legs Syndrome

Calming the Kicks

People who have restless legs syndrome often have a hard time describing the symptoms to their doctors. They say they have things like "tingly legs," or they're "writhing with worms" or "crawling with ants." In some cases, they say it feels as if irritating electricity is flowing through their muscles every time they go to bed.

This condition is unlikely to be a serious health threat, but people who have the attacks night after night can go months or even years without a good night's sleep. The resulting fatigue can make it nearly impossible for them to hold down jobs or function at full alertness during the day.

Doctors still don't know what causes restless legs syndrome (RLS). What they do know is that people who have this mysterious condition experience their symptoms only when they're lying down or are otherwise immobile. As soon as they move their legs vigorously, the symptoms go away. When they lie quietly again, the irritating feelings return.

RELAX YOUR LEGS

There aren't any definitive tests for RLS. Your doctor, probably a neurologist, will take a look at blood flow and nerve functions to make sure that your symptoms aren't caused by something else. Even if you appear to be perfectly fine—most people with RLS have no obvious health problems—the doctor may prescribe medications to relax the muscles and help you sleep.

Most people, however, don't need drugs. "Almost all restless leg patients can get very good relief from their symptoms and live a normal life," says Mark Buchfuhrer, M.D., a sleep specialist in Downey, California, and medical director of the Southern California Support Group for RLS. So before you deplete your checking account for questionable "cures," here are the best ways to keep your legs calm and get a better night's sleep.

Stretch or stand. When your legs start aching or tingling, sometimes just standing up will make the sensation go away. It's not uncommon, in fact, for people with RLS to get out of bed and read while standing. Stretching your legs also seems to help, so you might try doing some deep knee bends, rising up on your toes, or flexing your thighs, calves, and ankles. Some people report that stretching before going to bed makes attacks less likely.

Get a grip. The next time you're tossing

and turning because of restless legs, reach down and firmly massage the areas that are bothering you. While massage won't cure the condition, it does seem to ease symptoms for some people.

Be anti-antihistamine. Drugstore shelves are loaded with over-the-counter sleep aids, many of which contain antihistamines that promote sleepiness. Unfortunately, antihistamines tend to make restless legs worse, says Dr. Buchfuhrer. "When people with RLS can't sleep, they sometimes take one of these drugs, and that only makes things worse," he says. It's best to consult a physician who's familiar with RLS before trying any sleep medication.

Soak away the tingles. Some people with RLS find that heading from the bed to the bathtub calms their restless legs. A soak in warm water will sometimes reduce symptoms enough to let you get to sleep.

Let the water flow. While soaking in warm water is a common strategy for calming restless legs, some people do better when they alternate heat and cold. Soak a towel in warm water and drape it over your

Iron It Out

Even though the cause of RLS isn't known, there may be a link between restless legs and low levels of iron in your body. "Every patient with RLS should have a serum ferritin level test," says Mark Buchfuhrer, M.D. "It's a super-sensitive test for iron."

If your ferritin level is less than 45 micrograms per deciliter (45 mcg/dL) of blood, your doctor may advise you to take supplemental iron intravenously. Oral iron supplements help only about 20 to 30 percent of the time, says Dr. Buchfuhrer, and you shouldn't decide to take supplements on your own.

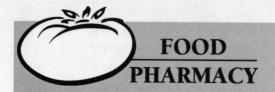

FOOD PHARMACY

Don't Scream for Ice Cream

Many people with RLS find that ice cream makes their problem worse, and no one knows why. "For some reason, ice cream just tends to bother a very high percentage of people with RLS," says Mark Buchfuhrer, M.D.

leg. After a minute, replace it with a towel soaked in cool water. Keep doing this for both legs until they feel better.

Watch what you drink. Both caffeine and alcohol seem to cause an increase in RLS symptoms. As a general rule, limit yourself to one or two daily servings of either alcoholic or caffeinated beverages. If you still have trouble, you may want to give them up entirely to see if things improve.

Get your legs moving. People who exercise regularly often find that their RLS symptoms improve. Even a daily walk seems to help. "It's best not to exercise right before going to sleep," adds Dr. Buchfuhrer. "You should do it at least a few hours before going to bed."

But don't overdo it. While moderate exercise can ease RLS symptoms, people who really exert themselves may find that their symptoms flare up. "Vigorous exercise can be a problem," says Dr. Buchfuhrer. "I have several younger patients who train to run marathons, and invariably, they get into trouble when they're really training hard."

Change your schedule. Depending on when your symptoms tend to occur, you may be able to make schedule changes that will help you cope. You might take a later shift at work, for example, so you won't be going to bed until after the time your symptoms usually flare up. Or you might schedule an afternoon walk for the time when you often have trouble.

Sciatica

No More Nerve Pain

■

If you've ever experienced sciatic pain (also called sciatica), you know that size really does matter. The sciatic nerve is your body's biggest nerve, and it can produce one of its biggest pains. Anyone who's had back problems is all too familiar with sciatica. It can be merely irritating if you're lucky, and devastating if you're not.

Sciatica is the main reason that people have back surgery, but most folks who have it don't necessarily need to book an appointment with a high-priced surgeon. It turns out that often, the most qualified person to cure your sciatica is you.

Anything that pinches or irritates your sciatic nerve has the potential to cause real trouble. Sciatica can produce symptoms as mild as a slight backache or as severe as shooting pains through your buttocks and legs.

Sciatica is often caused by muscle injuries. When muscles tighten or become inflamed, they can put painful pressure on this all-important nerve. It can also occur when one or more of the spinal disks, the shock absorbers between the vertebrae, squeeze out of the spinal column and jam against the nerve. The

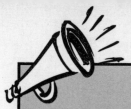

spinal bone spurs that occur with arthritis can cause sciatica as well.

EASE THE PRESSURE

It's essential to see a doctor at the first hint of sciatica. In the majority of cases, though, the pressure and pain will go away on their own. Here's the catch: Nerves are very slow to heal, so it may be weeks or months before all the pain is completely gone.

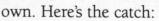

"The body has an inherent capacity to heal itself," says Boyd R. Buser, D.O., associate dean at the University of New England College of Osteopathic Medicine in Biddeford, Maine. Once you eliminate some of the factors that interfere with healing and do more of the things that help it along, sciatica will often disappear on its own. Here are a few tips you may want to try.

Apply cold fast. Even in this age of high-tech medicine, ice is still one of the best treatments for back and nerve pain. When you apply ice immediately after an injury, there's a lot less swelling and inflammation, which means there's less pressure on the vulnerable nerve.

At the first sign of sciatica, apply a cold pack to your lower back, as close to the origin of the pain as you can get. Hold it there for 20 minutes, remove it for 20 minutes, then repeat the cycle. Keep applying cold for at least 24 hours, says Dr. Buser.

Switch to heat. After applying cold for a day or two, use a warm compress or a heating pad set on low. "Heat's very helpful for relieving pain and relaxing those tight muscles," says John Nowicki, N.D., a naturopathic physician in Issaquah, Washington. Another benefit is that heat increases blood flow, which helps flush pain-causing chemicals from the area and promotes the flow of healing nutrients.

Knock out inflammation. The inflammation of the nerve is a major cause of leg pain, says David Borenstein, M.D., a rheumatologist based in Washington, D.C. Take nonsteroidal anti-inflammatory drugs such as aspirin or ibuprofen to decrease inflammation surrounding the disk and nerve. This will help reduce pain and shrink swollen tissues.

Hit the sack on your back. Prop a pillow under your knees or rest on your side with a pillow placed between your knees. Both positions take your weight off the inflamed nerve and decrease pressure on the spinal disks, says Dr. Borenstein. If you still can't sleep because of sciatic pain, lie on your back on a rug on the floor, with your feet and calves elevated on a chair so your knees are bent at a 90-degree angle.

FAST FIX
Helping Hams

Stretching is always good for sciatica, but don't focus on just your back muscles. It's just as important to stretch your hamstrings, the muscles at the backs of your thighs that often press on the tender nerve, says John Nowicki, N.D. Here's a good stretch: Lie on your back with your knees slightly bent. Grab your right thigh just above the knee with both hands and gently pull your leg toward your head. Raise it as close to vertical as you comfortably can, hold for a moment, then relax. Repeat with your other leg.

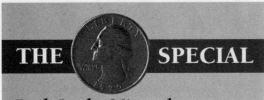

Pack In the Minerals

Supplements that contain both calcium and magnesium are like a magic bullet for sciatica because they help tight muscles relax. Check with your doctor first, then look for a supplement that provides 500 to 800 milligrams of each and take it daily until the pain is gone. Capsules tend to work better than tablets because they're easier for the body to break down, doctors say. Magnesium may cause diarrhea in some people. If this occurs, reduce the dose.

Walk on the mild side. As soon as possible, start walking on flat surfaces. Take it slow and easy, and gradually increase your distance. Climb stairs with caution, however, so your weakened leg doesn't cause a fall.

Oil your back. A combination of arnica oil, St. John's wort oil, and castor oil can help relieve the pain of inflammation. Combine equal parts of each oil and gently massage some onto the nerve track: Begin at your buttocks and go down the back of your leg. If you have a disk problem, massage the oil into that area as well. Arnica is for external use only; don't use it on broken skin.

Get some handwork. Sometimes it's a good idea to let someone grab your butt. No kidding: When you have sciatica, massaging your buttocks can reduce muscle tension that puts painful pressure on the nerve, says Lanika Buchanan, N.D., a naturopathic physician in the Puget Sound area of Washington.

Fidget more. People with sciatica are liable to be uncomfortable standing or sitting for long periods of time. "For most people, prolonged sitting is a problem, although some people have trouble with standing," says Dr. Buser. One way to keep pain at a minimum is to change positions frequently. If you're taking a long drive, for example, stop at least once an hour to get out and stretch. If you're working at a desk, set the alarm on your watch or a clock to remind you to get up and walk around.

Don't be a twister. You don't want to do anything to increase pressure on the irritated nerve. Obviously, this means no heavy lifting and a minimum of bending. In addition, try not to twist your torso too much to avoid increasing muscle spasms, which can put a lot of pressure on the nerve.

Fight pain with fish oil. The essential fatty acids (EFAs) in fish and fish oil block your body's production of chemicals that promote pain and inflammation. You can get plenty of EFAs by eating fish several times a week. If you're not a fish fan, try some ground flaxseed. It's loaded with EFAs, and you can sprinkle it on cereal or salads for a pleasantly nutty crunch.

Stretch it out. There are two main muscle groups, called the gluteal and piriformis groups, that contribute to sciatica pain. One of the best ways to ease sciatica—and prevent it— is to keep those muscles long and limber by stretching.

Lie on your back on the floor with your knees bent and your feet flat on the floor. Put your left ankle over your right knee, then use both hands to pull your right leg toward your shoulder. You should feel a good stretch on your left side. Switch legs and stretch the other side.

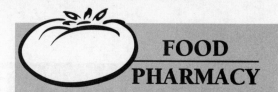

FOOD PHARMACY

Spice It Up

People with sciatica who like spicy foods should definitely seek out recipes that contain turmeric. This fragrant herb has powerful anti-inflammatory effects that help counteract sciatica flare-ups. You'd have to eat a lot of turmeric to get enough of the active ingredient, though, so a more practical approach is to get turmeric in capsule form at a health food store. Check with your doctor first, then start with about 250 milligrams three times daily, preferably with food.

Seasonal Affective Disorder

Erase Those Winter Blues

Millions of retirees have the right idea. Each year, these intrepid folks say goodbye to the dismal days of winter and embark for Florida, Mexico, or other sunny climes. They come back with cool souvenirs, great tans, and not a trace of seasonal affective disorder (SAD), a type of depression that often descends with the coming of colder (and darker) seasons.

The symptoms of SAD, sometimes called winter depression, are similar to those of other depressive disorders and include lethargy, a change in appetite or weight, and lack of interest in social situations. No long-term research has yet been completed, but doctors do know that SAD is a very real disorder. It affects more women than men and, logically, more people in the north than in the south. In fact, SAD is *seven* times more common in Washington State than in Florida, according to the American Academy of Family Physicians.

TURN ON THE LIGHT

Fortunately, wherever you live, there's a lot you can do to keep winter from making you too blue. Here's how to begin.

Start with a checkup. SAD is more than just a case of the blahs, says Gila Lindsley, Ph.D., a psychologist in Massachusetts. The symptoms, like those of any type of depression, can affect your entire life and sense of well-being. Some people, she says, even experience suicidal thoughts. So take your winter blues seriously and ask your doctor to refer you to a psychiatrist or psychologist, who can evaluate the disorder and recommend medication if it's necessary. If you think of suicide even once, immediately go to an emergency room.

Order a BLT to go. In this case, BLT is not a sandwich. It's a remarkably simple yet effective treatment called broad-spectrum light therapy. BLT involves simply sitting in front of a desktop light box equipped with special, high-intensity bulbs for about 30 minutes each day, generally in the morning. If the therapy works for you, your doctor will probably recommend that you continue it throughout the winter. The timing and length of exposure are highly individual, however, so be sure to ask your doctor for guidance.

Plan active events ahead of time. While it's easy to have fun in the summer sun, be sure to plan vacations, trips, or special events that will keep you happier

Tea Time

Mood-Lifting Tonic

You'll feel better fast when you sip a tea made with equal parts of St. John's wort, passionflower, betony, and vervain (all available at health food stores). Steep 1 teaspoon of the mixture in 1 cup of hot water for 15 minutes, then strain. Drink two cups daily. If you are taking antidepressants, check with your doctor before using St. John's wort.

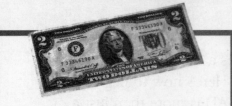

The $2 Deal

Feel Better with Flax

People who are depressed often have low levels of essential fatty acids. Unless you're taking aspirin or blood thinners, take 1 tablespoon of flaxseed oil, which has lots of these beneficial fats, once or twice daily during the winter to head off the cold-weather blues.

in the winter months, too. Make firm commitments well in advance, so you'll have something to look forward to when the blahs set in. And if you can, take your annual vacation in winter rather than summer, then head for the sun.

Light up your life. Use as much light indoors as your budget allows, suggests Dr. Lindsley. You might even try full-spectrum lightbulbs, which include all the colors of the rainbow. Their light is much more like natural daylight, and they can lift your home's indoor mood. They're energy-efficient, too, so although they cost more, they last much longer than standard bulbs.

Push back the dark. The temptation to hug the fireplace and become a couch potato in winter can overwhelm you if you prefer warmth and sun. If you're not up to joining winter sports lovers on the slopes or frozen ponds, head for the warmth and light of your local fitness center. If you get 30 minutes of regular exercise a day to keep those endorphins circulating, it will be easier to combat the depression of a long, cold, dark winter. Just be sure to begin your physical activity before the blahs hit, warns Dr. Lindsley.

Avoid tanning salons. Don't choose a tanning salon for do-it-yourself light therapy. The light sources used for tanning are high in ultraviolet rays and can cause serious harm to your eyes and skin, warns the American Academy of Family Physicians.

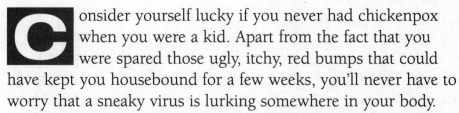

Shingles

Leave 'em on the Roof!

Consider yourself lucky if you never had chickenpox when you were a kid. Apart from the fact that you were spared those ugly, itchy, red bumps that could have kept you housebound for a few weeks, you'll never have to worry that a sneaky virus is lurking somewhere in your body.

You see, the virus that causes chickenpox never goes away altogether. It just goes into hiding. Sooner or later, it may reappear and cause a painful, blistering disease known as shingles.

PAINFULLY UGLY

If you've had chickenpox, there's about a 40 percent chance that you'll eventually have an attack of shingles. The virus that causes the original infection isn't completely destroyed by your immune system. Instead, it slips deep into the nerves and remains there in a dormant state. In some people, it stays dormant; in others, it wakes up, travels up the nerves to the skin, and causes a painful, blistery outbreak. The sores usually appear in a band across the torso or buttocks and sometimes on the face.

A fast way to reduce the itching and pain of shingles is to wrap a few ice cubes in a washcloth or small towel and hold them against the tender spots. Ice acts as a local anesthetic by temporarily numbing the skin, explains Priscilla Natanson, N.D.

If you have trouble keeping the ice pack in place, make a cold "slush pack" that conforms to the shape of your body. Mix 1 part rubbing alcohol with 4 parts water, fill a few plastic zipper-lock bags with the mixture, and put them in the freezer. After they're chilled, take one out to use on your shingles. When that bag warms up, put it back in the freezer and replace it with a cold one.

When you first come down with shingles, you may have a fever or other flulike symptoms. In most cases, you'll be completely recovered in a few weeks, and you can consider yourself cured once all the blisters have healed. If you're over age 50, however, there's a good chance that nerve damage caused by the virus will cause lingering pain known as postherpetic neuralgia.

A RASH APPROACH

Shingles can be extremely painful, so it's worth getting in to see your doctor right away. You may need painkillers or other medications to tide you over. In addition, there are drugs that can shorten the duration of attacks if they're given within 24 hours of the start of blisters.

The good news is that shingles isn't dangerous in most cases, and it does clear up on its own. To reduce discomfort in the meantime, take the following tips to heart.

Be serious about cleaning. Wash the blisters twice a day with regular soap and water to prevent infection. Resist the urge to cover them up with a bandage. And hang in there—the rash usually runs its course in three weeks or so.

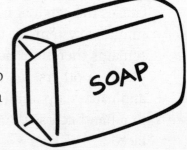

Rub away the itch. If the touch of clothing against your skin drives you crazy, here's a way to defuse the sensitivity, courtesy of the docs at the Mayo Clinic: Rub the area with a clean towel for several minutes—after you've gotten the okay from your doctor.

Nix nerve pain. St. John's wort oil may reduce any nerve pain that lingers once the shingles have cleared up. Apply the oil directly to the skin two or three times daily.

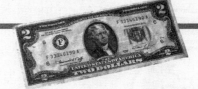

Pop a few aspirin. Over-the-counter remedies such as aspirin and ibuprofen can help control shingles pain.

Add some vitamin C. When you're battling the shingles virus, extra vitamin C is helpful as long as you don't have kidney or stomach problems. "Vitamin C is a great immune booster," says Priscilla Natanson, N.D., a naturopathic physician in Plantation, Florida. Check with your doctor about the amount that's right for you.

Check out the chick. Don't let the name fool you: The herb chickweed is no mere weed. "It's a wonderful anti-itch herb," says Dr. Natanson. You can buy creams or salves made with chickweed at health food stores.

Look pretty in pink. It's been on drugstore shelves almost forever,

The $2 Deal

Fight Back with Echinacea

It's one of the most powerful herbs for strengthening the immune system, and it will gear up your defenses to fend off the virus. Echinacea is more effective in the early stages, so start taking it as soon as you notice symptoms. It's available in capsule form at health food stores and drugstores; follow the label directions. Don't take it if you have an autoimmune disease such as rheumatoid arthritis, lupus, or multiple sclerosis, or if you're pregnant or nursing.

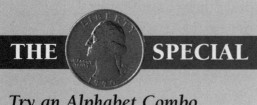
Try an Alphabet Combo

A potent nutrient combo that will strengthen your immune system and help shingles blisters heal more quickly includes vitamins A, C, and E, plus the mineral zinc. Look for a supplement that contains each of these important nutrients and follow the label directions.

and with good reason. Calamine lotion, best known for its vivid pink hue, can ease the itch of shingles and reduce pain as well. Apply the lotion after a shower or bath and several more times during the day.

Pepper away pain. Rubbing hot-pepper ointment on your shingles may not sound as though it would put out the fire, but apparently it does. The American Academy of Dermatology says that ointments made with capsaicin, the element that provides the heat in hot peppers, can help some people with shingles. Apply it three or four times a day, and within one to two weeks, the pain should gradually ease. Check with your doctor about what strength to buy, and when you apply it, be careful not to get it near your eyes or any area of broken skin.

Sleep well with valerian. This herb sedates the nervous system and helps put a damper on the pain of shingles. This is especially useful when you are having difficulty sleeping because of the pain. To make a tea, steep 1 heaping teaspoon of herb in 1 cup of hot water for 10 minutes, then strain. Drink one cup after dinner and before bed. Do not use valerian with pain relievers or anti-anxiety or antidepressant medications.

Soak in oats. A warm bath spiked with a cup of colloidal oatmeal can help keep itchy shingles from driving you crazy.

You can buy it at most drugstores and supermarkets. Or you can fill a sock with regular dry oatmeal, fasten the sock to the faucet with a rubber band, and let the water run through it as you fill the tub. If you don't have oatmeal, add a cup of baking soda to the water.

Baby those blisters. Shingles blisters are a lot more painful than the kind you get from too much hiking or working in the yard. They can be so sensitive, in fact, that even the pressure from heavy clothes can be agonizing. Until they're gone, get in the habit of wearing loose, light clothing.

Don't be a Typhoid Mary. Shingles blisters are packed with live viruses that can potentially cause chickenpox in people who haven't had it. Don't let anyone touch the blisters, and take the time to clean them every day with soap and water.

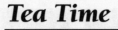

Tea Time

Help from Hips

Hot tea made with rose hips not only tastes good, it's good for you when you have shingles. "It's high in vitamin C," explains Priscilla Natanson, N.D. Plus, taking the time to enjoy a cup of tea will help you relax and maintain optimal immunity. Drop a teaspoon of dried herb into a cup of freshly boiled water. Steep for about 15 minutes, then strain out the herb and enjoy your tea.

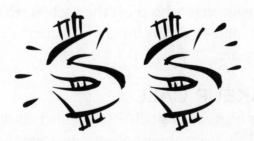

Shinsplints

Mendin' Your Tendons

If you've always been a casual athlete—you enjoy staying in shape but aren't exactly fanatical about it—you'll probably never get shinsplints. Serious athletes, on the other hand, get them all the time. Some even consider them a badge of honor. As if there's anything honorable about agonizing pain!

The term *shinsplints*, incidentally, isn't a medical term. Doctors don't even know how this particular pain in the front of the lower leg—pain that's invariably aggravated by exercise—got its name. They do know what causes it, though. What probably happens is that you strain or slightly tear one of the tendons in your lower leg. This usually happens at either end of the athletic spectrum: Elite athletes who push themselves really hard often get shinsplints, and so do beginners who aren't quite as fit as they think they are.

YOUR WAKEUP CALL

Shinsplints hurt, but usually not as much as a serious sprain or strain—and the pain almost always goes away once you get a little rest. Consider the pain of shinsplints to be a warning that it's time to take things a bit easier. In the meantime, try these tips to recover more quickly and prevent future problems.

Lie low for a while. You're likely to get shinsplints only when you're dishing out more stress than your body is able to handle, says Thomas Ayers, D.C., team chiropractor for Sprint Capital USA, a training center for world-class athletes in Raleigh, North Carolina. "We often see shinsplints in weekend warriors who go out and push themselves too hard," he says.

The solution, obviously, is to rest. For most recreational runners (shinsplints are a problem mainly for runners), taking a week off is enough to eliminate the pain.

Do the cube cure. Ice cubes are your best friends when you're coping with shinsplints, since putting cold on your lower leg will help reduce swelling as well as pain.

Apply a cold pack or ice cubes wrapped in a washcloth or small towel to the area that hurts. Keep it in place for about 20 minutes and repeat the treatment every hour or two until you're feeling better.

Get new shoes. Running shoes that are badly worn are a common cause of shinsplints, says Dr. Ayers, so plan on replacing your shoes about every 300 miles. In addition, don't settle for shoes that don't fit perfectly, because they give

FAST FIX
The Sour Solution

Moist heat is a great treatment for shin pain, and adding vinegar to the mix increases the anti-inflammatory power. Heat a mixture of equal parts vinegar and water, soak a small towel, wring it out, and apply it where you hurt. Leave it on for about 20 minutes. If you don't have any vinegar in the house, you can get similar results with castor oil. Rub the oil onto your sore shin, cover the oil with plastic wrap, then top that with a hot, moist towel. Leave it on for about 20 minutes, then wash off the oil with soap and water.

poor support and put excessive strain on the muscles and tendons in your lower legs.

Stay level. One of the quickest solutions for shinsplints is simply to run on level ground—a running trail, for example, or the track at a local high school or college. Runners who stay off rocky or uneven terrain often improve right away and stay pain-free in the future.

Go half-and-half. You're more likely to get shinsplints if you run every day. A better approach, especially if you're just beginning a workout program, is to run one day, take a day or two off, then run again. Giving your muscles a little recovery time means that you'll be less likely to limp home with shinsplints.

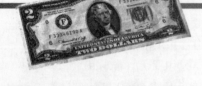

The $2 Deal

Protect Your Arches

If you have flat or fallen arches, you may be at risk for shinsplints. One of the easiest solutions is to drop by a drugstore and pick up some orthotic shoe inserts, which will support your feet and help keep your lower legs pain-free. You can also visit an orthopedic doctor to be fitted for custom inserts.

Walk into a wall. Well, stretch into one, anyway. If ice and pain pills don't make you feel better, you may want to try some gentle stretching. It helps the muscles relax and flushes away waste products that contribute to the pain.

Here's a stretch that will help: Stand in front of a wall with your legs shoulder-width apart and one foot a step or two in front of the other. Bend the knee of your front leg while keeping your rear leg straight, then lean into the wall, keeping both heels flat on the floor. Hold the stretch for 5 to 10 seconds, then switch leg positions and repeat.

Purge the pitch. A lot of runners

who practice on treadmills adjust the machines so they slant upward. While running uphill provides a great workout, it can also lead to shinsplints if your legs aren't ready for the strain.

While you're training, you may want to reduce the pitch or even make it completely level. Once you build up more leg endurance and strength, you can return to uphill running.

Tap away trouble. The underlying cause of shinsplints is often muscle weakness—especially in the shin muscle, says Timothy Tyler, a physical therapist at the Nicholas Institute of Sports Medicine and Athletic Trauma at Lenox Hill Hospital in New York City.

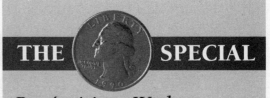

THE SPECIAL

Put Aspirin to Work

Most nonprescription pain relievers, including aspirin and ibuprofen, are very effective at easing the pain of shinsplints, says Thomas Ayers, D.C. Take them every 4 hours, following the label directions.

"When you run, that muscle has to pull really hard," he explains. You can make the muscle stronger simply by tapping your toes. No kidding, it's as easy as it sounds. A few times a day, sit in a chair and tap your toes up and down, keeping your heels on the floor. Continue until you feel a slight burn in the muscle at the front of your shin. "That's how we prevent shinsplints," says Tyler. "It works."

Walk before you run. A great way to loosen up your legs and prepare them for an injury-free run is simply to walk for a few minutes. It gets your muscles nice and warmed up before strenuous exertion.

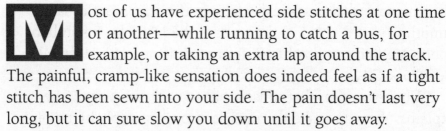

Side Stitches

Fixes for Painful Glitches

Most of us have experienced side stitches at one time or another—while running to catch a bus, for example, or taking an extra lap around the track. The painful, cramp-like sensation does indeed feel as if a tight stitch has been sewn into your side. The pain doesn't last very long, but it can sure slow you down until it goes away.

Side stitches are something of a mystery to doctors, since no one really knows what causes them. It could be a cramp in your diaphragm, the muscle that moves up and down to fill and empty your lungs as you breathe, or perhaps a muscle cramp in your side or somewhere in your respiratory tract. Other theories are that side stitches are caused by gas bubbles in your intestine or even the weight of your liver pulling on your diaphragm.

UNSTITCH THE PAIN

For reasons that aren't clear, side stitches occur more often on the right side than on the left. They never last very long, and they're never serious. The one sure cure is to rest, but there are a few other things you can do to make the pain go away more quickly.

Slow down, hands down. The quickest way to cut a side stitch short is to slow down, take some deep breaths, and let your hands drop to your sides.

"This helps stretch the diaphragm, which often helps relieve the pain," says John Nowicki, N.D., a naturopathic physician in Issaquah, Washington. Once the stitch is gone, you can go back to whatever it was you were doing.

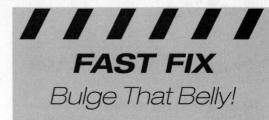

FAST FIX
Bulge That Belly!

The quickest way to stop a side stitch may be simply to take a deep breath. But don't just fill your lungs—let your abdomen expand as you breathe in. This technique, called belly breathing, seems to stretch the diaphragm and make side stitches less intense.

Reach and stretch. Stretching the side of your body that's stitched will often bring relief. If the pain is in your right side, for example, raise your right arm over your head and bend your torso to the left. Hold the position (called a side stretch) for about 30 seconds, then switch to the other side. By the time you've finished, the stitch will be gone.

Quit pushing yourself. Decreasing the intensity of your activities or workouts is a fairly reliable way to cut down on the frequency of side stitches, Dr. Nowicki says. "No one knows exactly what a side stitch is, so I can't say for sure that it's a clear sign that you're working too hard. But decreasing the intensity does seem to help."

Fill up on fluids. If your body is properly hydrated, you're

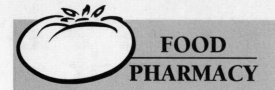
Bubbles Are Trouble

Your favorite carbonated beverage is best left in the fridge if you're trying to avoid side stitches. The bubbles tend to cause excess gas, which some experts think leads to side stitches or cramps. Stay away from fizzy drinks immediately before or right after intense activities.

less likely to get cramps of all sorts, side stitches included. On average, you need between 64 and 80 ounces of water a day. "Add 8 to 16 ounces for each hour of exercise," says Dr. Nowicki.

Give yourself a hand. One way to deal with a side stitch is to rub it out, says Dr. Nowicki. "Deep pressure on the affected area can help," he says. Just press against the painful spot for several seconds, then release. Repeat the pressure until the stitch is gone.

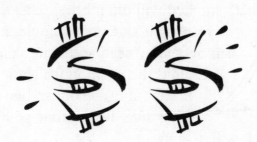

Sinusitis

Drain Away Pain

Has anyone ever told you that you have holes in your head? We usually use this humorous expression when someone's a little absent-minded, but there's also some literal truth to it. We do have holes in our heads. They're called sinuses, and they're simply empty spaces above and below the eyes and on either side of the nose.

Actually, life would be better sometimes if the sinuses really were empty, but that's not always the case. All too often, the mucous membranes that line the sinuses provide a safe haven for harmful bacteria. The resulting infection can cause fever, facial pain, and unbelievably painful headaches.

The sinuses normally produce a steady flow of mucus that traps dust particles and other airborne irritants and keeps them out of

Tea Time

Horse Around

Nothing clears your sinuses faster than a bite of horseradish root. If that's too intense, make a tea by grating 1 teaspoon of fresh root into 1 cup of hot water. Steep for 5 minutes, then strain. Drink three cups a day.

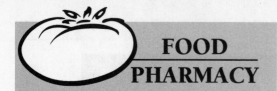

FOOD PHARMACY

A Peachy Cure

If you've come down with sinusitis, pick up a peach. One small study found that people with sinusitis may not be getting enough glutathione, an antioxidant compound found in peaches and other delicious fruits, such as watermelon and oranges.

the lungs. When you have a cold or allergies, however, the resulting congestion can prevent mucus from getting out. Bacteria love all that stagnant fluid, and they multiply like crazy. That's about when you start holding your head and looking for a quiet place to lie down.

SAVE YOUR SINUSES

In most cases, sinusitis clears up on its own, usually within a week. If you're sick for longer than that, check with your doctor. You may need antibiotics to clear up the remaining infection. In the meantime, though, the trick to beating sinusitis is to restore the normal flow of mucus. Here's what doctors advise.

Whack it with wasabi. This powerful Japanese horseradish, which could blow the lid off a manhole, will empty your sinuses. It's available at Asian restaurants and grocery stores, as well as some health food stores. Use it as a dip for sushi—or take it straight, if you dare!

Snort some salt. Use a saline nasal spray several times a day to remove mucus that could harbor bacteria. If you can find one that contains eucalyptus, so much the better, since eucalyptus kills bacteria.

Apply deep heat. When your sinuses are acting up, place a hot, damp towel over the top half of your face and let the heat penetrate into your nasal cavities. Leave it there for 15 minutes, then repeat three or four times a day to promote drainage and increase blood flow to the area.

Breathe tropical air. Inhaling steam is one of the best ways to clear clogged sinuses. Boil a pot of water and remove it from the stove. Drape a towel over your head to trap the steam, lean over the pot (being careful not to scald yourself), and breathe in the steam. Adding a few eucalyptus leaves will boost the penetrating power.

Add some oils. To open your nasal passages, use a sinus oil once or twice daily. First, soak a washcloth in hot water and apply it to your face to increase circulation to the area. Keep the cloth in place for 5 minutes, resoaking it to keep it as hot as you can tolerate. Then apply a thin layer of olive oil to your frontal bone, above your eyes and cheekbones, below your eyes, and on the bony part of your nose. Next, place a couple of drops of eucalyptus oil on your fingers and rub it into the same areas. Finally, place the hot cloth over your face again and rest for 15 minutes.

Fry up some salt. It sounds strange, but it's a traditional Russian remedy for sinusitis. Heat some salt in a frying pan, then spread it on a towel or clean cloth. Fold the cloth and put it over the bridge of your nose. The heat will open your sinuses.

Put water to work. Drink at least eight glasses a day to thin out your nasal mucus and improve its ability to drain.

Be a dairy delinquent. Dairy foods thicken mucus, and since you already have enough of that clogging up your sinuses, avoid milk and milk products until you're better.

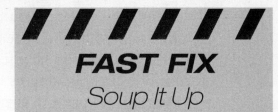

FAST FIX
Soup It Up

Nose clogged up so you can't breathe? Heat up a can of tomato or minestrone soup and toss in a few diced cloves of garlic and a generous sprinkle of chopped chile pepper. The combination of soup and spices acts as a natural decongestant that will help you breathe easier.

Clear the air. Keep your environment as dust-free as possible with an air-filtering system. If you can, keep your home and car air-conditioned to help filter out the pollens and allergens in the outside air. Your sinuses will thank you for it.

Plug up. Chlorine in swimming pools can be irritating to your nasal membranes, so don't go in the water without nose plugs.

Take care of allergies. If your sinusitis is usually a by-product of allergies, dry up the drip with antihistamines before it can clog you up.

Cover your sneezer. When it's cold outside, always wrap a wide scarf around your neck and lower face to cover your nose. This will keep your mucous membranes from drying out and also prevent a painful rush of cold air from reaching your tender sinuses.

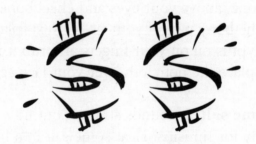

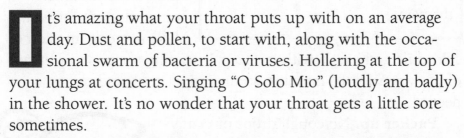

Sore Throats

Soothe Your Swallow

It's amazing what your throat puts up with on an average day. Dust and pollen, to start with, along with the occasional swarm of bacteria or viruses. Hollering at the top of your lungs at concerts. Singing "O Solo Mio" (loudly and badly) in the shower. It's no wonder that your throat gets a little sore sometimes.

You'll want to see a doctor if your sore throat lasts longer than about a week. That's a pretty good sign that you could have a bacterial infection that won't go away unless you take antibiotics. Fortunately, most sore throats get better on their own, but they can make you mighty miserable in the meantime. Here are some time-tested remedies that really work wonders—and won't empty your wallet.

Load up on lozenges. Use throat lozenges or hard candies to keep your throat moist. Look for cherry lozenges with benzocaine to numb your throat temporarily and help with swallowing. Slippery elm lozenges work well, too.

Shhh. The less work your throat muscles and membranes have to do, the better you will feel. Save the speeches until your

Tea Time

Go for the Green

Green tea, that is. It's among the best sore throat remedies because it's loaded with bioflavonoids. If green's not your cup of tea (and as long as you're not allergic to ragweed), try chamomile—it's a traditional remedy for sore throat pain. And don't forget to add honey. It coats your throat and helps numb the pain.

throat has healed. Better skip the choir rehearsals, too.

Quell it with calendula. For a speedy end to soreness, paint your throat with fresh calendula juice or tincture. Simply dip a cotton swab in the calendula juice and apply it thoroughly to the back of your throat, paying particular attention to the sides. Too unpleasant for you? Make a strong infusion of calendula and gargle with it. Steep 1 heaping teaspoon in ½ cup of hot water for 10 minutes, strain and let cool, and use as needed.

Pucker up. No cough drops or candy handy? Soak half a lemon in saltwater, then suck on it for a while. This treatment moistens your throat and relieves soreness.

Ease it with violet. Violets are not only beautiful, they're medicinal, too, helping to ease the pain of a sore throat caused by a cough. Simply steep 1 heaping teaspoon of violet flowers in 1 cup of hot water for 10 minutes, then strain. Drink two or three cups a day, sipping slowly to bathe your throat.

Take the ocean potion. Your grandmother was right: The quickest way to soothe a sore throat is to gargle with saltwater. Mix 1 teaspoon of salt in a cup of warm water and gargle with the solution for about 30 seconds. Spit it out, then gargle again.

The relief usually lasts anywhere from 15 minutes to an hour, and you can repeat as often as necessary.

Swig some juice. If you own a juicer, now's the time to rev it up. Juices are a great source of the extra fluids and natural healing substances your body needs to help a sore throat. All fruit juices are beneficial, but papaya, orange, and pineapple are good choices because they're loaded with vitamin C. Other throat-comforting produce includes carrots, spinach, blueberries, and dark cherries. The juice will be especially soothing if you warm it slightly before drinking it. If the flavor is too intense, just add a bit of water.

Ace it with A and C. Both nutrients strengthen immunity and increase the activity of specialized cells that fight infection. Take a multivitamin that contains both—plus (if you don't have stomach or kidney problems) 500 milligrams of vitamin C twice a day.

Gobble garlic. This herb is one of the best remedies for sore throats as well as for colds and flu. It has anti-inflammatory, antiviral, and antibacterial properties, says Jane Hopson, N.D., a naturopathic physician in Hillsboro, Oregon. The problem with garlic, of course, is that you'd have to eat a fair amount to take advantage of its healing properties—and that can give you a powerful aroma. To get the benefits

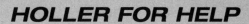

HOLLER FOR HELP
The Strep Trap

If your sore throat is accompanied by white spots in your mouth and throat or by difficulty swallowing, see your doctor immediately. You may have a strep infection, which can lead to serious complications if not treated appropriately.

without the stink, Dr. Hopson recommends taking odor-free garlic capsules. Look for a supplement that provides about 10 milligrams of allicin, the active ingredient.

If you're a real garlic fan, though, go ahead and enjoy the real McCoy. Plan on eating one or two cloves a day. Raw or lightly steamed garlic provides more allicin than garlic that has been thoroughly cooked, Dr. Hopson adds. Just don't decide to visit with the neighbors until you've showered and brushed your teeth.

Enlist echinacea. The herb echinacea is like an inspirational general who rallies the troops: It stimulates immune cells that fight off throat-burning infections. You can brew echinacea tea, but it's easier to take capsules. 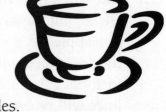 The recommended dose is 350 milligrams three times a day. Don't take echinacea if you have an autoimmune disease such as rheumatoid arthritis, lupus, or multiple sclerosis, or if you are pregnant or nursing.

Zap it with zinc. It may be at the end of the mineralogical alphabet, but zinc comes first when you need to soothe a sore throat. "It makes your throat feel better, and it boosts the immune system," says Dr. Hopson. She recommends sucking on zinc gluconate lozenges, available at most drugstores.

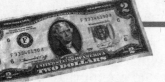

The $2 Deal

Lick It with Licorice

Licorice root is loaded with natural chemical compounds that soothe inflammation anywhere in your digestive tract, including your throat. Don't bother with licorice candy, though; it has only licorice flavor, not real licorice. What you want is licorice capsules, so visit your local health food store, then take 100 milligrams three times a day. Since a substance in licorice called glycyrrhizic acid can cause high blood pressure in some people, look for deglycyrrhizinated licorice (DGL) products.

Ax those allergies. If you tend to get sore throats during ragweed season (ragweed is one of the most common allergy triggers), you may want to take herbal supplements that contain nettle. The herb blocks the action of histamines, natural chemicals that fire up allergic reactions. Take 200 milligrams three times daily until your allergies—and your sore throat—are better.

Simmer some soup. Your throat will heal faster if you don't overuse it swallowing food. And if you happen to have a cold, you'll bounce back faster if your body doesn't expend a lot of energy in digestion. In other words, this is the best time to eat a bland diet—plenty of liquids and easy-to-digest foods. "Broths are a great choice," says Dr. Hopson. "No heavy, fatty meals; keep them light and liquid."

An important bonus of a diet that's heavy on liquids is that it will help make mucus thinner and more watery, so it will drain more easily and cause less throat irritation.

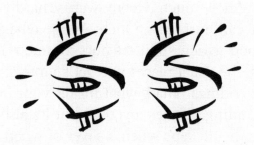

Splinters

Quick Fixes for a Thorny Problem

Y ou don't have to be a carpenter to have a close encounter of the splintery kind. The danged things are everywhere—on worn windowsills, old garden tools, and Grandma's old table, to name just a few possibilities. And it's amazing how much a teeny-weeny, hardly-nothin', sliver-of-somethin' can hurt. Yow. Ouch. And maybe even *$#@!!

There's a good reason splinters hurt so much. It's because your fingertips, the usual places you get splinters, are filled with sensitive nerve endings. That's what makes your fingers so deft at knitting or putting puzzles together, but it's also what makes them sting like the dickens when a sliver of wood gets under your skin.

FIRST-AID BASICS

Splinters aren't exactly a medical emergency. Unless the area is badly infected or the splinter is lodged under a nail or somewhere else where you can't get at it, there's no reason to call a doctor. You can remove most splinters in the time it takes to read this chapter. But read it anyway, just to be sure that you get the nasty thing out—or not, in some cases—with a minimum of discomfort.

Ignore it. If the splinter is lodged close to the surface of the skin, and the area isn't bleeding or painful, it's okay to ignore it, says Lisa Arnold, N.D., a naturopathic physician in Orleans, Massachusetts.

"Your body will generally work it out of there on its own," she says. Just keep an eye on it to be sure it isn't digging deeper into the skin or getting infected.

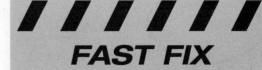

FAST FIX
Soak Away Pain

The skin where a splinter was embedded hurts the most right after the sliver's been removed. For quick relief, soak the area in warm water for 10 to 15 minutes. You can also use warm soaks to help propel difficult-to-remove splinters to the skin surface.

Tweeze to please. Don't use a needle to root out a splinter. Tweezers work better, says Dr. Arnold. Wash the area around the splinter with soap and water, sterilize the tweezers with rubbing alcohol, then grip and pull.

Here's a helpful piece of advice: If you can, pull the splinter out of the hole at the same angle that it went in. This will reduce the chances that it will break off in the skin.

Move it out with marshmallow. Marshmallow ointment can coax a stubborn splinter to the surface of your skin. Dab some ointment on the site, bandage it, and leave it alone for a few hours. When you remove the bandage, the splinter will have inched close enough to the surface for you to easily pluck it out.

Apply a potato poultice. Strange as it may sound, you can get a splinter out with a potato. Use a potato poultice or, in the case of a finger or toe, simply carve or hollow out the potato for a custom fit. Leave the spud on overnight, and you'll be able to

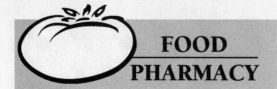

FOOD PHARMACY

Pop It Out with Plantain

If you don't feel up to splinter surgery, an herbal poultice can do all the work for you. Plantain is one of the best herbs to use. "It will actually draw the splinter out of the skin," says Lisa Arnold, N.D.

You can buy fresh or dried leaves at many health food stores. Chop or grind the herb and add enough water to make a paste, then slather it over the splinter. Cover it with a bandage and replace the poultice daily until the splinter comes out.

remove the splinter easily the next day.

Rub away the pain. If a splinter hurts like the dickens, but you can't find a way to remove it right away, simply press or rub the skin close to the sliver, advises Sean Sapunar, N.D., a naturopathic physician and clinical faculty member at the Bastyr Center for Natural Health near Seattle. "The pressure signals travel faster than pain signals," he explains. They get to the brain first and get all the attention, so you feel less pain.

Clean like crazy. Once the splinter's been removed, be sure to keep the skin around the injury clean. Wash the area gently with soap and water once or twice a day and cover

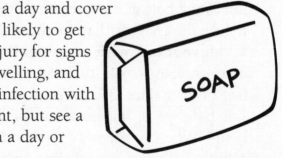

the area with a bandage if it's likely to get dirty. Check the site of the injury for signs of infection—redness, pus, swelling, and so on. You can treat a minor infection with some triple antibiotic ointment, but see a doctor if it doesn't clear up in a day or two.

Soothe with a soak. To promote healing and ease the sting of splinters, try this triple herbal wash. Combine equal parts of dried calendula, echinacea, and comfrey, which you can find at health food stores. Add a heaping tablespoon of the mixture to a pint of freshly boiled water and steep for 20 minutes. Strain the liquid, let it cool, and use it to wash the area thoroughly.

Ask about tetanus. Had a tetanus shot lately? Probably not. Do you need one? Probably, says Laura Pimentel, M.D., chair of emergency medicine at Mercy Medical Center in Baltimore.

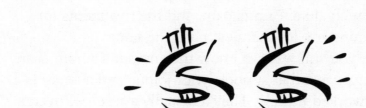

"Any sort of break in the skin could be an entrance for tetanus," she says. The tetanus germ can cause painful and potentially fatal muscle spasms, and it tends to live on wood or rusted metal. If you haven't had a tetanus shot in the past 10 years, you're probably due, she says.

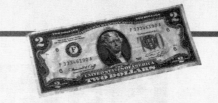

The $2 Deal

Take the Aspirin Initiative

The powerful salicylic acids in wart removers can also help you get rid of a splinter. The superficial layers of skin break down and become soft from contact with the acid. Use wart remover disks; they have a higher salicylic acid content than liquid wart removers do.

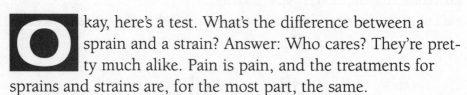

Sprains and Strains

Muscle Out the Pain

Okay, here's a test. What's the difference between a sprain and a strain? Answer: Who cares? They're pretty much alike. Pain is pain, and the treatments for sprains and strains are, for the most part, the same.

Just in case you still want to know the answer, a sprain is an injury to the ligaments that support your joints, and a strain is a pulled or overworked muscle. They're usually a result of overextending or twisting your arm or leg beyond its normal range of motion. You end up with pain when you move the limb, as well as swelling and pain in the involved joint. It feels tender to the touch, and you'll probably get black and blue.

HALT THE HURT

Strains and sprains almost always get better on their own, usually within a week or two. Here's what you need to do in the meantime.

Start with RICE. It stands for rest, ice, compression, and elevation. In other words, stop the activity and rest the injured body part. Apply ice wrapped in a towel or a cold compress to decrease swelling. Wrap the injured limb in an elastic bandage or use a splint or sling. And keep the injured part elevated above the level of your heart. Don't use heat until at least 24 hours after the injury, when the swelling is gone. And by all means, seek medical attention if the pain or swelling is severe.

Add herbs to ice. For a cooling, warming, and healing experience all wrapped into one, add herbal oils to your cold pack. First, fill a bowl with ice-cold water. Sprinkle several drops of oil into the water—try camphor, eucalyptus, chamomile, or rosemary. Next, soak a clean washcloth in the bowl and wring it out well. Lay it over the sprained area and cover with an ice pack. Limit the ice treatment to 10 to 20 minutes to avoid frostbite.

Heat it up. Once the swelling is gone, you can apply a heating pad set on low or a warm compress. The warmth will penetrate into the tissue and help improve the flow of nutrients into the area while promoting the outflow of pain-causing substances.

Keep up the pressure. If you have leg swelling that persists for more than a few days, you may want to get a compression stocking from your doctor or a medical supply store (the ones sold in drugstores aren't measured as precisely). It won't come loose and require rewrapping the way bandages do.

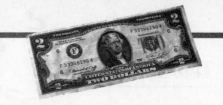

The $2 Deal

An Anti-inflammatory Duo

Bromelain and turmeric are powerful partners when it comes to reducing inflammation and pain. Take 250 to 500 milligrams three times daily between meals. People who are taking blood thinners or are sensitive to pineapple should avoid bromelain.

Tea Time

Sip the Witch

Witch hazel can help shrink the swelling from a sprain or strain. Brew a tea (minus any spooky spells) by tossing 1 teaspoon of dried leaves or 2 inches of root into 1 cup of boiling water. Steep for 10 to 15 minutes, then strain. Soak a clean washcloth in the cooled tea and apply it to the affected area several times a day.

Compression stockings provide different amounts of pressure, says Chris Miller, a physical therapist near Riverside, Connecticut. Get one labeled "25-35," which provides about the same amount of pressure as an elastic bandage.

Get comfort with comfrey. Comfrey wraps work wonders for speeding recovery. Blanch two to four leaves and place them on the injured area. You can apply an elastic bandage over the leaves and keep the wrap on all day.

Drain the fluid. A lot of the pain of sprains can come from the buildup of fluids in the area. A quick way to reduce swelling is to gently move the area through its full range of motion now and then. Keep going for a minute or two, but don't push yourself to the point of severe pain. Try it a few times a day while you're recovering. "It helps pump fluids out of the area," explains Miller.

Fish for relief. The essential fatty acids (EFAs) found in the oils of cold-water fish such as salmon and tuna help suppress inflammation and speed recovery. These oils also stabilize cell membranes that may have been damaged by the injury. It's a good idea to eat fish three or four times a week until you're feeling better. If you aren't a fish fan, you can get healing amounts of EFAs by eating a tablespoon of ground flaxseed daily. Try sprinkling it on cereal or mixing it with yogurt.

Stomachaches

Get Gut-Level Relief

Most stomachaches don't occur in your stomach at all, even though that's where the trouble usually begins. For various reasons, your stomach doesn't always do a great job of digesting its contents. When undigested food travels into the intestine, you're likely to experience cramps or painful gas. Thus, a stomachache is really an intestine ache—one that occurs when your bowel has to deal with your stomach's unfinished business.

A stomachache isn't always a routine problem. In fact, there's a long list of medical conditions that cause pain somewhere in the belly, and some of them are serious. You'll want to see your doctor if your stomachache lasts more than a day or two. In most cases, though, you can get relief without fancy tests or high-priced consultations.

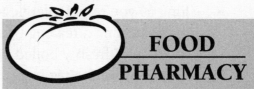

FOOD PHARMACY

Lemon Aid

To prevent stomachaches from getting started, squeeze a little lemon juice into a glass of water and sip it before meals. It will stimulate digestive secretions and get your stomach ready for action.

It's tempting to curl up on the couch after a big meal, but making a beeline from the kitchen to the sofa could leave you with a stomachache. A walk, combined with the effects of gravity when you're standing up, will prevent many stomachaches from getting started, says Andrew Parkinson, N.D.

Here are a few things that are sure to help.

Mix a "lawn salad." Dandelion greens are a traditional remedy for stomach problems of all kinds. Eaten before a meal, the pleasantly bitter leaves stimulate digestive secretions and curb cramps.

Be sure to pick your greens from an area that hasn't been treated with chemicals. The leaves are most tender when they're picked just before the flowers bloom.

Get real with chamomile. It's one of the world's most popular teas, and for good reason: It's been used as a stomach soother for centuries. Just be sure to wait 15 minutes after meals before drinking it. Otherwise, the liquid will dilute the acids needed for proper digestion. As long as you're not allergic to ragweed, you can make tea by adding a tea bag or a teaspoon of dried herb to a cup of freshly boiled water. Steep for 10 minutes, remove the tea bag or strain out the herbs, and drink.

Sniff and settle. Sometimes all it takes to settle an upset stomach is the right scent. The next time your gut's in a knot, scratch the peel of an uncut lemon and take a few whiffs, or open a bottle of peppermint oil and take a deep sniff. The odors travel to your brain and appear to help keep your stomach from going topsy-turvy.

Get extra enzymes. If your stomach's not

doing an effective job of digesting your meals, you're sure to get heartburn or a stomachache. Supplemental digestive enzymes can help, says Andrew Parkinson, N.D., a naturopathic physician and faculty member at the Bastyr Center for Natural Health near Seattle.

Many different digestive enzymes are available at health food stores, including bromelain and papain. It doesn't really matter what kind you get; they're all helpful. Take them before you eat, following the directions on the label. "They're particularly good for reducing that after-meal bloated feeling," says Dr. Parkinson. Don't use bromelain if you take blood thinners, though.

Hold off on the liquids. If you tend to get stomachaches after eating, you may want to give up drinking water or other liquids with your meals, because they dilute the stomach's acid secretions, says Dr. Parkinson. The acid, of course, helps you digest food.

Boost beneficial bugs. Your gut is loaded with beneficial bacteria that break down and digest food. Sometimes these bacteria get depleted—if you've been taking antibiotics, for example—resulting in painful abdominal cramps.

An easy way to boost their numbers back to healthful levels is to take supplements that contain acidophilus. One or two acidophilus capsules is often all you need to calm the upset feeling.

Dip into yogurt. A serving of

HOLLER FOR HELP

More Than Belly-Achin'

Stomachaches are rarely serious, but there are plenty of exceptions. The basic rule is this: A stomachache that clears up within a day probably isn't a problem. If the pain lingers, is accompanied by fever or vomiting, or keeps coming back, see your doctor. You'll probably need some tests to find out exactly what's going on.

yogurt is another great way to load your gut with more beneficial bacteria. Look for brands that contain live cultures. "It's not something you need on a daily basis, but it's a good idea to try to replenish those bacteria from time to time," says Dr. Parkinson.

Listen to Kitty. Everyone knows what catnip does to our feline friends. In humans, however, the herb is actually quite soothing. "It has a mild sedating quality, calms the gastrointestinal tract, and decreases cramping," says Dr. Parkinson. He recommends taking catnip in capsule form when you have a stomachache, following the directions on the label. Or make a tea by adding a teaspoon of dried herb to a cup of freshly boiled water. Steep for 10 minutes, strain, and drink. Both forms are available at health food stores.

Add some heat to your diet. Many pungent spices can help relieve stomach problems. "Ginger, turmeric, cumin, coriander, clove, cinnamon, and garlic all promote good digestion," says Dr. Parkinson. And you don't have to eat tons of these herbs to get the benefits.

Give up on antacids. While they're great for occasional bouts of heartburn, antacids won't do you any good when you have a stomachache. In fact, they can cause side effects, including constipation or diarrhea, that will make you feel even worse.

Drop the dairy. If you tend to get stomachaches after drinking milk or eating other dairy products, it's probably because you don't produce enough of the enzyme needed to digest lactose, a sugar found in dairy products.

One solution, of course, is to give up dairy altogether. Another is to buy reduced-lactose dairy foods at a supermarket. In addition, having small servings—say, half a glass of milk instead of a full pint—may allow your stomach to handle dairy foods without discomfort.

Stress

Tame It Now

Prices rise, roofs leak, cars break down, kids get sick. Bosses yell, bills mount, deadlines fall, keys get lost. Sound familiar? Stress is unavoidable in modern life. Always has been; always will be. A survey by the Gallup and Harris organizations reported that 25 percent of people participating in the survey said the stress in their lives was bad enough to put them on the verge of losing their temper—if not actually going postal!

While a little stress can improve productivity, the hormones generated by extreme or chronic stress can damage physical and emotional health. "It's difficult to think of any disorder in which stress could not play an aggravating role," says Paul J. Rosch, president of the American Institute of Stress. In fact, studies show that your risk of a heart attack

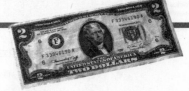

The $2 Deal

Get Out the Godiva

Research has shown that chocolate—yes, chocolate!—helps release endorphins, those brain chemicals that lift your mood.

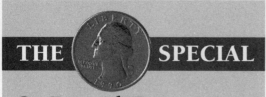

THE SPECIAL

Get Ease with Teas

Choose one of the following herbs to make your own tension-tamer tea: lemon balm, chamomile, passionflower, vervain, wood betony, or skullcap. Try them each for a week at a time until you find your favorite. Then, every time you feel stressed, steep 1 teaspoon of your preferred herb in 1 cup of hot water, covered, for 10 minutes, then strain, Drink one to three cups a day. Avoid chamomile if you're allergic to ragweed.

is tripled within 2 hours of an extremely stressful incident or major meltdown. What's more, the flood of stress hormones can actually warp your brain!

AVOID A MELTDOWN

Since we can't eliminate all stress from our lives, the smart approach is to change the ways we respond to it. Here's what experts advise.

Put it in perspective. Suppose that the IRS just informed you that it wants to audit your taxes for the past five years. Now that's stressful! Redford B. Williams, M.D., director of behavioral research at Duke University in Durham, North Carolina, suggests asking yourself these questions whenever you're in a tough spot.

- Is this really important to me?
- Would a reasonable person be this upset?
- Is there anything I can do to fix the situation?
- Would fixing it be worth the cost?

If you answer yes to all the questions, then take action, says Dr. Williams. But if you answer no one or more times, just take a deep breath and ride out the stressful situation.

Switch mental gears. If you are strumming your fingers on your desk as you pore over a report that is already late and not as good as you'd like it to be, get up and walk away from it. Just take a break and shift to something mindless—even if you're on deadline. You'll come back less stressed and better able to concentrate.

Rub it out. Get a professional massage whenever you can, even once a month, if you can afford it. According to researchers at the University of Miami, massage can cut cortisol levels, lower blood pressure, and boost immunity. To find a licensed therapist near you, contact the American Massage Therapy Association at www.amtamassage.org.

Get moving. Studies have consistently found that even a single exercise session can make you feel less stressed. A simple morning walk at a brisk pace enhances the flow of brain chemicals that block the effects of stress. In a pinch, even a dash up and down some stairs will help.

Unclench. Lots of people clench their teeth when they're uptight. Here's an easy exercise to relax your jaw, face, and neck, courtesy of Elaine Petrone, a Connecticut fitness and stress expert. Take a deep breath and drop your jaw right now. Next, open your mouth and exhale with a long "haaaaaaa" sound. Finally, gently close your lips. Repeat this exercise throughout the day. You'll soon become aware of how often your jaw clenches—and how that tightness moves tension down into your neck and shoulders.

Visualize relief. When you feel your stress level rising, close your eyes, breathe deeply, and visualize a peaceful scene from nature. Keep the scene in your mind for 15 to 20 minutes. You'll find that you feel a lot more relaxed afterward.

Strokes

Stop the Threat

There's one thing that the human brain needs more than anything else—more than mental stimulation, more than intriguing dreams, even more than a wake-up cup of coffee in the morning. It needs blood, and any shortfall can have extremely serious consequences.

When you have a stroke, blood can't get to specific parts of the brain. This happens when a blood vessel ruptures (hemorrhagic stroke) or is clogged by a clot or fatty deposits (ischemic stroke).

The prospect of a having stroke—either for you or someone you love—is immensely frightening. But here's something important to keep in mind as you face down those fears: There are only half as many strokes today as there were 30 years ago. Why? Because scientists have finally learned how to prevent this devastating problem.

MAINTAIN THE FLOW

The vast majority of strokes are the ischemic kind. They're frequently heralded by mini-strokes—what doctors call transient ischemic attacks (TIAs)—in which blood flow to the brain is blocked for only a few moments, then resumes.

The main risk factors for this type of stroke are smoking, high blood pressure, high cholesterol levels, and a family history of stroke. Fortunately, people who have strokes these days are frequently able to recover, but it's typically a long road back. That's why the best way to deal with a stroke is to prevent it in the first place. Here's how.

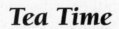

Tea Time

Get Blood Moving with Ginkgo

This herb can reduce platelet stickiness and increase microcirculation in the brain—both of which can help you avoid a stroke. To make a tea, steep 1 teaspoon of ginkgo in 1 cup of hot water for 10 minutes, then strain. Drink one cup a day. Avoid ginkgo if you're taking blood-thinning medications or aspirin therapy.

Eat plenty of apples. One study showed that men and women who munched an apple every day had a lower risk of embolic stroke (the kind caused by a tiny blood clot blocking an artery in the brain) than those who were halfhearted in their pursuit of the Isaac Newton special.

Don't forget the apricots. They're rich in potassium, the mineral that lowers blood pressure and reduces the risk of some kinds of strokes. In a Harvard study of more than 40,000 men, those who got the most potassium had about 40 percent less chance of having a stroke than those who consumed the least.

Take your tea black. A number of studies associate black tea—that's the regular kind you find in the supermarket—with reduced risk of heart disease and stroke. According to a report in the journal *Archives of Internal Medicine*, more than 800 elderly Dutch men who drank

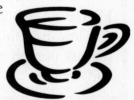

4 or more cups of black tea a day had a 69 percent lower risk of stroke than those who consumed less than 2.6 cups a day. Scientists believe black tea works because the antioxidants in it maintain the health of the circulatory system and reduce the risk of blood clots.

Raise a stink. This folk remedy is backed by solid science. Garlic stimulates circulation, reduces cholesterol, and decreases the stickiness of platelets—all of which may help prevent stroke. Chop some garlic, let it sit for 10 minutes, then sprinkle it onto your favorite food. Eat one to three raw cloves a day.

Start your workouts now! The more you move your body, the stronger your cardiovascular system gets—which helps prevent stroke. Being sedentary only adds to your risk. Begin by getting your doctor to give you a clean bill of health, then take off by going for a brisk walk every day. You don't have to go far—just to the corner and back. Gradually increase your distance and time until you're exercising for 15 to 20 minutes a day. Then try other activities, such as running, biking, swimming, or even dancing.

Get extra Bs. Homocysteine, an amino acid your body makes as it digests protein, has been linked to stroke and heart attacks for a long time, but new evidence is coming to light. A report presented at a meeting of the American Stroke Association revealed that homocysteine is

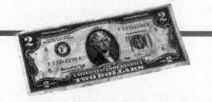

The $2 Deal

Slice Up Some Melons

Cantaloupe is a great source of potassium, and, according to the FDA, diets rich in potassium and low in sodium may reduce the risk of high blood pressure and stroke.

involved in actually causing a stroke, not just making you more vulnerable to one.

One way to lower homocysteine is to increase your intake of foods high in the B vitamins, specifically folate, B_6, and B_{12}. A major study—Vitamin Intervention for Stroke Prevention (VISP)—is now under way to find out if these vitamins ward off new strokes in people who have already had them. In the meantime, however, it can't hurt to get some more of those big Bs—whether or not you've already had a stroke. Eat lots of lean meats, whole grains, poultry, legumes, and fresh fruits and vegetables.

Keep your spuds covered. A potato baked in its skin packs 903 milligrams of stroke-preventive potassium—tons more than any other food. Take away the skin, and you'll get only 641 milligrams. So buy organic potatoes, scrub them well, bake them in their jackets, and eat every bite.

Fill your tank with fish oils. Results of the 14-year-long Nurses' Health Study, published in the *Journal of the American Medical Association*, revealed that women who ate fish two to four times a week reduced their stroke risk by a whopping 27 percent. Fish that are rich in beneficial omega-3 fatty acids include salmon, tuna, halibut, cod, and flounder.

Drink moderately. A drink a day may keep stroke at bay. In

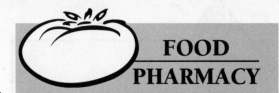

FOOD PHARMACY

Crunch More Crucifers

Eating broccoli, brussels sprouts, and other cruciferous vegetables may be as effective as controlling blood pressure and engaging in physical activity for preventing stroke, says Ralph Sacco, M.D., a stroke researcher at Columbia University in New York City and a spokesperson for the American Heart Association. One study showed that eating at least five servings of fruits and veggies daily, especially citrus fruits and members of the cabbage family, can lower your chance of stroke by about 30 percent.

fact, a report published in the *New England Journal of Medicine* revealed that light to moderate alcohol consumption reduced the risk of stroke for both men and women. A second study, published in the *Journal of the American Medical Association*, found that having up to two drinks a day helps prevent stroke. Too much alcohol, however, can actually increase your risk; experts recommend no more than one drink daily for women and two for men. If alcoholism runs in your family, don't add even a drop of alcohol to your diet.

Bring down the pressure. If you're not keeping your blood pressure under control, start now. It's crucial for preventing a hemorrhagic stroke. Work with your doctor to monitor your blood pressure, take any medication regularly, and make all the lifestyle changes necessary to keep your blood pressure off the ceiling.

Dump the smokes. Smoking constricts your blood vessels and only adds to your problems, especially if you already have high blood pressure. Join a support group, get medication from your doctor, use the patch—try everything you can to quit. Most experts say the best approach is a combination of behavioral techniques and medication.

Sunburn

Turn Down the Heat

The source of sunburn is no big mystery, but here's something you might not know. The brilliant rays of the sun that you see on a bright, sunny day aren't really the ones to worry about. Most of the damage comes from the invisible ultraviolet rays. They pack so much energy that even brief exposure causes your skin to darken—or, if you stay out too long, turn a painful, blistering red.

It almost goes without saying that severe burns—whether you get them in the kitchen or on the beach at Acapulco—always need to be treated by a doctor. Most sunburns aren't this serious, of course. Here's what you need to do to ease the pain and, more important, avoid getting fried in the future.

This enzyme is fine. An enzyme called photolyase, which

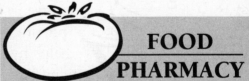

FOOD PHARMACY

Be Cucumber Cool

A quick way to soothe sunburn is to place chilled cucumber slices on your simmering skin. A dab of cold yogurt or a splash of vinegar will do the job, too.

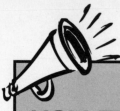

HOLLER FOR HELP

Burns That Go Too Far

Most sunburns are only minor annoyances, but sometimes they're serious enough to require emergency care. If your skin blisters or develops open sores, or you feel dizzy or nauseated, go to a doctor immediately. Severe sunburn can also cause chills or fever, which are early signs that you may be going into shock.

is made from ocean algae and added to some sunburn products, is said to be the magic elixir for a painful sunburn, reversing some of the critical DNA damage caused by soaking up too much ultraviolet light. In fact, studies have shown that photolyase reduced redness and DNA damage by as much as 45 percent.

Pop an analgesic. Aspirin, ibuprofen, or other pain relievers won't help heal your sunburned skin, but they're very effective at reducing pain while

nature takes its course.

Soak and cool. Cool water is a refreshing treat for sunburned skin. As soon as you can, soak a washcloth, wring it out, and apply it to the burned area, or simply lounge in a cool bath or shower. Apart from providing nearly instant relief, cool water helps hydrate the skin and prevents it from drying out.

Get extra C. If you're a sun worshiper, vitamin C is the one nutrient you need most. For one thing, your body uses it to build healthy skin that's at least somewhat resistant to the sun's burning rays. Vitamin C is also an antioxidant that blocks the damaging effects of free radicals, harmful oxygen molecules that are produced in profusion when the sun toasts the skin. Finally, C helps repair sunburn damage.

As long as you don't have stomach or kidney problems, you

should already be taking supplemental vitamin C every day. The Daily Value is 60 milligrams, which is enough under normal circumstances, but not if you've gotten burned. Then you'll need a lot more; your doctor can tell you exactly how much and the best way to take it.

Add some E. Another sun lover's nutrient is vitamin E. Like vitamin C, it's a protective antioxidant that helps prevent, or at least minimize, skin damage. Take 800 IU daily when you're nursing sunburn. You can also apply vitamin E cream or oil to the burned areas. They'll heal more quickly, and you'll be less likely to have permanent scars.

Slather on a moisturizer. Moisturizers pump healing fluids back into the skin and create a temporary cooling sensation, says Richard Wagner, M.D., professor of dermatology at the University of Texas Medical Branch in Galveston. "Make sure it's fragrance-free, or your skin may be irritated by an allergic reaction," he says. "That would make the sunburn worse."

Let the soap slide. For the first day or two after getting burned, don't use soap on the painful areas. It dries the skin and can make the pain worse. Of course, you may have to use soap if the area is dirtier than usual. Better to have a little irritation than to risk infection.

Drink and drink some more. Sunburns remove part of your body's natural moisture barrier, so you'll need to drink plenty of water to compensate. "It helps to offset fluid loss," says Dr. Wagner. Drinking water also helps your body repair the

The $2 Deal

Take the Capsule Cure

For mild sunburn, mix your own soothing oil by adding the contents of six capsules each of vitamin A and vitamin E to ¼ cup of flaxseed oil. Apply frequently to the burned areas. You may also add this combination to ¼ cup of aloe juice and smooth it over your skin.

burn and keeps your immune system in good shape to repel any bacteria that invade through the damaged skin. Drink as much as you can hold—anywhere from four to eight glasses a day, depending on your size and how active you are.

Wallow in aloe. The aloe plant may have been put on Earth just to help heal sunburned skin. Aloe thrives in any container, in any room, in any part of the country. If you get burned, break off a leaf, squeeze out the gel, and apply a generous amount. You can also slit a leaf lengthwise and tape the open area against your skin, says Heidi Weinhold, N.D., a naturopathic physician in the Pittsburgh area.

Buy the right screen. Did you get burned even though you slathered on sunscreen? It's possible that you used the wrong product. Most sunscreens protect against UVA and UVB, the sun's two types of burning rays, but they don't necessarily give all the protection you need, says Min-Wei Lee, M.D., a dermatologic surgeon and director of East Bay Laser and Skin Care Center in Walnut Creek, California.

When you buy sunscreen, buy only products that contain zinc oxide or Parsol 1789 (also called avobenzone). They provide optimal protection against both types of rays. Choose a sunscreen with a sun protection factor (SPF) of 30 or higher. Use a waterproof brand if you'll be swimming or you perspire heavily. Reapply sunscreen every 2 hours, no matter what it says on the label.

THE 25¢ SPECIAL

The Spritz Fix

Lavender is an antiseptic, cooling herb that can relieve burning and protect against secondary infections. Fill an 8-ounce spray bottle with cold water and add 6 drops of lavender oil. Shake well, then spray on the sunburned area.

Temporomandibular Disorder

Stop That Jaw from Poppin'

If it sounds like someone's cracking walnuts every time you open your mouth, or if your jaw occasionally freezes in either the open or closed position, you almost certainly have temporomandibular disorder. This condition, also known as TMD, isn't always painful, but no one likes going through life hearing clicking and popping sounds every time they yawn.

The temporomandibular joint is the hinge that allows your jaw to move up and down. Like any other joint in the body, it's vulnerable to things such as arthritis and sprains. The joint can also be looser than it should be, which can make it jump out of place on occasion.

Because TMD can be caused by so many different things, it's always worth checking with your doctor if the joint is sometimes painful or seems to be grinding instead of moving smoothly. Even if you don't have jaw-related problems, you should suspect TMD if you have frequent headaches, neck pain, or earaches, all of which are sometimes linked to problems with the jaw joint.

You can't always rub out TMD, but you can almost always rub it the right way. When you first notice pain, put your fingers on the side of your jaw, then open and close your mouth. The thick muscle that you feel is the one that controls your jaw. Put one finger on either side of the muscle and knead it gently, working all the way from your ear to your jaw. This is one of the best ways to prevent—or ease—painful spasms.

LUBE THAT HINGE

If TMD is causing you a lot of pain, or your jaw is locking up with some regularity, you may need surgery to repair the joint. In the vast majority of cases, however, you don't have to pay out big bucks to treat TMD. You can usually ease or even eliminate it with creative home care. Here's how to do it.

Pack in the vitamin C. This helpful vitamin is an antioxidant nutrient that helps prevent harmful molecules called free radicals from damaging your joints. It also promotes the growth of collagen, a tissue that helps keep joints healthy, says Gerald J. Murphy, D.D.S., director of publications for the American Academy of Craniofacial Pain. He tells people to take 3,000 milligrams of vitamin C daily. Doses this large may cause diarrhea or other side effects, and they may be harmful for people with stomach or kidney problems, so check with your doctor before you start. You can minimize digestive problems by taking the total amount in divided doses at different times during the day. Taking vitamin C with food also helps.

Have a cuppa ice. Flare-ups of TMD are usually accompanied by inflammation, which is what causes pain and swelling. Probably the quickest way to reduce inflammation is to immediately apply cold to your jaw to make blood vessels constrict, or narrow, which reduces swelling. "Fill some paper cups with water and keep them in the freezer," Dr. Murphy advises.

When TMD strikes, tear off part of the cup or push out an inch or two of ice, then apply it right where it hurts. Apply the ice for about 20 minutes every few hours throughout the day.

Warm your jaw. You don't want to apply heat to your jaw joint right away because it can increase swelling. After a day or two of cold treatments, though, heat will increase circulation and help remove any buildup of fluids and painful toxins. Soak a washcloth in hot water, wring it out, and hold it to your jaw until it cools. Then dip the cloth again and repeat the treatment as often as necessary for relief.

Sleep with a splint. Don't worry, it sounds worse than it really is. One of the most successful strategies for easing TMD is to use an oral splint that guides the jaw back into its proper position, says Dr. Murphy. The splints are custom-made by doctors and dentists, and they're usually worn only at night—although if your TMD is serious, you may have to wear a splint night and day for a while.

It takes time to get used to a splint, but it works very quickly.

HOLLER FOR HELP
The Key to Jaw Lock

Most people with TMD don't experience jaw lock, but it can happen, and when it does, there are usually some warning signs. If you notice that your jaw is getting increasingly stiff or sore, or it seems to be getting harder to move, see your doctor right away. If you're lucky, the problem can be corrected before your jaw takes itself totally out of action.

What do you do if you're caught by surprise? For starters, don't panic! Your jaw won't stay closed permanently, honest. What you want to do is move it carefully as much as you can—a little bit from side to side or a little bit up and down. Flex and relax the muscles. The more you do this, the more your jaw will relax. Sooner or later, it should start moving normally again. If it doesn't get better within an hour or two, though, you should see a doctor right away.

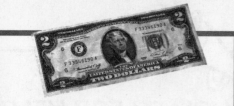

The $2 Deal

Supplement the Joint

Two over-the-counter dietary supplements, glucosamine and chondroitin, encourage the growth and repair of cartilage and other protective tissues in the joints. They may also help prevent age-related joint damage that can lead to TMD. The recommended dose is 500 milligrams of either (or both) three times daily. Most drugstores carry combination supplements, but avoid them if you're allergic to shellfish.

"In a week, most people don't want to do without them because their jaws are feeling so much better," says Dr. Murphy.

Nibble, don't chomp. When TMD is acting up, it's important to give your jaw a rest, just as you'd stay off your feet after spraining your ankle. Stick to foods that are easy on your chops and avoid those that require a lot of jaw action, such as apples and corn on the cob. And by all means, let the silverware do the work. Cut food into small pieces so you don't have to chew as much.

Pull those shoulders back. And no slumping while you work! "Postures that create the least stress on your upper body will also produce the least stress on your jaw," says Dr. Murphy. This means standing and sitting up straight and always making an effort to keep your head and neck in line with the rest of your body. It really does help!

Knock down the tension in your life. Any kind of emotional stress makes TMD worse because it makes muscles tense. It also increases levels of body chemicals that aggravate pain. Whatever it is that you do when you relax, do it even more often when TMD is acting up. "Things like meditation, yoga, or just getting away for a while can make a big difference," says Dr. Murphy.

Tennis Elbow

Ace the Pain

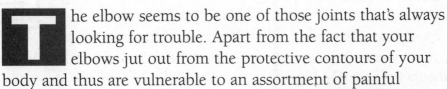

The elbow seems to be one of those joints that's always looking for trouble. Apart from the fact that your elbows jut out from the protective contours of your body and thus are vulnerable to an assortment of painful knocks, they also do an awful lot of bending. Raise a glass, pull a weed, or scratch your head—then thank your elbows for doing all the hard work.

All that constant movement comes with a price, however. Even if you've never picked up a racket in your life, you've probably experienced tennis elbow. Here's what happens: The strain of repetitive movements causes the muscles or tendons to become inflamed, causing pain that can range from a dull throb at your elbow to an ache that

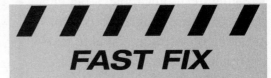

FAST FIX
Cream It with Calendula

Want fast, natural relief from an ouchy elbow? Grab a jar of calendula cream, available at health food stores, and rub $1/2$ teaspoon into the muscles surrounding your elbow. It can reduce the ache and help you heal more quickly.

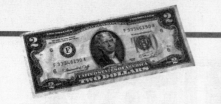

The $2 Deal

Pop a Pineapple Pill

Pineapple does more than add delicious sweetness to fresh fruit platters. It's also rich in bromelain, a substance that acts as a natural painkiller, says Kevin Conner, N.D. In fact, bromelain has been shown to reduce the swelling around muscles and tendons that causes the pain of tennis elbow. Since you can't get healing amounts of bromelain by eating fresh pineapple, a better approach (as long as you're not taking blood thinners) is to take supplements; the usual dose is 375 milligrams three times a day. Don't take them with meals, though, because your digestive juices destroy the active ingredient.

radiates down your arm. Often, the pain starts off as a minor twinge, and it may or may not flare into major agony. It all depends on what you do next.

AX THE ACHE

In extreme cases, tennis elbow will go away only if you take powerful drugs to reduce the inflammation. Occasionally, it's necessary to have steroid injections or physical therapy to get things working properly again. Unless your symptoms persist for a few weeks or more or steadily get worse, though, you can almost always treat tennis elbow at home simply by putting down the tennis racket (or whatever it was that caused the pain). In the meantime, here are a few quick ways to reduce the discomfort and help the muscles and tendons heal more quickly.

Freeze it fast. As soon as the pain starts, reach for an ice pack (with the other arm). You can't beat ice for reducing inflammation and numbing pain. For the first few days after the injury, apply it for 20 minutes at a time every few hours.

Stop the bends. Since moving your elbow too much is what causes tennis elbow, it makes sense that keeping it still will help it get better. You may want to pick up an arm brace at a drugstore or medical supply store to protect the injured joint and keep it from moving in an inappropriate (and painful) direction.

Wait it out. You shouldn't rush back into action as soon as your pain is gone. Wait a few days or a week to be sure you're really better, advises Kevin Conner, N.D., a naturopathic physician and faculty member at Bastyr University near Seattle. "The tissue's still healing," he says. "You don't want to aggravate it."

Rebuild with protein. When you're recovering from tennis elbow, you need a lot of protein, the nutrient that your body uses to repair muscle damage. The usual rule is to get 0.8 gram of protein for each kilogram of body weight. Here's an easy way to figure out how much you need: Divide your body weight by 2.2 (there are 2.2 pounds per kilogram), then multiply that number by 0.8 to get your daily target for protein. Thus, if you weigh 150 pounds, you'll need 54 grams of protein. That's roughly the amount you'd get in a cup of tuna salad, a cup of long-grain white rice, and a cup of milk.

Reach for omega-3's. Essential fatty acids, especially the omega-3 fatty acids in cold-water fish such as salmon and tuna, help suppress the inflammation that causes the pain. You can also get plenty of omega-3's

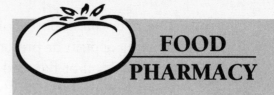

FOOD PHARMACY

Feel Berry Better

Dark berries, such as blueberries, blackberries, and boysenberries, contain natural chemicals called bioflavonoids that relieve pain and inflammation. It's also a good idea to eat plenty of other fruits and vegetables while you're healing to pump even more bioflavonoids into your system.

by eating a few tablespoons of ground flaxseed or—unless you're taking aspirin or prescription blood thinners—taking 1 to 3 grams of fish oil or flaxseed oil.

Heed the signals. You probably remember this old joke: A patient says to his doctor, "It hurts when I do this," and the doctor says, "Well, don't do that." Okay, it's a groaner, but there's a lot of truth behind it. "The single best thing you can do is find the movements that cause or aggravate the injury and then quit doing them," says Dr. Conner. Pain from tennis elbow tends to be very specific: It hurts when you move your arm one way, and it doesn't hurt when you move it a different way. Limit your movements to the nonpainful ones, and let the healing begin.

Stretch it out. Some slow, gentle stretching will help your aggrieved elbow heal and strengthen. First, extend your arm straight in front of you, palm down, and slowly bend your wrist so the back of your hand moves toward you. Then lower your hand and flex your wrist so that your fingers point down.

You can do a similar exercise with your elbow. Hold your arm out, palm up, and slowly bend your elbow so your palm moves toward you. Repeat both stretches a few times a day, but quit if they cause real pain. It's okay for stretches to be slightly uncomfortable, but they shouldn't hurt. If they do, you're overdoing it.

Weed the garden. Two common garden plants, chickweed and comfrey, are traditionally used to relieve swelling and pain. Pick a handful of chickweed and one or two large comfrey leaves. Blanch them in hot water and apply to your elbow, using chickweed as the first layer and holding it in place with the comfrey leaves.

Try indirect massage. When you have tennis elbow, direct pressure may make the sore area hurt even more, but massaging the surrounding area is fine.

Get a drop on pain. St. John's wort oil is an excellent pain reliever that can be applied directly to the aching area. For an extra boost, add 4 to 6 drops of arnica oil and 2 or 3 drops of wintergreen oil. Do not use arnica on broken skin.

Heat is neat. Smooth some hot-pepper cream over your sore joint, and you'll begin to feel relief. The heat from capsaicin, the stuff that gives peppers their bite, brings more blood circulation to the area. You can buy a cream containing 0.025 to 0.075 percent capsaicin at drugstores. Use it up to three times a day, but be careful not to get it in your eyes or on areas of broken skin.

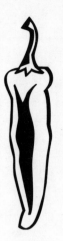

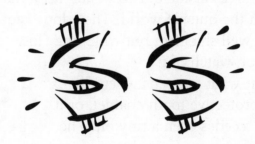

Toothaches

Stop Them Fast

It's a wonder we all don't get toothaches more often, since the tiny nerves inside our teeth are just a fraction of an inch from the outside world. They don't cause any pain as long as they're well shielded, but when they lose some of their protective armor, watch out!

Think about what happens when there's a breach in the protective tooth enamel, or if your gum line recedes even a tiny bit. The incredibly sensitive nerves are then exposed to air—or, in some cases, assaulted by inflammation or infection. They let you know what's happening immediately by causing excruciating pain.

ACHE NO MORE

It's not unusual for toothaches to disappear on their own, but you can bet that the pain's going to come back—probably sooner rather than later. You may as well bite the bullet and make an appointment to see your dentist. Toothaches are often caused by decay, explains Richard Price, D.M.D., a dentist in the

Boston area and consumer advisor for the American Dental Association. There's a good chance you'll need a filling or even a root canal. Once the damage is repaired, the toothache will be gone for good.

There's a curious thing about toothaches, though. It seems that they never happen when it's easy to see your dentist. They have an unfortunate way of cropping up late at night or at the beginning of three-day weekends. When that happens, you have to find ways to ease the agony until you can get some help. Here are a few terrific tips to try.

Fight it with floss. Sometimes a toothache is caused by a particle of food lodged between your teeth or between your teeth and gums. It's worth it to take a few minutes to gently floss the area to see if anything pops out.

Don't quit brushing. Even if it hurts a little when you brush, it's essential to keep your teeth clean until you can see a dentist. "Food and debris can collect on your tooth and make the pain worse," says Dr. Price.

Swish with salt. Thoroughly rinsing your mouth with a saltwater solution—made by mixing about 1/2 teaspoon of salt in a cup of warm water—will often reduce the pain of a toothache, says Dr. Price. The relief doesn't last very long, but you can repeat the swishing as often as necessary.

Spread on some spice. Relief from a raging toothache may be as close as your spice rack. Folk healers often advise people to spread a little ground ginger or

Tea Time

Rinse with Chamomile

Brew some chamomile tea by steeping 1 teaspoon of dried herb (available at health food stores) in a cup of hot water for 10 to 20 minutes. Strain the tea and let it cool, swish some around in your mouth for about 30 seconds, then swallow it or spit it out. Keep rinsing your mouth until you've used up all the tea. Avoid chamomile if you're allergic to ragweed.

Clove oil has been used for generations for easing toothaches, and there's good evidence that it works, says Flora Stay, D.D.S., author of *The Complete Book of Dental Remedies*. Buy the oil at a health food store or drugstore, then dip in a cotton swab and rub the oil on the sore tooth. In many cases, the pain will disappear almost instantly.

red pepper around the tooth. Add a little water to the spice to make a paste, then spread it liberally all around the point of pain. You may notice relief in as few as 5 minutes.

Hit it with ice. You wouldn't think that placing a cold pack—or a washcloth wrapped around some ice cubes—on the outside of your mouth would have much effect on a toothache, but it does seem to help. Hold it against the tender area for 15 to 20 minutes every few hours until you can see your dentist.

Take a painkiller. The analgesics in your medicine cabinet are more effective than you might think. Acetaminophen can sometimes ease a toothache as effectively as mild prescription drugs, and as long as you're not sensitive to them, aspirin and ibuprofen may be even better. "They reduce inflammation and stop the body's production of pain-causing prostaglandins," says Dr. Price.

Wet your mouth. Toothaches can get worse when your mouth is dry. Until the pain is gone, it's important to drink a lot of water to keep your mouth lubricated. Have a glass of water handy at all times and keep taking small sips, Dr. Price advises.

If your mouth is always a little dry, it's probably time to make a list of all the medications you're taking and review them with your dentist. Anywhere from 200 to 400 common drugs, such as antihistamines, heart drugs, and anti-anxiety medications, cause dryness, says Dr. Price.

Ulcers

Soothe the Sores

■

ere's a little factoid that boggles the mind: The digestive acids in your stomach are nearly as strong as battery acid. How is it that these acids are strong enough to dissolve the heaviest meal into a digestible soup of nutrients, but somehow they don't digest the stomach at the same time?

Nature, it turns out, designed the stomach to withstand constant acid onslaughts by giving it a thin, protective lining that prevents damage to the tender tissue underneath. Of course, this system works only if the protective barrier is intact.

That's where germs come in. *Helicobacter pylori*, a type of bacterium that commonly inhabits the stomach and intestine, digs into this protective lining. If you're infected with *H. pylori*, the lining may be pitted with tiny holes that permit stomach acid to leak through. The result: small, painful little sores known as ulcers.

INFECTION PROTECTION

Most people with ulcers experience a burning sensation from time to time, usually between meals, when their stomachs are empty. Don't ignore the pain; see your doctor. Ulcers that aren't treated can bleed, and sometimes they bleed a lot. It's not uncommon, in fact, for people with ulcers to become anemic because of blood loss.

In most cases, ulcers can be eliminated with a relatively simple, two-part treatment: Antibiotics to kill the bacteria and medications to lower levels of stomach acid. Along with treatment, however, there are a few lifestyle approaches that do make a difference—and they're a lot cheaper! Here's what doctors recommend.

Don't depend on antacids. When the burning pain of ulcers flares, your natural instinct is probably to pop a few antacids. There's certainly nothing wrong with this approach in some cases, but some doctors suspect that quenching stomach acid with antacids may make ulcers worse in the long run.

"You need stomach acids to obliterate microorganisms," says Christie C. Yerby, N.D., a naturopathic physician in Sanford, North Carolina. "Lowering the acidity of the stomach makes it easier for ulcer-causing bacteria to survive."

Soothe with cinnamon. This aromatic spice appears to help knock out ulcer-causing germs, so the next time an ulcer flares, try a cup of cinnamon tea. The German Commission E, which studies herbal medicines in Europe, says it really works.

Say hello to aloe. Aloe vera is one of nature's great healers, and

HOLLER FOR HELP

Drugs to Watch Out For

Some ulcers are triggered by the prolonged use of pain relievers, including aspirin and ibuprofen. If you take these drugs on a regular basis, call your doctor if you experience any kind of stomach pain. Ulcers caused by these drugs can be extremely serious. In most cases, your doctor will be able to give you a different pain reliever that doesn't have stomach-damaging side effects.

it's especially good for ulcers because it coats irritated tissues and may promote faster healing. You can buy aloe juice at health food stores, or if you grow aloe at home to treat minor injuries, just break open a leaf and squeeze some juice into your mouth, Dr. Yerby suggests. You can take aloe up to a couple of times a day.

Get extra nutrients. If you don't eat a lot of fruit, vegetables, and other plant foods, you may not be getting enough of a few key nutrients—mainly vitamins A, C, and E—that are needed to repair damaged tissues throughout your body, including the stomach lining. If you have a history of ulcers, it's a good idea to take daily supplements that provide the recommended daily amounts of each of these important nutrients.

Take a fish pill. Doctors and nutritionists almost beg Americans to eat more fish, in part because it's a rich source of essential fatty acids that help quell inflammation. If you have ulcers, however, eating too much fish may cause an increase in stomach acid—and pain, says Dr. Yerby. Instead of eating fish, she recommends that people with ulcers take fish-oil supplements. Unless you take aspirin or prescription blood thinners, pick up some capsules at a drugstore or health food store, then follow the label directions.

Load up on licorice. This sweet-tasting herb (not the candy) is powerful medicine. It reduces

Tea Time

Protect with Slippery Elm

The herb slippery elm soothes the lining of the digestive tract. This may protect small ulcers from further acid damage and may help them heal more quickly. Slippery elm is available in powdered form at health food stores. Add a teaspoon of powder to a glass of water or juice and drink one or two glasses daily when ulcers flare up.

inflammation and appears to help ulcers heal more quickly. You can buy licorice-root tea bags or powder at health food stores. As long as you don't have high blood pressure, you can drink two or three cups of tea a day to ease the pain of ulcers and help keep them from coming back.

Also look for chewable DGL tablets, which are made from licorice that's had the blood pressure–raising compound removed. Chewing these tablets between meals will speed pain relief and aid in healing an ulcer. Follow the package directions.

Peel some relief. Having an ulcer is no reason to hold the onions. In fact, it's all the more reason to add them to salads, sandwiches, soups, and so forth. Onions contain compounds that seem to help eliminate ulcer-causing bacteria, so try to include them in at least one meal a day.

Hide the hooch. And while you're at it, give up cigarettes if you're a smoker. Alcohol and tobacco tend to make ulcer pain worse, and they inhibit your body's ability to heal the damage. People who smoke and drink are also more likely to get ulcers than those who don't indulge.

Chill. Even though emotional stress doesn't cause ulcers, it does increase levels of stomach acid, which can make the pain worse. Stress reduction should be part of every anti-ulcer strategy, says Dr. Yerby.

When you feel your stress levels rising, close your eyes, breathe deeply, and visualize a peaceful scene from nature, she advises. Keep the scene in your mind for 15 to 20 minutes. You'll find that you feel a lot more relaxed afterward—and you'll have less discomfort.

Urinary Tract Infections

Purge Those Pesky Germs

There are plenty of things men will never understand about women—why their dress pants never have pockets, for example, or why they need three or four shampoos and conditioners when the average guy gets by with the same brand year after year.

They also have a hard time relating to urinary tract infections (UTIs). Men rarely get them, but they're among the most common, and annoying, health issues women deal with. About a third of American women will get urinary tract infections at some point in their lives, and some women get them over and over again.

EASY ACCESS

Most UTIs occur when bacteria that normally live in the area surrounding the anus make their way inside the urethra. Once they get into that warm, moist environment, they quickly multiply, and sometimes they even work their way up to the bladder.

Men sometimes get UTIs, but their extra inches of anatomy make it harder for bacteria to get inside. Women don't have that protection, so they're a lot more vulnerable.

The infections can occur anywhere in the urinary tract, but they usually affect the urethra, the tube through which urine leaves the body, or the bladder. The main symptom is a burning sensation, along with urinary urgency—the sudden, overwhelming need to go to the bathroom.

"I used to have five or six infections a year," says Crystal Abernathy, N.D., a naturopathic physician in Charlotte, North Carolina. "It's a very irritating thing to deal with." Although it took some time, Dr. Abernathy eventually discovered how to keep the pesky infections under control. She hasn't had one in years—and the advice she shares here will work just as well for you.

NO MORE INFECTION

If you think you have a UTI, or even if you're sure you do (women who get them know the symptoms all too well), see your doctor right away. You're going to need antibiotics to knock out the germs and relieve the symptoms. In the meantime, now's the time to think about ways to prevent future infections and take steps to keep your current discomfort to a minimum. Here's what to do.

Spoon up some blueberries. They're bursting with tannins, compounds that boot out the bacteria responsible for UTIs. Researchers have found that tannins prevent the germs from attaching to the bladder wall, where they thrive.

Fight back with cranberries. Harvard scientists have found that women who drink a little more than a cup of cranberry juice daily for a month may be only 42 percent as likely to have a UTI as women who don't. Look for a drink that's 27 percent cranberry juice, preferably one without too much added sugar.

Cut the sweets. Sugar can be a real problem if you get frequent UTIs. It encourages the growth of bacteria, and it reduces the ability of your immune system to battle infection. "It's sort of a double whammy," says Dr. Abernathy.

Remember, too, that it's not only sweets such as candy that cause problems but all sources of sugar, including the sugar in packaged foods. Read labels so you know what you're getting.

Imbibe less. The bacterial colonies that cause UTIs love alcohol because it's converted into sugar in your body. Give up the drinks until the infection is gone.

Load up on protein. You need plenty of protein to keep your immune system healthy. To make sure you're getting enough, divide your weight by 2.2 to get your weight in kilograms, then eat 1 gram of protein daily for each kilo-

HOLLER FOR HELP
Stop the Spread

Most urinary tract infections are merely uncomfortable. Call your doctor immediately, however, if your infection is accompanied by fever, blood in the urine, or back pain. These are signs that you may be developing a kidney infection, which can be life-threatening without prompt treatment.

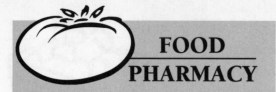

FOOD PHARMACY

Stock Up on 'shrooms

Most supermarkets offer several tasty varieties of gourmet mushrooms. You should definitely stock up on them when you have a UTI, because they boost the ability of your immune system to combat infections. "Different mushrooms stimulate different aspects of the immune system, so it's good to combine them and get a broad spectrum of effects," says Crystal Abernathy, N.D. The types to look for include shiitake, reishi, and maitake.

gram of body weight.

As long as you eat a healthy diet that includes plenty of whole grains, legumes, and lean meat and fish, you're almost guaranteed to get enough protein to boost your defenses against UTIs.

Take the C cruise. "Vitamin C is helpful because it supports the immune system," says Dr. Abernathy. When you have a UTI, plan on taking 500 milligrams of vitamin C every 2 hours, she suggests.

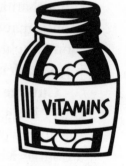

Vitamin C in large amounts may cause diarrhea. If you're having problems, cut back on the dose until you find a level that works for you. If you have kidney disease or stomach problems, discuss using vitamin C with your doctor before giving it a try.

Try an herbal combo. "I use a combination of four different herbs to treat urinary tract infections," Dr. Abernathy says. "It tends to be pretty effective; people usually start getting relief in 1 to 4 hours."

The herbs she uses are uva-ursi (sometimes called bearberry), buchu, echinacea, and goldenseal, which are available at health food stores. Take 200 milligrams of each three times daily for a week, she advises. Skip the echinacea, though, if you have an autoimmune disease such as rheumatoid arthritis, lupus, or multiple sclerosis, or if you are pregnant or nursing.

Drink like a fish. The more water you drink, the more bacteria will be flushed from your bladder. "Drink at least 2 quarts of water a day," Dr. Abernathy suggests.

That may seem like a lot, but if you carry water and sip it throughout the day, you won't even realize how much you're drinking.

Clean from front to back. It's an unfortunate fact of anatomy—the proximity of the anus and urethra—that makes women vulnerable to bacterial invasions. If you always wipe from front to back after using the toilet, you'll be less likely to push bacteria somewhere where they can cause problems.

Take a bathroom break after sex. Some women find that they get UTIs after sex because intercourse can push bacteria where they shouldn't go. Urinating after intercourse can flush out any germs that may have worked their way into the urinary tract.

Don't hold it. When your body tells you it's time to find a restroom, do it. Holding urine in the bladder for too long gives bacteria the chance to multiply.

Boost your immune system. To help your body fend off UTIs, whip up a homemade immune system strengthener. Mix equal parts of dried echinacea, goldenseal, and licorice root, all available at health food stores. Put about a tablespoon of the mixture in a tea ball and steep in hot water for 10 to 15 minutes. Drink two or three cups daily until the infection is gone. Omit the licorice root if you have high blood pressure, and avoid echinacea if you have an autoimmune disease or are pregnant or nursing.

The $2 Deal

Protect with Citrate

If you take supplemental magnesium or calcium, be sure to get the citrate form, says Crystal Abernathy, N.D. Citrates are easier for your body to absorb, and they make the urine more alkaline, which can help prevent UTIs.

Varicose Veins

No More Leg Pain

Do your legs start hurting as the day goes by? Do you find yourself wearing long pants even on 95-degree days? Maybe you're one of the millions of Americans with varicose veins—and no matter what you hear, they're not just a cosmetic problem.

Even though nearly everyone has some varicose veins, there's a lot of confusion about what they really are. As doctors sometimes explain, they're nature's proof that gravity only pulls one way. Confused? Let's take a look.

AN UPHILL CLIMB

A varicose vein is simply a blood vessel that doesn't have quite enough strength to push its cargo of blood uphill and back into circulation. When blood leaves your heart, it's traveling at tremendous velocity. The initial speed, combined with gravity, means that blood doesn't have any trouble reaching the blood vessels in your legs.

Now consider the return trip. This time, the blood has to go uphill, without the heart's pumping action to help it along. As it moves upward from veins in your legs—assisted by the pumping action of your leg muscles—the blood passes through tiny one-way valves, which snap shut behind it at intervals. Basically, it moves uphill in stages.

Sometimes, the valves aren't strong enough to support the weight of the blood, so it slips backward, forming pools inside one or more veins. After a while, the accumulated blood causes the vein to swell, resulting in a varicose vein.

Varicose veins can make your legs feel tired and achy. That's the most common problem, but there's also a risk that the poor circulation that accompanies varicose veins can cause ulcers on your lower legs. Less often, the swollen veins can promote the formation of blood clots that are potentially serious.

FOOD PHARMACY

Fight Back with Flavonoids

Strong, healthy veins are less likely to become varicose. One way to strengthen yours is to get more bioflavonoids in your diet. These natural plant chemicals, found in most fruits and vegetables, make the vein walls stronger and better able to push blood uphill. Most researchers recommend at least five servings of fresh fruit and vegetables a day.

GET THAT BLOOD MOVING

You can see, then, that you have to do something when you have varicose veins. If you really hate the way they look, or they're causing a lot of physical discomfort, surgery and other techniques can remove them. In most cases, however, you can bolster your veins with some simple home strategies that cost little or nothing to do. Here are a few things you ought to try.

Firm up with stockings. Snug-fitting hose, called compression stockings, are available from drugstores and medical supply stores. They provide extra support to the walls of blood vessels in the legs, which helps keep blood moving upward, says Peter Beatty, M.D., an interventional radiologist at Legacy Meridian Park Hospital in Tualatin, Oregon, and national cochair of the Legs for Life Program. (You can visit www.legsforlife.org for information about free screening for leg circulation problems.) Your doctor should write a prescription for the right kind of hose for you. Over-the-counter compression stockings work well, but they may not provide the exact amount of pressure that you need.

Raise your legs. The blood in your legs has to fight gravity to climb all the way back to your heart. Why not reverse the situation and let gravity work for you? To do it, raise your feet above the level of your heart for a couple of hours each day, or sit with your legs propped up on pillows. About 10 minutes after you elevate your legs, the ache will go away.

Point your feet. Sleeping with your feet raised a few inches will give your veins a boost all night. You can prop your feet on a flat pillow or put some boards under the foot of your bed. Check with your doctor first, though, since this sleeping position may aggravate some health problems.

Sit and put your feet up. If you spend most of your day on

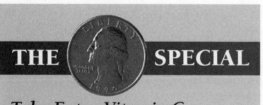

THE SPECIAL

Take Extra Vitamin C

Your body uses vitamin C to strengthen blood vessels, says Erica LePore, N.D. Unless you have stomach or kidney problems, she suggests taking 500 to 1,000 milligrams of vitamin C two or three times daily. Since taking this much vitamin C may cause diarrhea, it's a good idea to start with the lower dose and gradually work up from there.

your feet, your varicose veins may feel as if they're going to pop out of your legs by the time the day's over. Don't wait until you get home from work to give your legs a breather. Take breaks as often as possible. If you stand a lot, take some time to relax in a comfortable chair. Put your feet up on a desk if you can.

Dress loosely. Compression stockings are designed to give your veins the kind of pressure they need, but other garments that put pressure on your legs can interfere with circulation. Avoid tight panty hose, girdles, and other kinds of restrictive clothing.

Exercise often. Having varicose veins isn't an excuse for not exercising. In fact, it's all the more reason to be active. "Exercise is helpful in managing varicose veins," says Kimberly Beauchamp, N.D., a naturopathic physician in Wakefield, Rhode Island. The more fit you are, the better your circulatory system will be able to cope with the diminished capacity of your leg veins.

"It's best to do exercise like yoga, swimming, or walking, which doesn't put excessive pressure on the lower extremities," Dr. Beauchamp adds.

Beat the heat. You don't want your legs to get too hot when you have varicose veins, because it could result in tissue-damaging inflammation, says Erica LePore, N.D., a naturopathic physician in Wakefield, Rhode Island. You should avoid long, hot baths and other activities that make your legs hotter than usual.

Strengthen the veins. You can improve the pumping action of leg veins with a technique called contrast hydrotherapy, in which you alternate between hot and cold treatments. First, soak a cloth in hot water, wring it out, and place it over the area where you have varicose veins. Leave it in place for 3 minutes,

FAST FIX
Cool the Ache

Cold witch hazel is a cool solution to aching veins. Chill a cup of witch hazel in the refrigerator for about an hour, then soak a washcloth in the liquid and apply it to the parts of your legs that hurt. Keep the compress in place for about 15 minutes while also elevating your legs. Witch hazel has astringent properties, which means that it improves blood flow and eases pain.

then replace it with a cold cloth for 30 seconds. Repeat the cycle two or three times, always ending with the cold cloth. "It's helpful for strengthening blood vessels and promoting healthy circulation," says Dr. Beauchamp. And it makes your legs feel good!

Rub 'em right. There's nothing like a massage for soothing tired legs (or tired anything, for that matter). Besides making you feel good, massage can improve your circulation, which is a big plus if you have varicose veins. To help ease the ache even more, add a few drops of comfrey oil to a few tablespoons of olive oil, then give yourself a soothing oil massage. The comfrey will boost circulation and help the discomfort fade a lot faster.

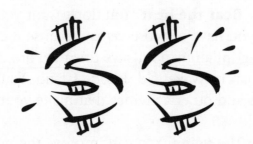

Warts

Victory over Viruses

In *The Adventures of Huckleberry Finn*, Tom and Huck debated about several ways to get rid of warts—most involving prowling around town at midnight. But the most effective, they agreed, was to take a dead cat to the grave of a recently deceased, "wicked" person. At midnight, they said, a devil would come to take the wicked person's body away. "You heave your cat after 'em and say, 'Devil follow corpse, cat follow devil, warts follow cat, I'm done with ye!' "

Folklore is full of such wart remedies, simply because the unsightly little bumps are tough to get rid of. There are more than 50 types of warts that can appear anywhere on your body, but the hands and feet are the most common sites. And, as if one weren't bad enough, they sometimes appear in groups. They're caused by the human papillomavirus, which stimulates rapid cell growth on the outer layer of your skin.

SAY GOODBYE TO BUMPS

Fortunately, warts appear less frequently as we age—possibly because we develop immunity to the virus that sprouts them. If

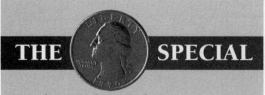
Bark Up the Right Tree

Folklore from Michigan suggests that you find yourself a nice birch tree and cut off a strip of bark. (You can also get birch bark in some health food stores.) Soak the bark in water until it softens, then tape it directly to your wart. Nobody knows why it works, but folks point out that birch bark contains salicylates, the basis of some FDA-approved wart treatments.

you do happen to get them, and dragging dead felines through a cemetery seems just a bit much, consider the following ways to get rid of them.

Keep your feet covered. The wart virus is everywhere, and you can pick it up easily by following in someone's footsteps in a shower, locker room, or public pool. These little growths are also acquired through direct contact with an infected person. Don't shower in the same stall with someone who has warts, and wear flip-flops or thongs when you're walking around in locker rooms or at public pools.

Leave them alone. Picking at a wart just spreads the virus that causes it. It will grow back anyway, so let nature take its course.

Ax 'em with acid. Warts will usually disappear on their own, but if you're impatient, head for the drugstore. An over-the-counter acid solution can help, say doctors at the Mayo Clinic. You'll have to apply the remedy twice a day for a few weeks, or it won't be effective. Look for a product that contains salicylic acid, which will peel off the infected skin, but be aware that the acid can be irritating. Try a 17 percent acid solution on your hands (or the end of your nose) and a 40 percent solution on your feet. If you're pregnant, ask your doctor if a wart remedy is safe to use.

Clobber them with cedar. Yellow cedar, also known as

thuja, contains potent oil in its leaves that makes an excellent wart remedy. Fill a small jar with thuja leaves and cover them with olive oil. Add the contents of a capsule of vitamin E oil. Let the jar sit in a sunny window for 10 days, shaking it well each day. Strain the oil, then store it in a cool, dark place. (If you keep it in the refrigerator, it will last for four to six months.) Apply the oil to the surface of the wart two or three times daily.

Boost your immunity. The development of warts can signal a weakened immune system. You can give yourself an antiviral boost with astragalus tea. To make it, simmer 1 heaping teaspoon of dried root in 1 cup of water for 20 minutes, then strain. Drink two cups daily.

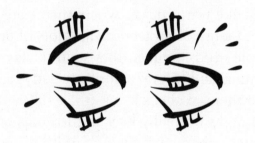

Yeast Infections

Fight the Fungi

In some ways, germs aren't a whole lot different from people. They like warm places where there's an abundance of moisture, plenty of protection, and lots of tasty treats. Once these basic needs are met, they tend to stay right where they are and multiply like crazy until the body's mechanisms step in to keep them in check.

The yeast fungus normally lives in the body, but under normal circumstances, there's not enough of it for you to notice. When something upsets the body's internal ecosystem, though, the fungus, called candida, may grow out of control. Thus, you can think of vaginal yeast infections as a sign that something's not quite the way it should be. Changing levels of hormones can allow it to thrive. So can changes in acidity. Women who take antibiotics often get yeast infections because the drugs kill beneficial organisms that normally keep the fungus in check.

Most women are all too familiar with the symptoms—usually pain, itching, or a bad odor—that accompany yeast infections. If you've never had one before and you experience any of these symptoms, check with your doctor just to be sure that what you have is really a yeast infection.

STOP THE YEAST FEAST

For the most part, your body is pretty good at getting this all-too-common problem under control, and most infections will clear up even if you do nothing. But why suffer? There are many over-the-counter treatments, and they're very effective. Since drugs don't work instantly, though, and they won't prevent future problems, take a look at the following remedies.

Unlike drugs, these strategies can help you get to the root of the problem and keep infections from recurring.

Switch methods. If you use oral contraceptives, they may be triggering yeast infections, says Jana Nalbandian, N.D., a naturopathic physician and faculty member at Bastyr University near Seattle. "Birth control pills are at the top of the list for causing vaginal yeast infections," she says.

You're more likely to have trouble with pills that contain a high percentage of estrogen, she says. If you have recurrent yeast infections, ask your doctor if you should try a different type of

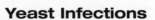

pill or even switch to a different form of birth control.

Heal with echinacea. Studies in Germany show that echinacea tea can prevent yeast infections. Make a cup of the tea by putting ½ teaspoon of dried echinacea in 1 cup of boiling water. Steep for about 10 minutes, then strain out the herb. Researchers found that the tea loses its effect after eight weeks, so stop for a month, then start drinking it again. Don't use echinacea if you have an autoimmune disease such as rheumatoid arthritis, lupus, or multiple sclerosis, or if you are pregnant or nursing.

Spoon up some yogurt. Whether you want to prevent a yeast infection or relieve an existing one, the solution may be in your refrigerator. Eating a cup or two of live-culture yogurt daily will replenish your body's healthful bacteria, which will help keep the bad bugs under control. "The bacteria make it difficult for the yeast to grow," says Dr. Nalbandian.

Change your diet. Recurring, recalcitrant, or unresponsive yeast infections may require even more drastic dietary changes. Eliminate all refined starches, such as bread and pasta, from your diet. Avoid foods that contain yeast or fungus, such as beer, leavened pastry products, aged cheeses, and mushrooms. You'll also want to give up fermented foods, such as vinegar, pickles, and sauerkraut.

Get tested. Women who get frequent yeast infections sometimes have underlying blood sugar

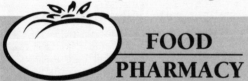

FOOD PHARMACY

Snack on Apricots

The beta-carotene in these sunny fruits may bolster your immune system enough to ward off infection. A study at Albert Einstein College of Medicine in New York City found that the vaginal cells of women with yeast infections had significantly lower levels of beta-carotene than did cells taken from women with no infections.

problems, Dr. Nalbandian says. Elevated blood sugar levels caused by diabetes can greatly increase the risk of infections, so if you keep getting them, ask your doctor for a diabetes test just to be sure.

Fix it with garlic. "Garlic, garlic, and more garlic." That's yeast-fighting advice from Dr. Nalbandian, who explains that garlic has powerful anti-fungal properties. Raw or lightly cooked garlic delivers the biggest kick. "I tell people to toss the garlic in after the food's off the stove," says Dr. Nalbandian. "Just chop it up and throw it in."

Keep cool. "Heat and hot water will aggravate a yeast infection," says Dr. Nalbandian. You may want to shower in lukewarm water until the infection is gone.

Dress for the heat. Summer's heat always makes yeast infections more uncomfortable, but even in winter, panty hose or tight clothing can trap heat and increase itching and other symptoms. It's a good idea to wear loose clothing made from cotton or other natural fibers, at least until the infection is gone.

Flush after sex. Some women tend to get yeast infections after intercourse. It's not really the man's fault, it's just that semen is a bit alkaline and can alter the acidity of the vagina. Less acid means more yeast. To help restore a normal chemical balance after sex, either urinate soon afterward or take a quick shower and flush out the area.

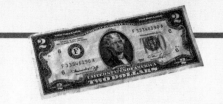

The $2 Deal

Tame It with Tea Tree

Peppermint and tea tree oils are powerful fungus fighters. You can buy capsules at a health food store, then follow the label directions. Be sure to buy oil that is meant for internal use, and don't put it anywhere but in your mouth.

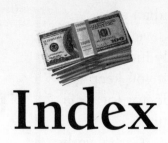

Index

Vacuuming, effect on asthma, 47
Valerian root
contraindications, 190–91, 294
as treatment for
anxiety, 32
back pain, 60
diarrhea, 190-91
insomnia, 294
shingles, 390
Vaporizers, avoiding, with bronchitis, 92
Varicose veins, 452–56
Vegetables
effect on
bad breath, 64
body odor, 84
breast pain, 89–90
chapped lips, 129
coughs, 161
intermittent claudication, 300
irritable bowel syndrome, 302
kidney stones, 308
macular degeneration, 322
muscle cramps, 342
stroke risk, 425
tennis elbow, 437
varicose veins, 453
raw versus cooked, 19
Vegetarians, anemia in, 18, 19
Vervain, for
chronic fatigue syndrome, 134
depression, 179
seasonal affective disorder, 385
stress, 420
Vibrations, effect on Raynaud's syndrome, 374
Viburnum. *See* Cramp bark
Vinegar
effect on
hives, 275
iron absorption, 19
as treatment for
athlete's foot, 53
colds, 142
dandruff, 168, 170
earaches, 208
insect bites and stings, 69

muscle cramps, 341–42
rashes, 366
shinsplints, 393
sunburn, 427
Violets, for sore throat, 404
Vioxx, for arthritis, 41
Vision. *See* Eye problems
Visualization, for
stress, 421
ulcers, 446
Vitamin A, for
acne, 3
age spots, 7
blisters, 74
bruises, 100
carpal tunnel syndrome, 122
dry skin, 202
shingles, 390
sore throat, 405
sunburn, 429
ulcers, 445
Vitamin B_6, for
bloating, 80
depression, 177–78
kidney stones, 308
memory problems, 327
menstrual pain, 332
stroke prevention, 425
Vitamin B_{12}, for
memory problems, 327
stroke prevention, 425
Vitamin C
contraindications, 249
effect on iron absorption, 19
for osteoporosis prevention, 353
side effects of, 99, 173, 249
as treatment for
age spots, 8
angina, 26
athlete's foot, 51
black eyes, 72
bruises, 99
bursitis, 114
carpal tunnel syndrome, 122
cataracts, 126
constipation, 154
coughs, 159–60
denture pain, 173
gallstones, 231
gingivitis, 240
headaches, 249

insect bites and stings, 69
memory problems, 327–28
Raynaud's syndrome, 373
shingles, 389, 390
sore throat, 405
sunburn, 428–29
temporomandibular disorder, 432-33
ulcers, 445
urinary tract infections, 450
varicose veins, 454
Vitamin D
sources of, 312
for arthritis, 40
for osteoporosis prevention, 352, 353
Vitamin E
contraindications, 328
as treatment for
age spots, 10
angina, 26
blisters, 74
breast pain, 90
carpal tunnel syndrome, 122
cold sores, 145
dry skin, 203
hot flashes, 277, 278
insect bites and stings, 69
intermittent claudication, 300
memory problems, 327–28
Raynaud's syndrome, 373
shingles, 390
sunburn, 429
ulcers, 445
warts, 459
Vitamin F, for dry skin, 201
Vitex, for breast pain, 90

W

Walking, for
arthritis, 38
asthma, 48
depression, 180
diabetes, 184
headaches, 247
sciatica, 382